No atrial activity present
(1) Sinus arrest
(2) Atrial arrest
(3) Junctional rhythm with P waves buried within QRS complexes

or interatrial conduction delay
(2) Ectopic atrial rhythm
(3) Reentrant rhythm with retrograde atrial activation
(4) Multifocal atrial tachycardia

Irregular
(1) Sinus arrhythmia
(2) Sinus pauses
(3) Sinoatrial exit block

Regular
(1) Regular sinus rhythm
(2) Sinus brady-cardia
(3) Sinus tachy-cardia
(4) Sinus node reentry tachy-cardia

PRINTED IN THE REPUBLIC OF SINGAPORE

a LANGE medical book

1989

Principles of Clinical Electrocardiography

Thirteenth Edition

Nora Goldschlager, MD
Professor of Clinical Medicine
University of California at San Francisco
Division of Cardiology
San Francisco General Hospital
San Francisco, California

Mervin J. Goldman, MD
Clinical Professor of Medicine
University of California at San Francisco
Department of Medicine
Veterans Hospital Medical Center
San Francisco, California

Prentice-Hall International Inc.

Table of Contents

Preface

The ECG is one of the most frequently performed tests in all of clinical medicine. Proper interpretation is therefore of great importance to physicians of all specialities. It is the intent of the authors to provide a thorough understanding of both the fundamental principles of clinical electrocardiography and, building upon these, more advanced concepts of interpretation. The material is therefore suited to the beginning student and to the house officer and practicing physician who may wish to review the subject or some aspect of it.

To achieve the aims of the authors, the first four chapters of the book consist of introductory material in which the recording of the ECG and electrophysiologic principles underlying cardiac electrical activity are described, the terms used in clinical electrocardiography are defined, and the depolarization sequence of the heart is reviewed. Chapters describing the normal ECG and its variants follow. Building upon the information contained in these early chapters, the subsequent four chapters define patterns of atrial and ventricular hypertrophy, normal and abnormal intraventricular conduction, and myocardial ischemia and infarction. In these chapters, emphasis is placed upon the diagnostic accuracy of the ECG and its limitations in certain clinical circumstances. Since the clinician is likely to encounter patients receiving various medications, a chapter describing the important effects of various drugs, especially cardioactive ones, on the ECG is included. And, in view of the large numbers of patients with cardiac pacemakers, a chapter defining the types and modes of function of these devices is included, which contains examples of normal and abnormal pacemaker function.

Two entirely new chapters have been included in this edition: exercise electrocardiography and ambulatory electrocardiographic monitoring. Exercise testing is so widely performed that an appreciation of the indications and contraindications and interpretation of results has become very important to all those who care for patients. Similarly, ambulatory electrocardiographic monitoring is now so widely employed that knowledge of the technique and the information it is capable of providing in certain patients is deemed necessary.

Finally, the reader has been provided with a new format in which to test this newly acquired knowledge. Test tracings are displayed, which are followed by specific questions pertaining to them. The questions are set out in a manner reflecting the organized approach to electrocardiographic analysis as introduced in the early chapters of the book. Answers are immediately available when the student has completed the analysis.

Tables and schematic diagrams are liberally used to facilitate the learning process. It is hoped that upon completion of this book, the student of electrocardiography will have acquired a thorough and practical working knowledge of the field.

Nora Goldschlager, MD
Mervin J. Goldman, MD

San Francisco
July, 1989

Note to the Reader

A principal goal of this book is to provide the reader with the ability to competently analyze and correctly interpret an ECG. Each of the following chapters addresses this goal. We believe, however, that the reader will be well served by having a compact reference source available when **a how-to, step-by-step overview of electrocardiographic interpretation** is needed. Chapter 21 is intended to provide this overview. While detailed discussions will be found in chapters preceding Chapter 21, the latter serves as a constantly available reference for the reader in need of a memory jogger or a rapid guide. The algorithms on the inside front cover serve the same function.

The Electrocardiogram: Fundamentals

The electrocardiogram (ECG) is a graphic recording of the electrical potentials produced by cardiac tissue. The heart is unique among the muscles of the body in that it possesses the properties of automatic impulse formation and rhythmic contraction. Electrical impulse formation occurs within the conduction system of the heart; excitation of the muscle fibers throughout the myocardium results in cardiac contraction. Formation and conduction of these electrical impulses produce weak electrical currents that spread through the body. The ECG is recorded by applying electrodes to various locations on the body surface and connecting them to a recording apparatus. The connections of the apparatus are such that an upright deflection indicates positive potential and a downward deflection negative potential.

Clinical Value of the ECG

The ECG is of diagnostic value in the following clinical circumstances: (1) atrial and ventricular hypertrophy; (2) myocardial ischemia and infarction; (3) pericarditis; (4) systemic diseases that affect the heart; (5) determination of the effect of cardiac drugs, especially digitalis and certain antiarrhythmic agents; (6) disturbances in electrolyte balance, especially potassium; and (7) evaluation of function of cardiac pacemakers. The ECG is of *considerable* diagnostic value in assessing (1) conduction delay of atrial and ventricular electrical impulses and (2) determination of the origin and behavior of dysrhythmias.

The ECG is a laboratory test, not a sine qua non of the diagnosis of heart disease. A patient with heart disease may have a normal ECG, and a normal individual may have an abnormal ECG. All too often, patients are told erroneously that they have cardiac disease solely on the basis of some abnormality on the ECG; on the other hand, a patient may receive unwarranted assurance of the absence of heart disease solely on the basis of a normal ECG. The ECG must *always* be interpreted in light of surrounding clinical circumstances.

RECORDING & MONITORING AN ELECTROCARDIOGRAM

BIPOLAR STANDARD LEADS

The bipolar standard leads (I, II, and III) are the original leads selected by Einthoven to record electrical potentials in the frontal plane. Electrodes are applied to the left arm (LA), right arm (RA), and left leg (LL). Proper skin contact must be made by rubbing electrode paste on the skin; alcohol sponges may also be used. The LA, RA, and LL leads are then attached to their respective electrodes. By turning the selector dial of the recording apparatus, the standard leads (I, II, and III) are recorded (Fig 1–1).

Electrocardiographic machines also have a right leg (RL) electrode and lead, which acts as a ground and plays no role in the production of the ECG.

Electrical Potentials

The bipolar leads represent the difference in electrical potential between 2 selected sites (Fig 1–2):

Lead I = Difference of potential between the left arm and the right arm (LA – RA).

Lead II = Difference of potential between the left leg and the right arm (LL – RA).

Lead III = Difference of potential between the left leg and the left arm (LL – LA).

The electrical potential recorded from any one extremity will be the same no matter where the electrode is placed on the extremity. Electrodes are usually applied just above the wrists and ankles. If an extremity has been amputated, the electrode can be applied to the stump. In a patient with a tremor, a satisfactory record may be obtained by applying the electrodes to the upper portions of the limbs. In exercise electrocardiography and in ambulatory electrocardiography, the electrodes are applied near or on the torso.

UNIPOLAR LEADS
(Extremity Leads, Precordial [Chest] Leads, Esophageal Leads, Intracardiac Leads)

Unipolar leads (VR, VL, and VF), precordial leads (V), and esophageal leads (E) were introduced into clinical electrocardiography by Wilson in 1932; unipolar intracardiac leads were introduced a decade later. The frontal plane unipolar leads (VR, VL, and VF) bear a definite mathematical relation to the standard bipolar leads (I, II, and III). The precordial (V) leads record poten-

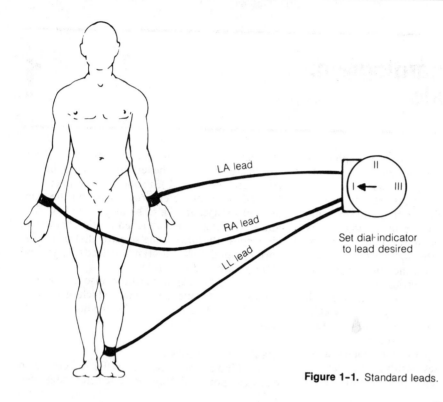

Figure 1-1. Standard leads.

Figure 1-2. Connections for bipolar standard leads I, II, and III. The relation between the 3 leads is expressed algebraically by Einthoven's equation: lead II = lead I + lead III. This is based on Kirchhoff's law, which states that the algebraic sum of all the potential differences in a closed circuit equals zero. If Einthoven had reversed the polarity of lead II (ie, RA - LL), the 3 bipolar lead axes would result in a closed circuit, and leads I + II + III would equal zero. However, since Einthoven did make this alteration in the polarity of the lead II axis, the equation becomes I − II + III = 0. Hence, II = I + III.

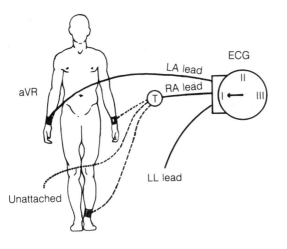

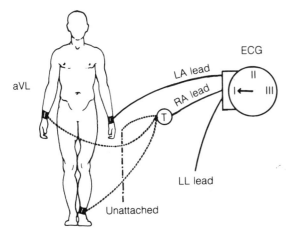

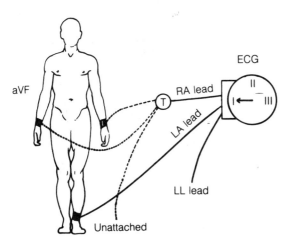

Figure 1-3. Augmented extremity leads. (T, terminal.)

tials in the horizontal plane without being influenced by potentials from an "indifferent" electrode. Any unipolar lead records not only the electrical potential from a small area of underlying myocardium, but also *all* of the electrical

events of the entire cardiac cycle as viewed from that site.

Augmented Extremity Leads aVR, aVL, & aVF (Fig 1–3)

By a technique automatically accomplished by all modern electrocardiographic machines, the amplitude of the deflections of VR, VL, and VF can be increased by about 50%. These leads are called augmented unipolar extremity leads and are designated as aVR, aVL, and aVF. The augmented unipolar extremity leads have replaced the nonaugmented leads because they are easier to read. Electrocardiographic machines are constructed so that the augmented extremity leads can be recorded using the same hookup as that used for standard leads, by turning the selector dial to aVR, aVL, and aVF.

Unipolar precordial leads are recorded by applying the chest lead and electrode to any desired position on the chest and turning the selector dial to the V position (Fig 1–4). Multiple chest leads are recorded by changing the position of the chest electrode. Unipolar esophageal leads are recorded by attaching the esophageal electrode to the chest lead and turning the selector dial to the V position. Unipolar intracardiac leads are recorded by attaching the intracardiac electrode to the chest lead and turning the selector dial to the V position.

UNIPOLAR PRECORDIAL LEADS

The unipolar precordial leads are obtained by turning the selector dial to V and recording from the various precordial positions. By convention, these precordial positions are as follows (Fig 1–5):

V_1:	Fourth intercostal space, right sternal border.
V_2:	Fourth intercostal space, left sternal border.
V_3:	Equidistant between V_2 and V_4.
V_4:	Fifth intercostal space, left midclavicular line. All subsequent leads (V_{5-9}) are taken in the same horizontal plane as V_4.
V_5:	Anterior axillary line.
V_6:	Midaxillary line.
V_7:	Posterior axillary line.
V_8:	Posterior scapular line.
V_9:	Left border of the spine.
V_{3R-9R}:	Right side of the chest in the same location as the left-sided leads V_{3-9}. V_{2R} is therefore the same as V_1.
$3V_{1-9}$:	One interspace higher than V_{1-9}; these are the third interspace leads. The same terminology can be applied to leads taken in other interspaces, eg, $2V_{1-9}$, $6V_{1-9}$, etc.

The usual routine ECG consists of 12 leads: I, II, III; aVR, aVL, aVF; and V_{1-6}.

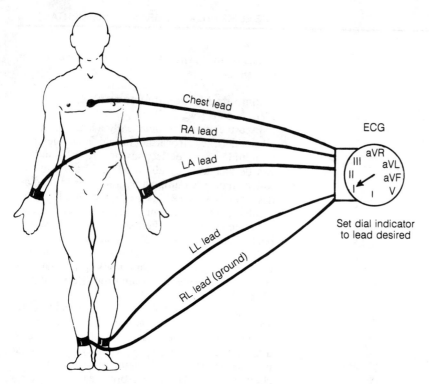

Figure 1-4. Unipolar leads.

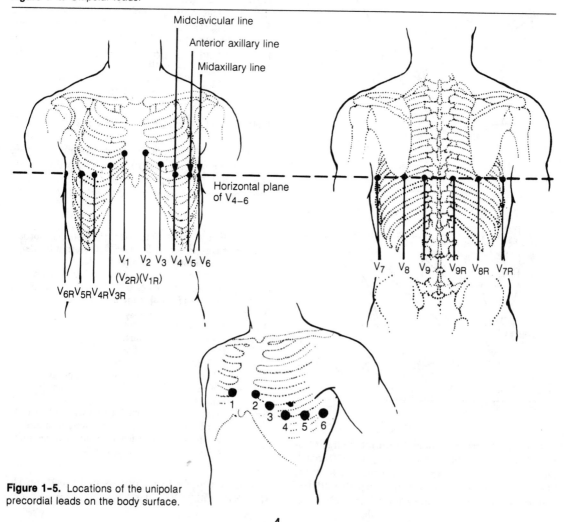

Figure 1-5. Locations of the unipolar precordial leads on the body surface.

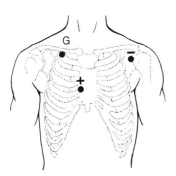

Figure 1-6. Modified chest lead (MCL₁) system for cardiac rhythm monitoring. The positive electrode is placed in the V₁ position, the negative electrode near the left shoulder, and the ground electrode at a remote area of the chest. By changing the placement of the positive electrode, any MCL lead may be recorded.

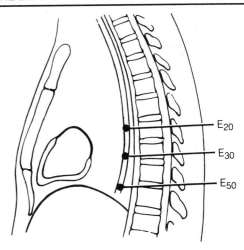

Figure 1-7. Diagrammatic sagittal view of the thorax illustrating positions of esophageal electrodes.

MONITOR LEADS

Although it is possible to use any lead for purposes of cardiac rhythm monitoring (or multiple leads if equipment is available) in a specialized patient care area such as a coronary care unit, it is more common to use a **modified bipolar chest lead.** The positive electrode is placed in the usual V_1 position and the negative electrode near the left shoulder. A third electrode is placed at a more remote area of the chest and serves as a ground (Fig 1-6). The recording thus obtained will be similar to a modified V_1 precordial lead (MCL₁). This lead is of value in evaluation of cardiac rhythm. However, if it is deemed necessary to monitor the patient for ST and T wave abnormalities due to myocardial ischemia, it is advisable to place the positive electrode in the V_4 or V_5 position (MCL₄ or MCL₅) or in any position that is expected or has been previously demonstrated to show the abnormality.

UNIPOLAR ESOPHAGEAL LEADS

Unipolar esophageal recordings **(esophageal electrograms)** are made by attaching an esophageal lead to the V lead of the machine. An electrode catheter is either swallowed or passed through the nares into the esophagus. Using this electrode as one terminal and the zero potential as the other terminal, a unipolar esophageal (''E'') electrogram can be obtained. The usual nomenclature of the lead is derived from the distance in centimeters from the nares to the electrode. Thus, E_{50} represents an esophageal electrode located 50 cm from the nares. Leads E_{40-50} usually record the posterior surface of the left ventricle; leads E_{15-25}, the atrial area; and leads

E_{25-35}, the region of the atrioventricular groove (Fig 1-7). Since these positions vary with differences in individual body size and shape and heart position, assessment of precise electrode location should not be made from a single esophageal lead; a series of low to high esophageal lead recordings must be made for proper evaluation. For more accurate localization of the position of the esophageal electrode, fluoroscopy may be used.

A bipolar esophageal lead has been developed in which the electrodes are encased in gelatin to allow easy swallowing by the patient. The gelatin capsule then dissolves, leaving the esophageal electrodes to record atrial electrical activity. The bipolar esophageal electrogram is recorded through the lead I channel of the electrocardiograph machine, simultaneously with surface lead II.

Esophageal leads are especially useful in recording atrial depolarization signals, which are greatly magnified at this location, and in exploring the posterior surface of the left ventricle.

UNIPOLAR INTRACARDIAC LEADS

Unipolar intracardiac recordings **(intracardiac electrograms)** are made by attaching an electrode catheter to the V lead and turning the selector dial to the V position. Unipolar intracardiac electrograms can be recorded from various cardiac chambers, depending upon the location of the catheter electrodes. Intracardiac electrography is of great clinical value in the assessment of dysrhythmias by amplification of atrial electrical activity (Fig 1-8) and in the proper positioning of a pacing catheter ''floated'' into the heart without fluoroscopic guidance. In the latter circumstance, the contour and relative sizes of the atrial and ven-

Figure 1-8. Unipolar intracardiac electrogram recorded from a catheter electrode positioned in the right atrium. The large, narrow diphasic complexes (arrows) represent atrial electrical activity, and the broad deflections that follow them represent ventricular electrical activity. Simultaneous recording of the intracardiac electrogram and a surface electrocardiographic lead can help to clarify the origin of the intracardiac deflections; this is of particular importance in dysrhythmia evaluation.

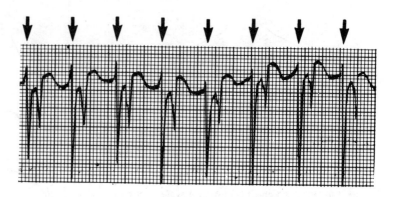

tricular deflections will help identify the location of the catheter tip, thus aiding in its proper positioning.

With appropriate electrode catheters inserted into the heart under fluoroscopic guidance, recordings can be made of electrical activity occurring at the bundle of His and proximal portions of the bundle branches (**His bundle electrography**). This technique, which is limited to the cardiac laboratory, has resulted in major advances in the understanding and interpretation of dysrhythmias and atrioventricular conduction. Intracardiac recordings from multiple sites during electrical stimulation of various areas of the heart can also be made in specially equipped laboratories (intracardiac **mapping** studies). These recordings are of value in determining the site of origin of tachycardias and their conduction pathways, elucidating the presence of accessory atrioventricular bypass tracts (see Chapter 15), and inducing clinically significant dysrhythmias so that the best form of treatment can be selected.

Attachment of the V lead to the metal hub of a pericardiocentesis needle, under sterile precautions, permits electrographic recording during this procedure. When the needle meets the epicardium, ST elevation will be recorded and is an indication for withdrawing the needle slightly and beginning aspiration.

In all situations in which an electrode is in direct contact with the myocardium, proper electrical grounding is essential. Currents as low as 10 μA can induce ventricular fibrillation.

TECHNICAL DIFFICULTIES AFFECTING THE ELECTROCARDIOGRAM

Attention to the following details will ensure against artifacts and technically poor records:

(1) The ECG should be recorded with the patient lying on a comfortable bed or table large enough to support the entire body. The patient must be relaxed in order to ensure a satisfactory tracing (Fig 1-9). It is best to explain the procedure in advance to an apprehensive patient in order to allay anxiety. Muscular motions or twitchings by the patients can alter the record (Figs 1-10 and 1-11).

(2) Good contact must exist between the skin and the electrode. Poor contact can result in a suboptimal record (Figs 1-12 and 1-13).

(3) The electrocardiographic machine must be properly *standardized* so that 1 millivolt (mV) will produce a deflection of 1 cm. Incorrect standardization will produce inaccurate voltage of the

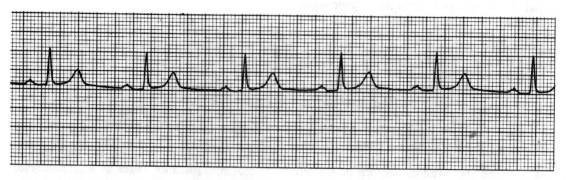

Figure 1-9. A technically good tracing.

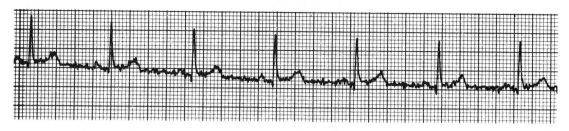

Figure 1-10. Effect of muscle twitchings.

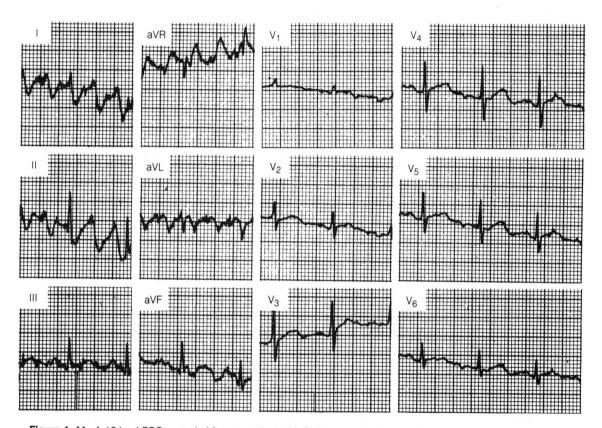

Figure 1-11. A 12-lead ECG recorded from a patient with Parkinson's disease. Artifacts due to muscular tremor may obscure both the rhythm and the morphology, or may resemble an arrhythmia (as in this example, in which atrial flutter is mimicked).

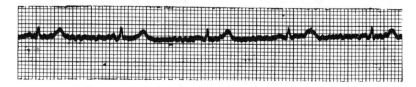

Figure 1-12. Effect of poor contact between skin and electrode.

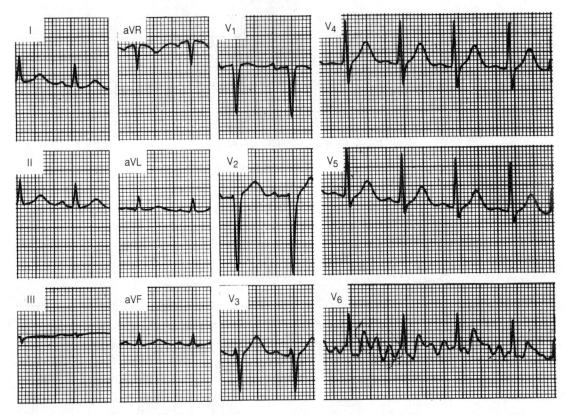

Figure 1-13. A 12-lead ECG illustrating faulty contact between the electrode in the V$_6$ position and the patient, resulting in baseline artifact in lead V$_6$ only.

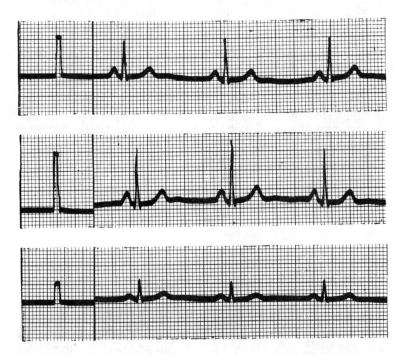

Figure 1-14. Effect of standardization. *Top:* Proper standardization: 1-cm deflection. *Middle:* Overstandardization: 1.4-cm deflection. This increases the voltage of the complexes. *Bottom:* Understandardization: 0.5-cm deflection. This decreases the voltage of the complexes.

complexes, which can lead to faulty interpretation (Fig 1–14).

(4) The patient and the recording machine must be properly grounded to avoid alternating current interference (Fig 1–15).

(5) Any electronic equipment in contact with the patient, eg, an electrically regulated intravenous infusion pump, can produce artifacts in the ECG (Fig 1–16).

THE ELECTROCARDIOGRAPHIC GRID

Electrocardiographic paper is graph paper with horizontal and vertical lines at 1-mm intervals. A heavier line is present every 5 mm. Time is measured along the horizontal lines: 1 mm = 0.04 s; 5 mm = 0.2 s (Fig 1–17). Voltage is measured along the vertical lines and is expressed as mm (10 mm = 1 mV). In routine practice, the record-

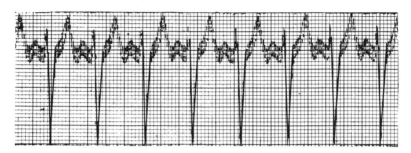

Figure 1–15. Effect of alternating current interference.

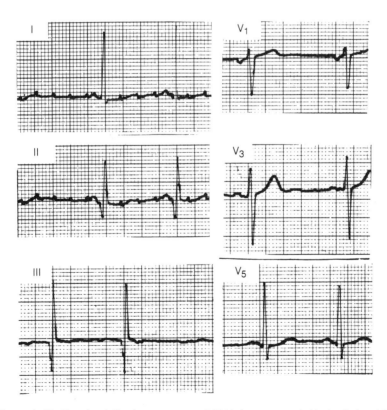

Figure 1–16. Regular deflections at a rate of 300/min are recorded in leads I and II, which could result in an interpretation of atrial flutter. However, lead III and the precordial leads indicate sinus rhythm. The deflections occurring at this rapid rate were due to an artifact from an intravenous infusion pump unit inserted into a right forearm vein.

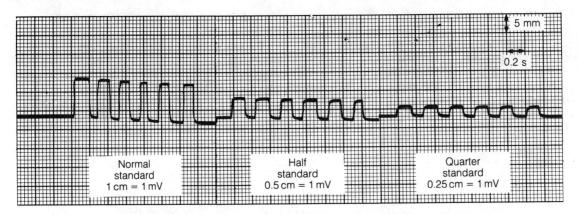

Figure 1–17. Electrocardiographic paper and 1-mV calibration signals.

ing speed is 25 mm/s. The usual calibration is a 1-mV signal that produces a 10-mm deflection. "Double standard" produces a 20-mm deflection, "half standard" produces a 5-mm deflection, and "quarter standard" produces a 2.5-mm deflection (Fig 1–17).

Many ECG machines in current use have a marker inscribed at 3-s intervals to facilitate determination of heart rate.

REFERENCES

Brody DA, Copeland DG: The principles of esophageal electrocardiography. *Am Heart J* 1959;**57**:3.

Damato AN et al: Recording of specialized conduction fibers (A-V nodal, His bundle, and right bundle branch) in man using an electrode catheter technic. *Circulation* 1969;**39**:435.

Hammill SC, Pritchett EL: Simplified esophageal electrocardiography using bipolar recording leads. *Ann Intern Med* 1981;**95**:14.

Shaw M et al: Esophageal electrocardiography in acute cardiac care: Efficacy and diagnostic value of a new technique. *Am J Med* 1987;**82**:689.

Electrophysiology of the Heart

2

Transmembrane Action Potentials

Much of clinical electrocardiography is based upon the behavior of transmembrane action potentials. The character of the transmembrane action potential varies with its site of origin and is different in different cell types and in different locations within the heart. Normal cardiac rhythm depends upon normal mechanisms of generation of cellular action potentials. Abnormally generated cellular action potentials may result in disturbances of cardiac rhythm (see Chapters 10 and 13). Faulty propagation—or delays in conduction—of electrical impulses generated by transmembrane action potentials can result in abnormalities of cardiac rhythm or in delayed depolarization of a cardiac chamber (see Chapters 8, 10, 12, and 13).

Four electrophysiologic events are involved in the genesis of the ECG: (10 **impulse formation** in the primary pacemaker of the heart (usually the sinoatrial node); (2) **transmission of the impulse** through specialized conduction fibers; (3) activation (**depolarization**) of the myocardium; and (4) **repolarization** (recovery) of the myocardium.

If a microelectrode is placed on the surface of a resting myocardial cell and a second (indifferent) microelectrode is placed in a remote location such as the extracellular space, no electrical potential (zero potential) is recorded because of the high impedance of the cell membrane. However, if the cell membrane is penetrated by a microelectrode, a negative potential will be recorded, which represents the potential difference between the inside and the outside of the cell. This potential is known as the **resting membrane potential** (Fig 2-1). The major factor that determines the resting membrane potential is the gradient of potassium ions (K^+) across the cell membrane; the resting potential is -80 to -90 mV in most cardiac cells, with the exception of those of the sinoatrial and AV nodal areas. The intracellular concentration of K^+ is about 150 meq/L, and the extracellular concentration is about 5 meq/L, resulting in a 30:1 concentration gradient. An opposite gradient exists for sodium ions (Na^+), resulting in a high extracellular Na^+ concentration relative to intracellular Na^+ concentration. However, because the cell membrane is considerably less permeable to Na^+ than to K^+, the Na^+ gradient does not alter the resting potential appreciably. These concentration gradients are maintained by an active ion transport mechanism, the **sodium pump.**

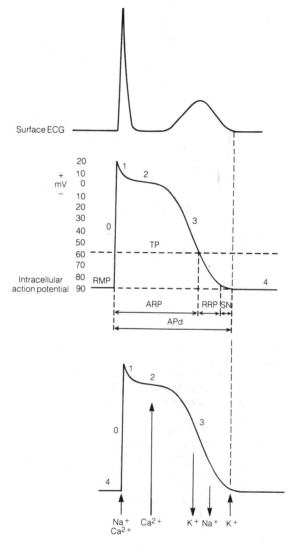

Figure 2-1. Diagrams of the action potential of a ventricular muscle cell. RMP = resting membrane potential; 0 = depolarization; 1, 2, 3 = phases of repolarization; 4 = diastolic phase; APd = duration of action potential; TP = threshold potential; ARP = absolute refractory period; RRP = relative refractory period; SN = supernormal period of excitability. Phase 4: Resting membrane potential = -90 mV. Phase 0: Rapid depolarization due to Na^+ (and Ca^{2+}) influx. Phase 1: Initial phase of repolarization. Phase 2: Plateau phase of repolarization in which there is a slow influx of Ca^{2+}. Phase 3: Efflux of K^+ resulting in slow return of intracellular potential to -90 mV. At the termination of phase 3 an active transport system extrudes Na^+ from the cell and pumps K^+ into the cell.

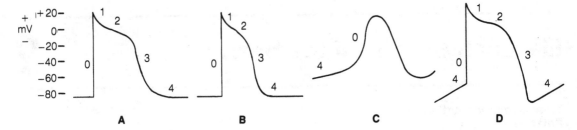

Figure 2-2. Diagrams of the action potentials of various cell types within the heart. *A:* Ventricular muscle cell. *B:* Atrial muscle cell. *C:* SA or AV nodal cell. *D:* Purkinje cell. Note the differences between the working myocardial cells (A and B), whose phase 4 is flat, and the cells (C and D) which have automaticity whose phase 4 rises toward activation threshold during diastole. This **diastolic depolarization** characterizes automatic cells, since once threshold is spontaneously attained, cellular activation occurs.

Cellular Depolarization & Repolarization. At the onset of depolarization of a myocardial cell, there is an abrupt change in permeability of the cell membrane to Na^+. Na^+ (and, to a lesser extent, calcium ions [Ca^{2+}] enter the cell through their respective channels and result in a sharp rise of intracellular potential to positivity (about $+20$ mV) (Fig 2-1). This phase of depolarization is designated **phase 0** and reflects the Na^+-dependent **fast inward current** typical of working myocardial cells and Purkinje fibers. The maximum rate of depolarization of ventricular cells is 200 V/s and that of atrial cells is 100–200 V/s. The maximum rate of depolarization of Purkinje cells is 500 V/s. Pacemaker cells in the sinoatrial (SA) and atrioventricular (AV) nodes are depolarized by a Ca^{2+}-dependent **slow inward current.** Under certain abnormal conditions, such as ischemia, cells whose fast inward current of Na^+ is inhibited are depolarized by slow inward currents of Ca^{2+}.

Following cellular depolarization, there is a gradual return of potential to the resting potential. This **repolarization** process is divided into 3 phases: **phase 1:** an initial rapid return of intracellular potential to 0 mV, largely the result of closing of the Na^+ channels; **phase 2:** a plateau resulting from the slow entry of Ca^{2+} into the cell; and **phase 3:** return of the intracellular potential to resting potential, resulting from extrusion of K^+ out of the cell. At the end of phase 3, the normal negative resting potential is reestablished; however, the cell is left with an excess of Na^+ and a deficit of K^+. A Na^+ pump, which removes Na^+ from the cell and permits the influx of K^+, then becomes effective. In Ca^{2+}-dependent cells (SA and AV nodal cells) the phases of repolarization are less well demarcated (Fig 2-2).

Relation of Cellular events to the surface ECG. The summation of all phase 0 potentials of atrial myocardial cells results in the P wave inscribed in the ECG. Phase 2 corresponds to the PR segment, which follows the P wave (see Chapter 4). Phase 3 corresponds to the T_a wave of atrial repolarization. The summation of phase 0 potentials of ventricular myocardial cells results in the QRS complex in the ECG. Phase 2 corresponds to the ST segment and phase 3 to the T wave (Fig 2-1).

Excitation & Threshold Potential

Excitation of a cardiac cell occurs when a stimulus reduces the transmembrane potential to a critical level known as the **threshold potential** (Fig 2-1). The threshold potential is about -60 mV in atrial and ventricular muscle cells and about -40 mV in SA and AV nodal cells. If the resting membrane potential is raised toward the level of the threshold potential, a relatively weak stimulus can evoke a response. Conversely, if the resting potential is lowered away from the threshold potential, a relatively stronger stimulus will be required to produce a response.

Refractoriness

The refractory period of myocardial cells and tissue is divided into the **absolute refractory period** (Fig 2-1), during which no stimulus of any intensity can evoke a response, and a **relative (effective) refractory period** (Fig 2-1), during which only a strong stimulus can evoke a response. The absolute refractory period includes phases 0, 1, 2, and part of 3 of the transmembrane action potential. During this time, the Na^+ channels, which were activated during depolarization, become inactivated. The relative refractory period begins at about the time the membrane potential reaches the threshold potential and ends just before the termination of phase 3. During the relative refractory period, increasing numbers of Na^+ channels become available for activation. The relative refractory period is followed by the period of **supernormal excitability** (Fig 2-1), during which a relatively weak stimulus can evoke a response.

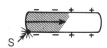

Resting muscle cell   Stimulated muscle cell   Depolarized muscle cell

Figure 2-3. Diagrams of resting, stimulated, and depolarized muscle cells. When the muscle is stimulated (S = stimulus), the surface of the stimulated portion of the muscle becomes electrically negative. As the impulse traverses the muscle, there is advancing negative charge. The portion of muscle that has not yet received the stimulus is electrically positive.

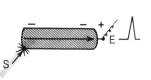 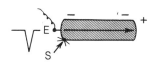 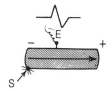

A. Upward deflection   B. Downward deflection   C. Diphasic deflection

Figure 2-4. Electrical deflections produced by muscle stimulation. *A:* The upward deflection is produced by the spread of the stimulus (S) toward an electrode (E) located at the positively charged end of the muscle. *B:* Downward deflection produced by spread of the impulse away from an electrode located at the negatively charged end of the muscle. *C:* Diphasic deflection, recorded by an electrode positioned at the mid portion of the muscle, produced by the initial advancing positive charge and subsequent passing negative charge.

Conduction Velocity

The speed at which electrical impulses spread through the heart varies considerably and depends upon the intrinsic properties of different portions of the conduction system and myocardium. Conduction velocity is most rapid in the His bundle and Purkinje system (about 2 m/s) and slowest in the SA and AV nodes (0.01–0.02 m/s); conduction within atrial and ventricular muscle is about 1 m/s.

The Electrogram

A recording of the electrical potentials of a stimulated muscle is analogous to a unipolar ECG recording and is termed an **electrogram.** There are 2 parts to an electrogram: depolarization (the deflection produced during passage of the electrical stimulus through the muscle) and repolarization (the deflection produced during return of the muscle to a resting state) (Fig 2–3). The direction in which a stimulus spreads through the muscle and the position of the recording electrode relative to the direction of spread of the impulse will determine its polarity in the recording (Fig 2–4). If muscles of different masses are stimulated, the electrical potentials recorded will reflect the net depolarization and repolarization (Fig 2–5).

The time required for the spread of the impulse from the stimulated end of a muscle to the opposite end can be measured on the electrogram from

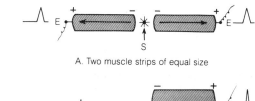

A. Two muscle strips of equal size

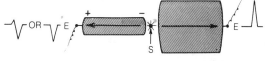

B. Two muscle strips of markedly different sizes

Figure 2-5. *A:* Muscles of equal size. If 2 muscle masses of approximately equal size are stimulated at a central point, a positive deflection (of depolarization) of equal magnitude will be recorded at both ends. *B:* Muscles of unequal size. If 2 muscle masses of markedly different sizes (analogous to the right and left ventricles) are stimulated at a central point, a large positive deflection will be recorded over the larger muscle mass, and a small positive deflection followed by a deep negative deflection (or an entirely negative deflection) will be recorded over the smaller muscle mass. This negative deflection is due to the fact that *net* deflection of depolarization is directed away from the smaller muscle mass.

the onset of the depolarization deflection to its peak. In clinical electrocardiography, an approximation of this time, measured from the onset of the inscription of the complex to its peak, is termed the **intrinsic (intrinsicoid) deflection** or **activation time;** the measurement is usually applied only to QRS complexes (Fig 2–6).

During repolarization, the muscle returns to its resting state. If repolarization occurs in a direction opposite to that of depolarization, the repolarization deflection will be in the same direction as that produced by the depolarization deflection (Fig 2–7A). If repolarization occurs in the same direction as that of depolarization, the repolarization deflection will be opposite to that of the depolarization deflection (Fig 2–7B). These concepts apply to isolated muscle strips and not to the intact human heart.

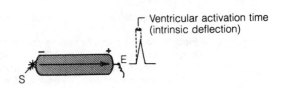

Figure 2–6. The intrinsic (intrinsicoid) deflection, or ventricular activation time, is a measure of the time taken by impulse propagation from one end of the stimulated muscle to the other.

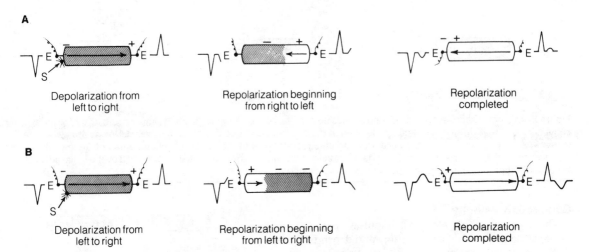

Figure 2–7. *A:* Depolarization from left to right and repolarization in the opposite direction. *B:* Depolarization from left to right and repolarization in the same direction.

REFERENCES

Cranefield PF: Action potentials, afterpotentials, and arrhythmias. *Circ Res* 1977;**41**:415.

Wit AL, Rosen MR: Pathophysiologic mechanisms of cardiac arrhythmias. *Am Heart J* 1983;**106**:798.

Wit AL, Rosen MR, Hoffman BF: Electrophysiology and pharmacology of cardiac arrhythmias. 2. Relationship of normal and abnormal electrical activity of cardiac fibers to the genesis of arrhythmias. *Am Heart J* 1974;**88**:515, 798.

Zipes DP, Jalife J (editors): *Cardiac Electrophysiology and Arrhythmias.* Grune & Stratton, 1985.

The Cardiac Vector

The term "cardiac vector" designates all of the electromotive forces of the cardiac cycle. A vector has **magnitude, direction,** and **polarity.** At any given instant during depolarization and repolarization, electrical potentials are propagating in many directions in space. Over 90% of these potentials are canceled out by opposing forces, and only the net force is recorded. The **instantaneous vector** represents the net electrical force at a given instant. The **mean vector** of a given portion of the depolarization-repolarization sequence (eg, the QRS complex) represents the mean magnitude, direction, and polarity for that time period (eg, the mean QRS vector). The mathematical symbol of a vector is an arrow pointing in the direction of the net potential (positive or negative); the length of the arrow indicates the magnitude of the electrical force. A vector can be drawn for atrial depolarization (P vector), ventricular depolarization (QRS vector), and ventricular repolarization (ST and T vectors).

FRONTAL PLANE VECTORS

The result of the electrical potentials of the entire cardiac cycle as reflected in the frontal plane of the body is the **frontal plane vector.** By combining the frontal plane bipolar leads I, II, and III (Fig 3-1) with the frontal plane unipolar leads VR, VL, and VF (Fig 3-2), a hexaxial reference system can be drawn that illustrates all 6 leads of the frontal plane (Fig 3-3).

By convention, the positive pole of lead I is designated as 0° and the negative pole as ±180°; the positive pole of VF as +90° and the negative pole as −90° (or +270°); the positive pole of lead II as +60°; the positive pole of lead III as +120°; the positive pole of VR as −150° (or +210°); and the positive pole of VL as −30°.

Polarity of Individual Frontal Plane Lead Axes

If a perpendicular is drawn through the center of a given lead axis, any electrical force (vector) oriented in the positive half of the electrical field will record an upright deflection in that lead; any force oriented in the negative half of the electrical field will record a downward deflection (Fig 3-4).

Direction of Mean Frontal Plane Axis

The mean QRS vector in the frontal plane can be approximated from standard leads by use of

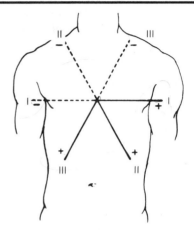

Figure 3-1. Frontal plane bipolar leads.

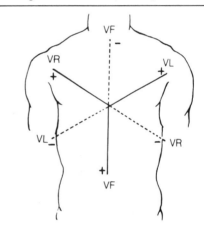

Figure 3-2. Frontal plane unipolar leads.

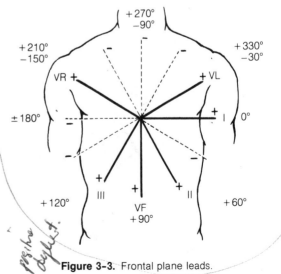

Figure 3-3. Frontal plane leads.

15

the hexaxial reference system (Fig 3–3). This approximation is determined by measurement of magnitude (voltage) alone; and true mean QRS vector must be determined from both magnitude and time.

There are 2 simple ways to calculate the mean frontal plane axis. In the first, the net magnitude and direction of the QRS complexes in any 2 of the 3 standard leads are plotted along the axes of the 2 standard leads selected. Perpendicular lines are then drawn at these points. A line drawn from the center of the reference system to the intersec-

tion of the perpendiculars represents the approximate mean QRS vector, and its angle represents the axis of the complex in the frontal plane. This method is only very rarely used. In the second method, the 1 lead of the 6 frontal plane leads which has a net QRS magnitude of zero is identified; the mean QRS vector will be perpendicular to that lead axis. Inspection of another lead (I or aVF) will tell in which half of this perpendicular the mean vector is located (Figs 3–5 and 3–6). If no frontal plane lead has a net QRS magnitude of zero, the mean vector can be interpolated and

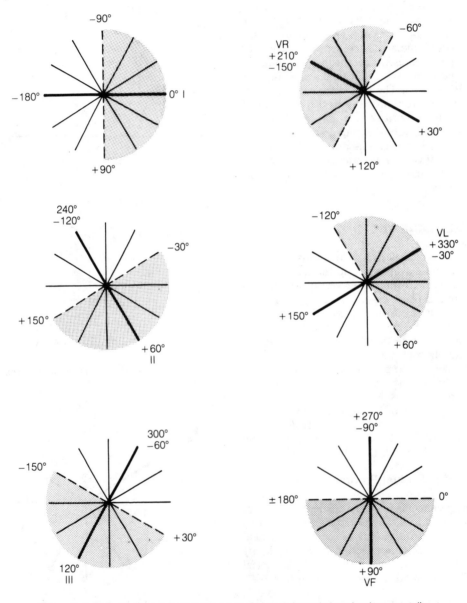

Figure 3-4. Polarity of frontal plane lead axis. For each frontal plane lead a perpendicular (dashed) line divides the regions of positive and negative vectors for that lead. Vectors in the stippled regions will evoke a positive (upright) deflection in that lead, and vectors in the clear region will evoke a negative deflection in that lead.

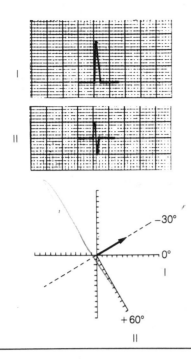

Figure 3-5. Lead II shows a QRS complex whose net magnitude is zero. The lead II axis is +60°. Therefore, the mean QRS vector in the frontal plane is perpendicular to +60° which is −30 or +150°. If the net QRS in lead I is positive, as it is in this example, the mean vector is −30°; if the net QRS in lead I is negative, the mean vector is +150°.

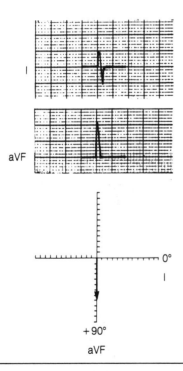

Figure 3-6. Lead I shows a QRS complex whose net magnitude is zero. The lead I axis is 0°. Therefore, the mean QRS vector in the frontal plane is perpendicular to 0°, which is +90 or −90°. If the net QRS in lead aVF is positive, as it is in this example, the mean vector is +90°. If the net QRS in lead aVF is negative, the mean vector is −90°.

estimated by inspection of several frontal plane leads. The frontal plane axis should be determined from the initial 0.04–0.06 s of ventricular activation rather than from the entire QRS complex.

By the same methods, the frontal plane axis of the P and T waves can be determined, as can the angle between the QRS complex and T wave.

Abnormal Axis Deviation

The angle of the mean frontal QRS vector determines its frontal plane axis. The normal QRS axis lies between 0 and +110°; left (superior) axis deviation between −30 and −90°, and right axis deviation between +110 and ±180° are generally abnormal. Leftward deviation of the frontal plane

QRS axis can occur with advancing age, in the absence of clinically overt heart disease. Within the range of normal, left (superior) axis deviation (0 to −30°) represents a normal horizontal heart position in unipolar terminology, and right axis deviation (+75 to +110°) represents a normal vertical heart position (Fig 3–7). Although the term left axis is traditional, a more accurate term would be **superior axis.**

The normal T wave axis usually corresponds to the normal QRS axis, and normally points in the same general direction. However, a 45° variation

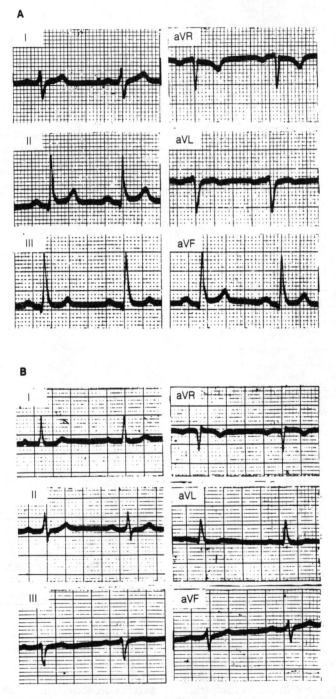

Figure 3-7. Examples of normal variations in frontal plane QRS axis. *A:* Frontal plane QRS axis = +96°; vertical heart position. *B:* Frontal plane QRS axis = −10°; horizontal heart position.

Figure 3-8. Lead axes in the horizontal plane.

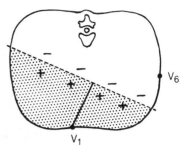

Polarity of V_1 axis

may be present in the frontal plane leads. Similarly, the normal P wave axis generally corresponds to the normal QRS axis.

HORIZONTAL PLANE VECTORS

The unipolar precordial leads represent approximations of the electrical potentials (vectors) in the horizontal plane (Fig 3-8).

Horizontal plane axes (Fig 3-9) are derived by adapting the same principles outlined for determination of frontal plane axes to the precordial leads; however, for practical purposes, they are rarely calculated.

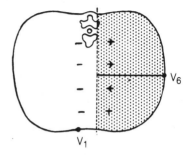

Polarity of V_6 axis

Figure 3-9. Polarity of V_1 and V_6 axes.

REFERENCES

Bachman S, Sparrow D, Smith LK: Effect of aging on the electrocardiogram. *Am J Cardiol* 1981;**48**:513.

Grant RP, Estes EH Jr: *Spatial Vector Electrocardiography.* Blakiston, 1951.

Lipman BS, Massie E, Kleiger RE: *Clinical Scalar Electrocardiography.* 6th ed. Year Book, 1972.

Figure 3-T1.
TEST TRACINGS

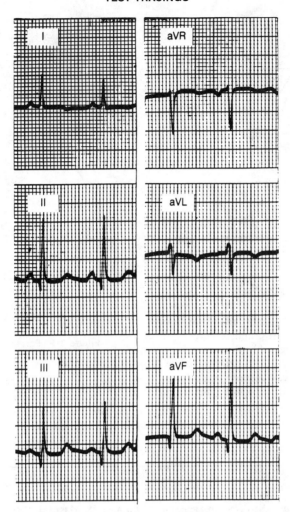

Is the mean frontal plane QRS axis horizontally or vertically directed?	Vertically.
What is the mean frontal plane QRS axis?	Since the net QRS magnitude best approaches 0 in lead avL, the QRS axis is either about +60° or about −120°. Since the QRS complex is mainly positive in the inferior leads II, III, and aVF, the QRS axis is positive. Since in aVL the QRS complex is slightly more negative than positive, the correct axis is slightly more vertical than +60°, and is about +75°.
Is the frontal plane QRS axis abnormal?	No. It is within the limits of normal.
Is the P wave axis in the frontal plane horizontally or vertically directed?	Vertically.
What is the P wave axis?	Since the net P wave magnitude is 0 in aVL, the P wave axis is either +60 or −120°. Since the P wave is positive in the inferior leads II, III, and aVF, the P wave axis is positive, and is +60°.
Is the P wave axis normal?	Yes. It is within the limits of normal.

Figure 3-T2.
TEST TRACINGS

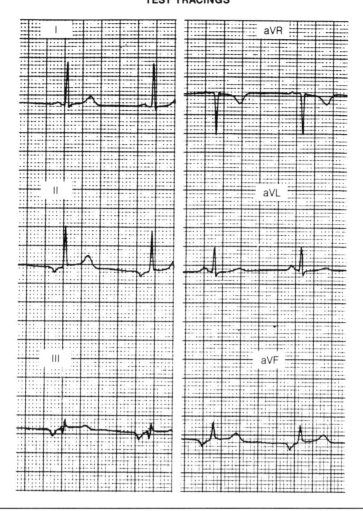

What is the QRS axis in the frontal plane?	Since the net magnitude of the QRS complex is 0 in lead III, the QRS axis is either +30 or −150°. Since the QRS complex is positive in leads I and II, its axis is positive in the frontal plane, at +30°.
Is the P wave directed inferiorly or superiorly in the frontal plane?	Superiorly, since it is negative in, and thus directed away from, the inferior leads II, III, and aVF.
What is the P wave axis?	The net magnitude of the P wave approaches 0 in lead aVR. The P wave axis is thus either −150 or +30°. Since the P wave is superiorly directed, the axis is about −150°.
Is the P wave axis normal?	No. It is abnormally superiorly directed. (In this tracing the P waves are probably originating in an ectopic focus rather than in the sinus node [see Chapters 6 and 10].)

Figure 3–T3.
TEST TRACINGS

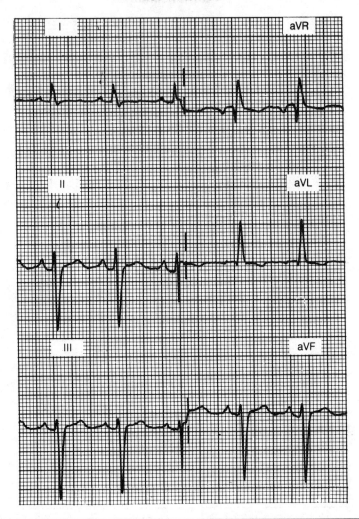

Describe the direction of the QRS axis in the frontal plane.	Leftward and superiorly directed, since the complexes are positively directed in leads I and aVL and mainly negatively directed in leads II, III, and aVF.
Is the QRS axis normal?	No. It is superior to −30° (−70°).
What is the P wave axis?	+60°.

The Normal Electrocardiogram

4

The ECG consists of complexes, intervals, junctions, segments, and waves. Each should be precisely described or measured when interpreting the tracing.

NORMAL ELECTROCARDIOGRAPHIC COMPLEXES

Atrial Activation

The **P wave** is the deflection produced by atrial **depolarization** (Fig 4–1).

The **T$_a$ wave** is the deflection produced by atrial **repolarization**. This deflection is not usually seen in the 12-lead ECG (Fig 4–1).

Ventricular Activation

The **Q (q) wave** is the **initial negative** deflection resulting from ventricular depolarization (Fig 4–2).

The **R (r) wave** is the **first positive** deflection resulting from ventricular depolarization (Fig 4–2).

The **S (s) wave** is the first negative deflection of ventricular depolarization that *follows* the first positive deflection (R) wave (Fig 4–2).

A **QS wave** is a negative deflection that does not rise above the baseline.

An **R′ (r′) wave** is the **second positive** deflection, that is, the first positive deflection during ventricular depolarization that *follows* the S wave (Fig 4–2). The negative deflection following the r′ is termed the s′ wave. If a clear s wave does not follow the initial R (or r) wave, this second positive deflection is still termed an R′ (r′) wave, and the QRS complex is described as an Rr′ (or rR′) complex.

Capital letters (Q, R, S) refer to relatively large waves (> 5 mm); small letters (q, r, s) refer to relatively small waves (< 5 mm).

Ventricular Repolarization

The **T wave** is the deflection produced by ventricular **repolarization** (Fig 4–3).

The **U wave** is the deflection (usually positive) seen following the T wave but preceding the next

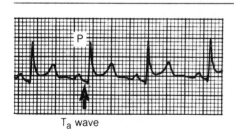

T$_a$ wave

Figure 4-1. The P and T$_a$ waves.

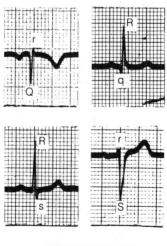

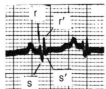

Figure 4-2. The QRS complex.

Figure 4-3. The T and U waves.

P wave. The cause of this wave is thought to be repolarization of the intraventricular (Purkinje) conduction system, although its precise mechanism of production is not entirely known (Fig 4-3). Inverted, or negative, U waves are occasionally seen, usually in patients with heart disease such as coronary artery disease with acute myocardial ischemia or hypertension.

NORMAL INTERVALS

The **RR interval** (Fig 4-4) is the interval between 2 consecutive R waves. If the ventricular rhythm is regular, the interval in seconds (or fractions of a second) between 2 successive R waves divided into 60 (seconds) will give the heart rate per minute. Thus, RR intervals of 0.2 s (interval

between 2 heavy lines on the ECG paper) = heart rate of 300/min; intervals of 0.4 s (interval between 3 heavy lines) = heart rate of 150/min; intervals of 0.6 s (interval between 4 heavy lines) = 100/min, etc.

If the ventricular rhythm is irregular, the number of R waves in a given period of time (eg, 6 s) should be counted and the results converted into the number of R waves per minute. For example, if 10 R waves that occur at irregular intervals are counted in a 6-s interval, the ventricular rate averages 60 per minute (10 × 6). The RR intervals should be measured from the onsets of the QRS complexes rather than at the peaks of the R waves.

The **PP interval** (Fig 4-5) is the interval between 2 consecutive P waves. In regular sinus rhythm, the PP interval will be the same as the RR inter-

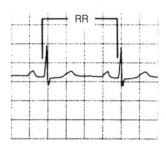

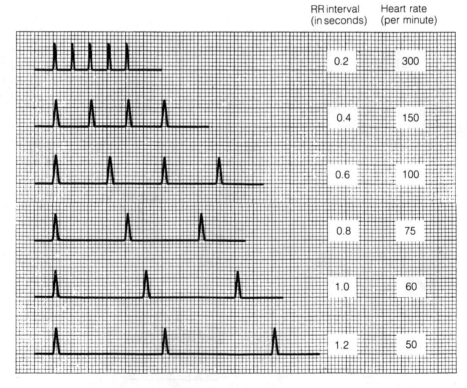

Figure 4-4. The RR interval.

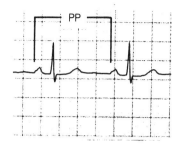

Figure 4–5. The PP interval.

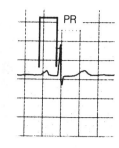

Figure 4–6. The PR interval.

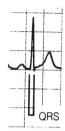

Figure 4–7. The QRS interval.

val. However, when the ventricular rhythm is irregular or when atrial and ventricular rates are regular but different from each other, the PP interval should be measured from the same point on 2 successive P waves (preferably at their onsets) and the atrial rate per minute computed in the same manner as the ventricular rate per minute.

The **PR interval** (Fig 4–6) is the interval between the onset of the P wave and the onset of the QRS complex. It measures the atrioventricular (AV) conduction time and includes the time required for (1) atrial depolarization, (2) the normal conduction delay in the AV node (approximately 0.07 s), and (3) the passage of the impulse through the bundle of His and bundle branches, to the onset of ventricular depolarization. The normal PR interval is in the range of 0.12–0.2 s and is related to heart rate; the slower the heart rate, the longer the PR interval.

The **QRS interval or duration** (Fig 4–7) represents the ventricular depolarization time. It is measured from the onset of the Q wave (or R wave if no Q wave is visible) to the termination of the S wave (or r′ or s′ wave if no S wave is visible). The upper limit of normal is 0.1 s in the frontal plane leads and 0.11 s in the precordial leads.

The **ventricular activation time** (VAT or "intrinsicoid" deflection) is the time it takes an impulse to traverse the myocardium from endocardial to epicardial surfaces. It is reflected in clinical electrocardiography by the interval measured from the beginning of the Q wave to the peak of the R wave (Fig 4–8). The VAT should not exceed 0.03 s in leads V_{1-2} and 0.05 s in leads V_{5-6}.

The **QT interval** (Fig 4–9) is measured from the onset of the Q wave to the end of the T wave and

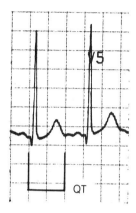

Figure 4–9. The QT interval.

represents the duration of electrical systole. The QT interval varies with the heart rate and with autonomic nervous system input. The QT interval may be corrected for heart rate (QT_c) (Fig 4–10), but this rate correction does not take into consideration autonomic tone, which may not vary directly with heart rate; thus the QT_c may not always have specific clinical significance. The normal QT_c usually does not exceed 0.42 s in men and 0.43 s in women.

On occasion, the end of the T wave is not well seen, or a U wave may be superimposed upon the T wave. Measurement of the QT interval under these circumstances cannot be made with precision. If a portion of the downstroke of the T wave is visible, extrapolation of a line of this slope to the baseline will give a reasonable approximation of the QT interval. The QT interval should be measured in those electrocardiographic leads that display the best-defined T waves.

In patients who have bundle branch block, the QT interval includes the abnormally prolonged QRS complex. In these patients, ventricular repolarization time is more accurately assessed by measuring the **JT interval,** from the J point (the beginning of the ST segment) to the end of the T wave.

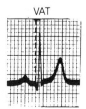

Figure 4–8. Ventricular activation time.

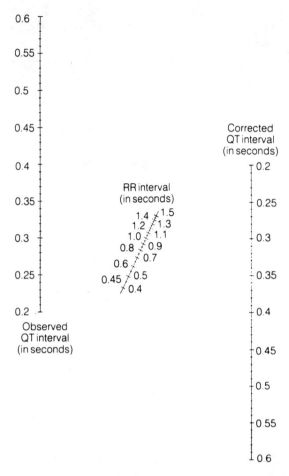

Figure 4-10. Nomogram for rate correction of the QT interval. Measure the QT and RR intervals. Mark these values in the respective columns of the chart. Place a ruler across these 2 points. The point at which the extension of this line crosses the third column is read as the corrected QT interval (QT_c). (Reproduced, with permission, from Kissin et al: *Am Heart J* 1948;**35**:990.)

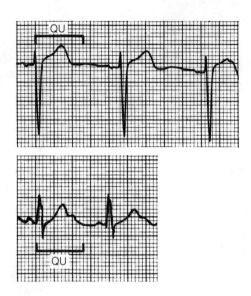

Figure 4-11. The QU interval.

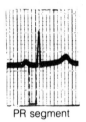

PR segment

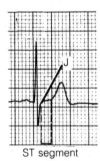

ST segment

Figure 4-12. PR and ST segments.

QU interval (Fig 4–11): This measures the interval from the beginning of the Q wave to the end of the U wave and represents total ventricular repolarization time, including that of the Purkinje fibers. When the end of the T wave is not well demarcated because of superimposition of a U wave, the QTU (or "QU") interval may be measured in place of the QT interval.

NORMAL SEGMENTS & JUNCTIONS

The **PR segment** (Fig 4–12) is that portion of the electrocardiographic tracing from the end of the P wave to the onset of the QRS complex. It is normally isoelectric.

The **J (RST) junction** is the point at which the QRS complex ends and the ST segment begins.

The **ST segment** is that portion of the tracing from the J point to the onset of the T wave. This segment is usually isoelectric but may vary from −0.5 to +2 mm in the precordial leads. It is determined to be elevated or depressed in comparison with that portion of the baseline between the end of the T wave and the beginning of the P wave (**TP segment**) or when related to the PR segment.

If neither of these is isoelectric, the point of onset of the QRS complex may be used.

The **TP segment** is that portion of the tracing between the end of the T wave and the beginning of the next P wave. At normal heart rates, it is usually isoelectric. At rapid heart rates, the P wave encroaches on the T wave, eliminating the isoelectric TP segment.

VOLTAGE MEASUREMENTS

The voltage of upright deflections is measured from the upper portion of the baseline to the peak of the wave.

The voltage of negative deflections is measured from the lower portion of the baseline to the nadir of the wave (Fig 4-13).

THE CONDUCTION SYSTEM OF THE HEART

Cardiac muscle has the property of automatic impulse formation and rhythmic contraction. Impulses are generated in specialized tissue that forms the atrioventricular (AV) conduction system. The conduction system consists of the **sino-atrial (SA) node** (which itself consists of P cells that form the impulse, **transitional cells** that transmit the impulse through the node, and collagen fibers), **interatrial conduction "pathways"** (or tracts), the AV node, the bundle of His, the right and left bundle branches, the fascicles of the left bundle branch (anterosuperior, inferoposterior, and septal), and the distal Purkinje system (Fig 4-14).

The rhythm of the heart normally originates in the SA node. The SA node is about 5 × 20 mm and is located at the endocardial surface of the right atrium at the junction of the right atrial appendage and the superior vena cava. The impulse formed in the P cells of the SA node is transmitted to atrial muscle via specialized cells, or "pathways" (although they are not clearly anatomically defined as such). The **anterior interatrial pathway** leaves the SA node anteriorly and curves around the superior vena cava and anterior wall of the right atrium, where it divides into 2 bundles: one goes to the left atrium and the other traverses the interatrial septum to the anterosuperior margin of the AV node. The **middle interatrial pathway** leaves the posterior margin of the SA node, curves behind the superior vena cava, and courses along the posterior portion of the interatrial septum to enter the superior margin of the AV node. The

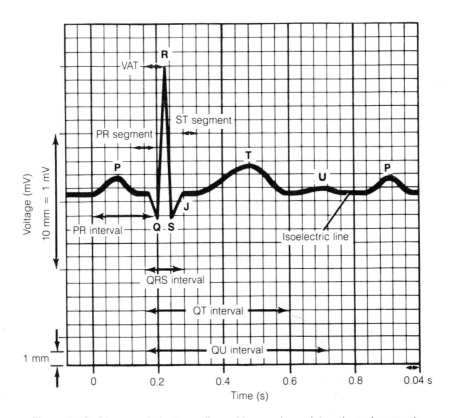

Figure 4-13. Diagram of electrocardiographic complexes, intervals, and segments.

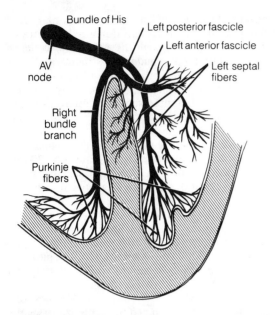

Figure 4-14. Illustration of the AV node–His-Purkinje conduction system.

posterior interatrial pathway leaves the posterior margin of the SA node and courses along the crista terminalis and eustachian ridge to enter the posterior margin of the AV node. Fibers from all 3 pathways converge before entering the AV node; some bypass the AV node to enter the His-Purkinje system distal to the node.

The AV node measures about 2×5 mm and is located on the endocardial surface of the right side of the interatrial septum just inferior to the os of the coronary sinus (Fig 4–14). The bundle of His is in direct continuity with the lower portion of the AV node. It is about 20 mm long and is located on the endocardial surface of the right side of the interatrial septum. The bundle of His is divided by collagen septa into longitudinal tracts, which continue into the bundle branches; thus, the bundle branches actually originate in the bundle of His.

The right bundle branch arises from the bundle of His and traverses the endocardial surface of the right side of the interventricular septum (Fig 4–10). It divides into Purkinje fibers quite close to the myocardium. The left bundle branch arises from the bundle of His and divides into 3 radiations, or **fascicles.** The more proximal is the inferoposterior fascicle, which spreads as a broad band of fibers over the posterior and inferior endocardial surface of the left ventricle. Just distal to the origin of the inferoposterior fascicle is the origin of the anterosuperior fascicle, which spreads as a narrower radiation of fibers over the anterior and superior endocardial surface of the left ventricle. Septal fibers, which do not constitute a well-defined fascicle, spread over the left side of the interventricular septum; there is considerable individual variability in the configuration of the septal fibers.

After traversing the bundle branches, the cardiac impulse enters the peripheral Purkinje system, which covers the endocardial surfaces of both ventricles. It spreads from endocardium to epicardium through the ventricular myocardium.

ATRIAL COMPLEXES

The P wave represents atrial depolarization. The normal P wave in standard, extremity, and precordial leads does not exceed 0.11 s in duration or 2.5 mm in height. Since the spread of excitation from the SA to the AV nodes is in a leftward and superior-inferior direction, the P wave is normally upright in leads I, II, aVF, and V_{3-6} and normally inverted in aVR (and frequently in V_1 and sometimes in V_2). It may be upright or inverted in lead III or aVL, depending upon the mean frontal plane P wave axis (Fig 4–15).

The T_a wave of atrial repolarization is usually best recorded in leads II, III, and aVF when the P waves in these leads are prominent. The T_a wave recorded in the inferior leads is a broad (up to 0.4 s), negative wave that can occasionally deform the ST segment. Most often, however, the T_a wave is inapparent in the ECG.

VENTRICULAR COMPLEXES

The QRS complex represents ventricular activation. Initial depolarization of the ventricles occurs from left to right across the mid portion of the interventricular septum. The impulse then passes down the right and left bundle branches and fascicles into the peripheral Purkinje system, initiating activation in the ventricles. The myocardium is depolarized from the endocardial to the epicardial surface. Since the muscle mass of the left ventricle is much greater than that of the right ventricle, there is a greater electrical potential spreading through the left ventricle compared to the right ventricle. The last portions of ventricular muscle to be depolarized are the posterobasal portion of the left ventricle, the area of the pulmonary conus, and the uppermost portion of the interventricular septum.

Repolarization follows depolarization and is a complex event that remains poorly understood. It is known that the ventricular cavities are negative during repolarization; the epicardial surface of the left ventricle is positive and that of the right ventricle is either positive or negative.

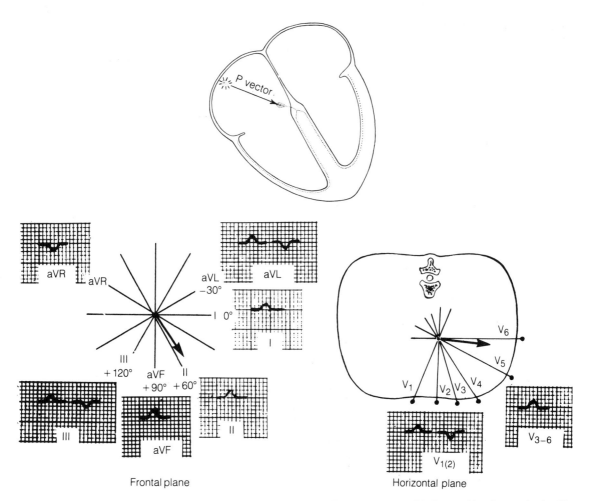

Figure 4-15. Direction of the normal frontal and horizontal plane P wave vectors with the resulting P wave in the 12-lead ECG. The normal P wave vector in the frontal plane is between 0 and +90°. A P wave vector between 0 and +30° will produce an inverted P wave in lead III. A P wave vector past +60° will produce an inverted P wave in lead aVL. The degree of anterior orientation in the horizontal plane will determine whether the P wave is upright or inverted in lead V_1.

(Text continues on page 30)

Septal Depolarization
(Fig 4–16)

Activation of the septum from left to right results in a vector oriented to the right and anteri-orly. The vector is of short duration (usually less than 0.01 s) and small magnitude (0.1–0.2 mV). It contributes to the normal small q waves in leads I and V_{5-6} and the r wave in V_{1-2}. The septal vector

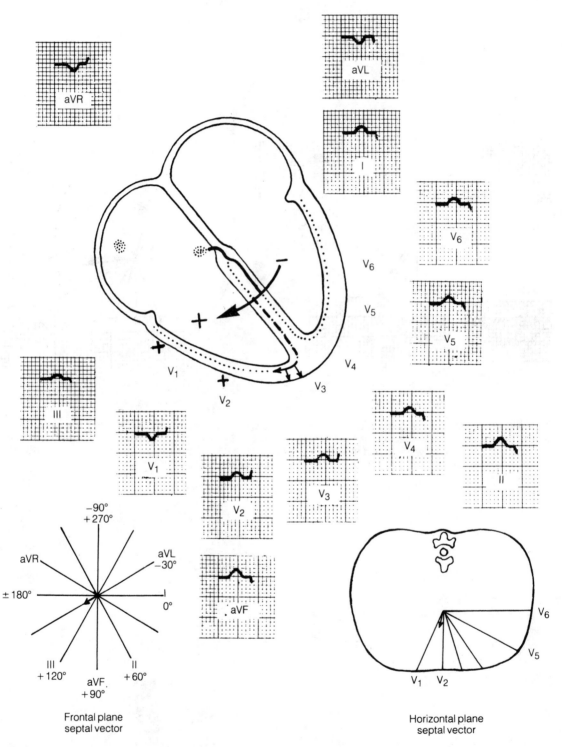

Figure 4-16. Septal depolarization. The vector of septal depolarization is directed rightward and anteriorly. This results in a positive deflection (r wave) in lead V_1 and a negative deflection (q wave) in left ventricular epicardial leads (such as V_5).

may be oriented inferiorly or superiorly; in the latter instance, a small q wave in aVF will be inscribed.

Early Activation of the Anteroseptal Region of the Myocardium
(Fig 4-17)

The resulting vector is oriented in a direction similar to that of septal depolarization. It is also of short duration and small magnitude and further contributes to the q wave in leads I and V_{5-6} and r wave in V_{1-2}.

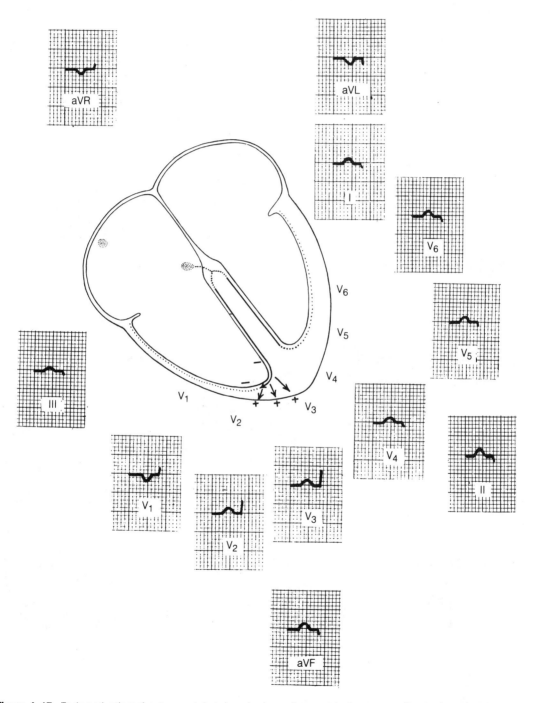

Figure 4-17. Early activation of anteroseptal region of myocardium, producing a mean force oriented to the right and anteriorly.

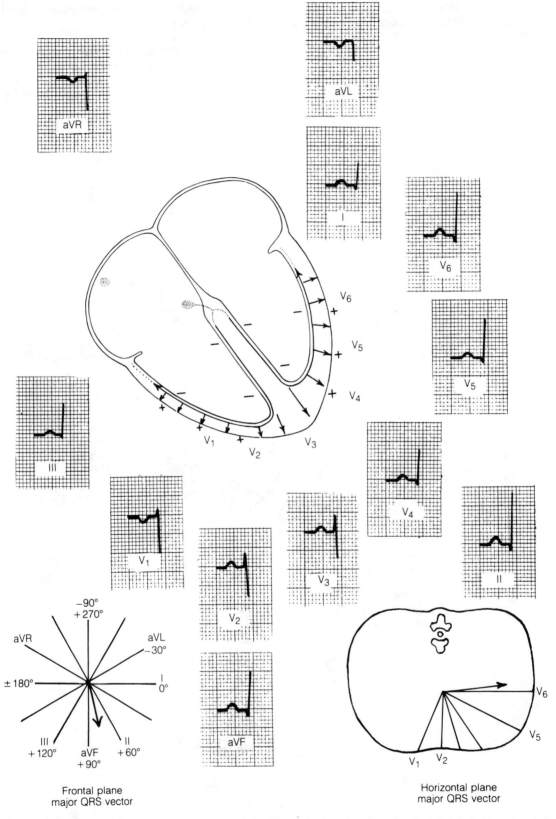

Figure 4-18. Major activation of left and right ventricles. The mean force is oriented to the left, inferiorly, and posteriorly.

Major Activation
of the Right & Left Ventricles
(Fig 4–18)

Since the left ventricle is dominant in the normal adult, the mean forces will be oriented to the left, posteriorly, and usually inferiorly. This vector will produce a dominant R wave in lead I and V_{5-6}. The actual morphology of the QRS complexes in leads II, III, aVL, and aVF will depend upon the frontal plane QRS axis. Lead V_1 will record a small r wave with a deeper S wave (R:S ratio less than 1). As one progresses from V_1 to V_6 the R waves become larger and the S waves smaller.

Late Activation
of the Posterobasal Portion
of the Left Ventricle, Pulmonary
Conus, & Uppermost Portion
of the Interventricular Septum
(Fig 4–19 on page 34)

The mean vector is often oriented to the right, producing small s waves in leads I and V_{5-6}. In 5% of normal adults it is directed anteriorly, producing small r′ waves in V_{1-2}.

Ventricular Repolarization
(Fig 4–20 on page 35)

In the normal adult, ventricular repolarization results in an isoelectric ST segment and a mean T wave vector oriented to the left, inferiorly (between 0 and $+90°$ in the frontal plane), and slightly anteriorly. This produces upright T waves in leads, I, II, and aVF and inverted T waves in aVR. The polarity of the T wave in leads III and aVL will depend upon the mean frontal plane T wave axis. If it is between 0 and $+30°$, it will normally be inverted in lead III; if it is between $+60$ and $+90°$, it will be inverted in lead aVL. The T wave may be upright or inverted in lead V_1 but is upright in leads V_{2-6}.

REFERENCES

James RN: The connecting pathways between the sinus node and A-V node and between the right and left atrium in the human heart. *Am Heart J* 1963;**66**:498.

James TN, Sherf L: Fine structure of the His bundle. *Circulation* 1971;**44**:9.

James TN, Sherf L: Specialized tissues and preferential conduction in the atria of the heart. *Am J Cardiol* 1971;**28**:414.

James TN, Sherf L, Urthaler F: Fine structure of the bundle branches. *Br Heart J* 1974;**36**:1.

Kishida H, Cole JS, Surawicz B: Negative U wave: A highly specific but poorly understood sign of heart disease. *Am J Cardiol* 1982;**49**:2030.

Millar RN et al: Studies of intra-atrial conduction with bipolar atrial and His electrograms. *Br Heart J* 1973;**35**:604.

Sherf L: The atrial conduction system: Clinical implications. *Am J Cardiol* 1976;**37**:814.

Titus JL: Normal anatomy of the human cardiac conduction system. *Mayo Clin Proc* 1973;**48**:24.

Watanabe Y: Purkinje repolarization as a possible cause of the U wave in the electrocardiogram. *Circulation* 1975;**51**:1030.

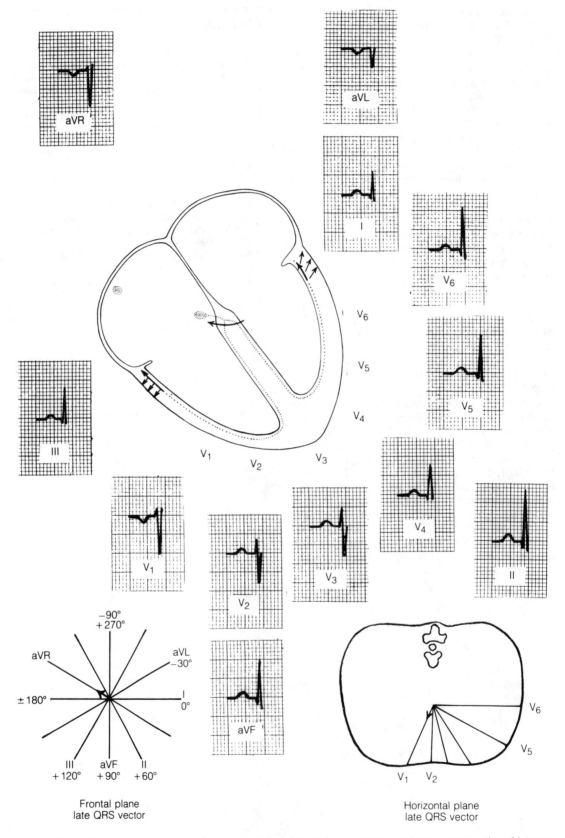

Figure 4-19. Activation of posterobasal portion of left ventricle, pulmonary conus, and uppermost portion of interventricular septum. The mean force is oriented rightward, superiorly, and anteriorly.

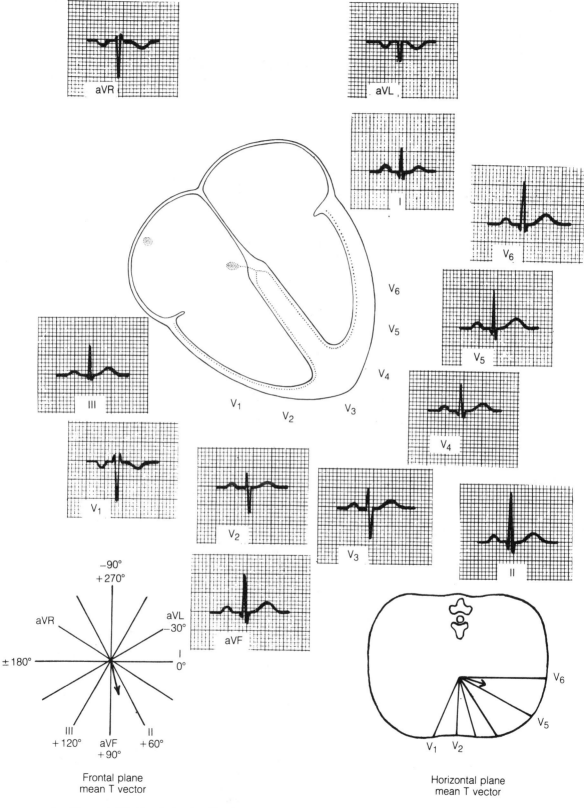

Figure 4-20. Repolarization. The mean T vector is oriented leftward, inferiorly, and anteriorly.

Figure 4–T1.
TEST TRACINGS

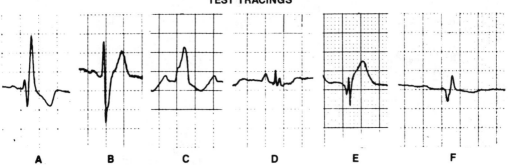

| A | B | C | D | E | F |

Describe the configuration of the QRS complexes.

A: rSR′; B: RS; C: notched R wave, or rR′; D: qRsr′; E: QRS; F: QR.

Figure 4–T2.
TEST TRACINGS

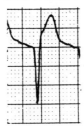

Is the J junction and ST segment normal, elevated, or depressed?

Elevated.

Figure 4–T3.
TEST TRACINGS

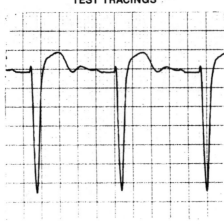

Measure the intervals of this P–QRSTU complex.

P wave duration = 0.11 s,
PR interval = 0.25 s,
PR segment = 0.16 s, QRS duration = 0.16 s,
QT interval = 0.45 s, QU interval = 0.66 s.

Figure 4-T4.
TEST TRACINGS

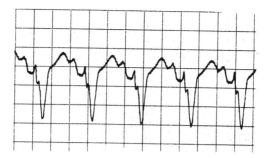

Is the PR segment normal, depressed, or elevated?

Due to the rapid heart rate, the TP segment, normally isoelectric, is obliterated. The PR segment cannot, therefore, be evaluated in relation to it. Although PR segment depression is suggested at first glance, absence of an isoelectric portion of the baseline makes this diagnosis likely to be erroneous. The PR segment cannot be properly evaluated from this tracing.

Figure 4-T5.
TEST TRACINGS

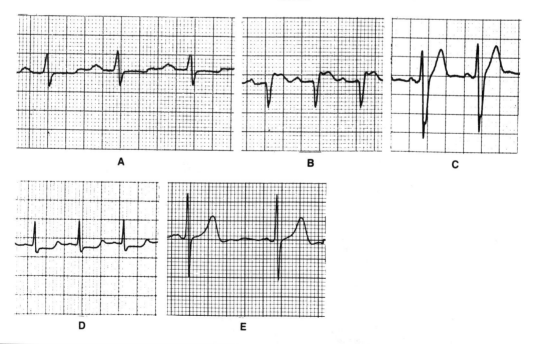

A

B

C

D

E

Describe the location of the J junction (isoelectric, depressed, or elevated) in the tracings.

A: isoelectric; B: depressed; C: elevated; D: elevated; E: isoelectric.

Variants of the Electrocardiogram in Normal Adults

"Normal" electrocardiographic measurements are determined from studies of large groups of clinically normal individuals. If a 100th percentile range for each measurement were used, the overlap between normal and abnormal measurements would render electrocardiographic interpretation practically worthless. Thus, arbitrary limits of "normality" are set in the 95th–98th percentile range; for any given electrocardiographic measurement, 2–5% of normal persons will have abnormal ECGs.

Causes of Variability in the ECG

Recognized sources of variability in the ECG include age, sex, body weight, chest configuration, position of the heart within the thoracic cage, race, food intake, ambient temperature, exercise, smoking, hyperventilation, and position of the precordial lead electrodes. Ideally, the patient should be at rest for 15 minutes prior to recording an ECG, should not have had a recent meal, and should not have smoked for 30 minutes. Reproducibility of precordial lead placement should be

Table 5-1. Definitions of functions of some clinical tests such as the ECG.

Sensitivity of the test for the abnormality	$= \dfrac{\text{Number of true positive results}}{\text{Number of patients with the abnormality}} \times 100$
Specificity of the test for the abnormality	$= \dfrac{\text{Number of true negative results}}{\text{Number of patients without the abnormality}} \times 100$
Pretest risk (probability of the abnormality in the patient undergoing the test, or *prevalence* of the abnormality)	$= \dfrac{\text{Number of patients in a given population having the abnormality}}{\text{All patients in the given population}} \times 100$
Posttest risk (probability of the abnormality in the patient undergoing the test, who has a given test result)	$= \dfrac{\text{Number of patients with a given pretest risk and the abnormality showing the given test result}}{\text{All patients with this test result}} \times 100$
	$= \dfrac{\text{Prevalence} \times \text{Sensitivity}}{(\text{Prevalence} \times \text{Sensitivity}) = + [(1\text{-prevalence}) (1\text{-specificity})]}$

Table 5-2. Some electrocardiographic abnormalities seen in asymptomatic subjects without heart disease.

(1) Abnormally tall P waves (P wave height is affected by heart rate, sympathetic tone, and position of the heart relative to the diaphragm).
(2) Notched P waves of normal duration.
(3) Abnormal Q waves (affected by body build, position of the heart in relation to the diaphragm, chest cage abnormalities such as kyphoscoliosis, and pulmonary conditions such as pneumothorax).
(4) Tall right precordial R waves (prominent anterior forces).
(5) Prominent precordial voltage (affected by ventricular muscle mass, distance of recording electrodes from cardiac muscle, and body build).
(6) Intraventricular conduction delay, notched QRS complexes, and bundle branch block patterns.
(7) AV nodal conduction delay and block (affected by vagal tone).
(8) Early repolarization.
(9) Isolated T wave inversions.

ensured by proper attention to correct positioning and, when indicated, by marking the precordial positions on the chest wall with ink.

The phrase "normal variant" of an ECG connotes a tracing recorded from a normal individual which displays some degree of variation, generally minor, in P–QRST morphology from the usual. Some normal persons may also exhibit pronounced electrocardiographic abnormalities, such as bundle branch block. The result of a specific test (such as the ECG), although outside the range of normal in itself, does not necessarily predict the presence of disease in the subject being tested. The predictive capability of any given test for the presence or absence of a disease will depend on the *prevalence* of that disease in the population being tested (Bayes's theorem) (Table 5–1): if the prevalence is low, the predictive accuracy of an abnormal test for the disease is also low; and conversely, if the prevalence is high, the predictive accuracy

of the abnormal test is also high. Thus, an abnormal ECG recorded in a healthy asymptomatic individual need not necessarily warrant diagnostic workup. Since abnormal ECG patterns that occur in normal subjects can mimic various forms of heart disease (Table 5–2), correlative clinical information is mandatory to accurate ECG interpretation. If heart disease is either not suspected or is known to be absent, the ECG interpretation should be limited to a precise description of the findings rather than suggesting a particular diagnosis.

ST SEGMENT ELEVATION

The J junction and ST segment may be elevated up to 2 mm in the precordial leads in normal persons. Occasionally, up to 4 mm of ST segment elevation can occur in left precordial leads (Fig 5–1).

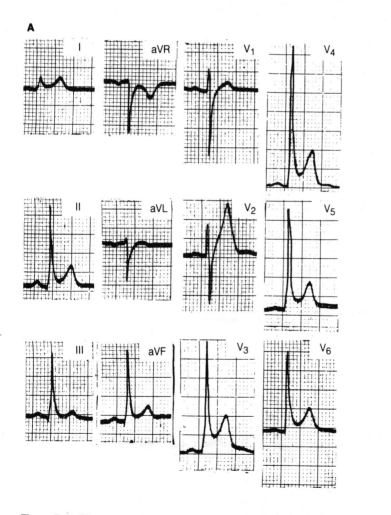

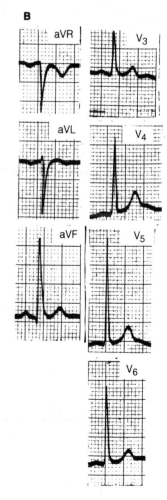

Figure 5–1. ST segment elevation in a normal person, occurring as a normal variant. *A:* The resting ECG shows marked ST segment elevation in V_{3-5} reaching 4 mm in V_{3-4}. *B:* After exercise, the ST segment approaches the isoelectric baseline.

The elevated ST segment occurring in a normal individual has an upward concave configuration, and the T wave is usually upright. During exercise, the elevated ST segments usually become isoelectric (Fig 5-1).

ST segment elevation in normal persons is considered to represent **early repolarization** of a portion of the ventricular myocardium, occurring before depolarization is completed in other areas of the myocardium.

ST SEGMENT ELEVATION WITH T WAVE INVERSION

As a further variant of the above pattern, late T wave inversion can be seen in those leads that record the ST segment elevation (Fig 5-2). This combination of ST-T wave abnormalities may simulate myocardial disease and therefore requires clinical correlation. For unknown reasons, ST elevation with T wave inversion is more common in black people. With exercise and the concomitant sinus tachycardia, these changes are normalized.

HYPERVENTILATION

In normal subjects who have episodic anxiety and hyperventilation, several abnormalities of the ECG have been described, including PR interval prolongation, sinus tachycardia, and ST segment depression with or without T wave inversion. These findings are most often recorded in leads II, III, aVF, and the left precordial leads. The electrocardiographic abnormalities may simulate myocardial ischemia but have been documented to occur in individuals with no heart disease and normal coronary arteriograms. The abnormalities have been considered to be due, at least in part, to imbalance of autonomic nervous system input. Drugs such as atropine, propranolol, and potassium can result in normalization of the ECG (Fig 5-3).

EFFECT OF FOOD INTAKE ON THE ELECTROCARDIOGRAM

Following a heavy meal, especially one of high carbohydrate content, ST depression or T wave

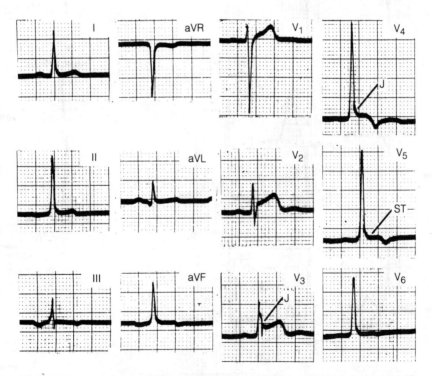

Figure 5-2. J junction and ST segment elevation with T wave inversion as a normal variant, recorded in a 23-year-old healthy black man. These ST–T wave abnormalities were not modified by mild exercise, beta-blocking drugs, hyperventilation, or vagal blocking agents. Whereas submaximal exercise may not result in normalization of the ST–T findings, maximal effort can temporarily abolish them. (From Goldman MJ: *Am Heart J* 1960;**59:**71.)

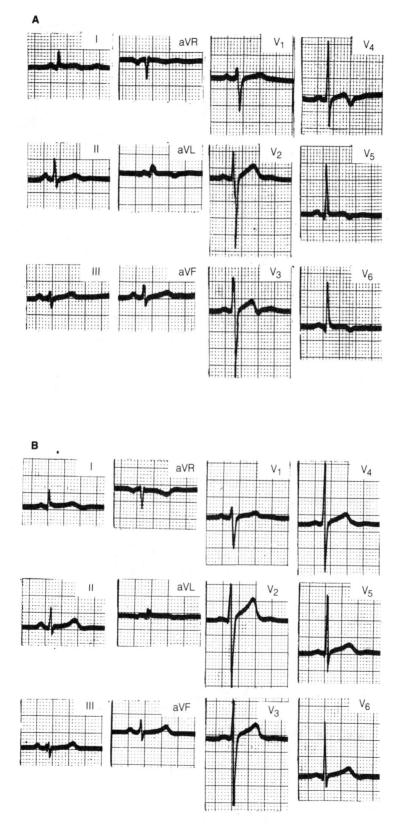

Figure 5-3. ECGs from a 26-year-old man without heart disease but with anxiety reaction and hyperventilation. *A:* Abnormal "resting" ECG shows inverted T waves in V_{4-6}. *B:* After intravenous atropine, the ECG is normal.

Figure 5-4. Nondiagnostic ST and T wave abnormalities in a healthy 30-year-old woman who had eaten a heavy meal 60 minutes earlier. A repeat ECG taken 3 hours postprandially was entirely normal.

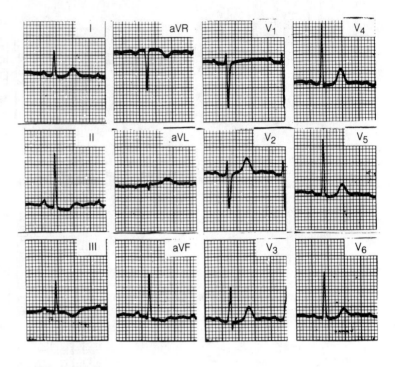

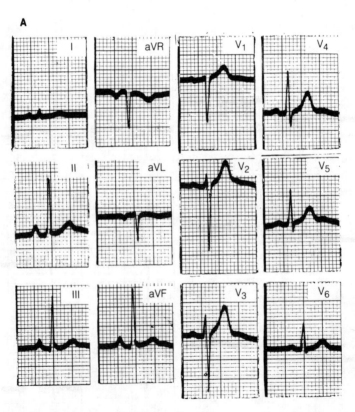

Figure 5-5. Effect of deep respiration on the ECG. *A:* Deep inspiration. The mean frontal plane QRS axis is +85°, and the heart position is vertical. *B:* Deep expiration. The heart position is now more horizontal, and the mean frontal plane QRS axis is +65°. There is greater QRS voltage in lead I, less negative voltage in aVF, and an increase in voltage in V_{4-6} during expiration.

inversion (or both) may occur. This represents a physiologic (not a pathologic) phenomenon and is due in part to an intracellular shift of potassium in association with intracellular glucose metabolism. Such electrocardiographic changes may simulate a variety of pathologic states (Fig 5–4).

EFFECT OF DEEP RESPIRATION ON THE ELECTROCARDIOGRAM

While not strictly speaking a "normal variant" of the ECG, substantial changes in individual electrocardiographic leads during deep respiration develop in some patients (Fig 5–5). These changes occur because the position of the heart within the chest cage becomes more vertical with deep inspiration and more horizontal with full expiration. Variations in right and left ventricular stroke volume during respiration may also play a role in these electrocardiographic changes. Occasionally, respiratory variation in QRS morphology can be quite marked in the precordial leads (Fig 5–6).

REFERENCES

Bachman S, Sparrow D, Smith KL: Effect of aging on the electrocardiogram. *Am J Cardiol* 1981;**48**:513.

Balady GJ, Cadigan JB, Ryan TJ: Electrocardiogram of the athlete: An analysis of 289 professional football players. *Am J Cardiol* 1984;**53**:1339.

Diamond GA, Forrester JS: Analysis of probability as an aid in the clinical diagnosis of coronary artery disease. *N Engl J Med* 1979;**300**:1350.

Frank S, Colliver JA, Frank A: The electrocardiogram in obesity: Statistical analysis of 1,029 patients. *J Am Coll Cardiol* 1986;**7**:295.

Proudfit WL, Heupler FA: Electrocardiographic evidence suggestive of myocardial infarction without significant organic heart disease. *Am Heart J* 1985;**110**:448.

Surawicz B: Assessing abnormal ECG patterns in the absence of heart disease. *Cardiovasc Med* 1977;**2**:629.

Zeppilli P et al: T wave abnormalities in top-ranking athletes: Effects of isoproterenol, atropine, and physical exercise. *Am Heart J* 1980;**100**:213.

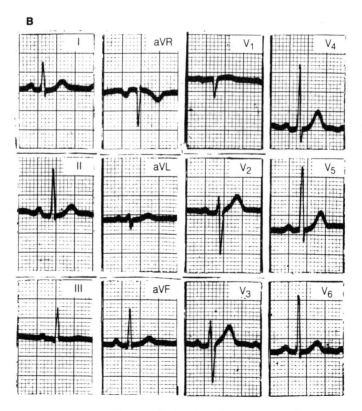

Figure 5–5. *(continued)*

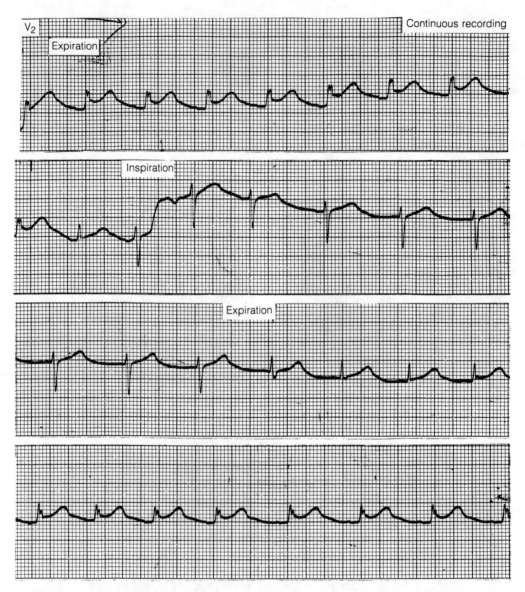

Figure 5–6. Continuously recorded lead V_2 in a patient without heart disease recorded during deep respiration. The QRS morphology has a notched R configuration during expiration, and an rS morphology during inspiration. These changes probably reflect the difference in heart position within the chest during these respiratory maneuvers, rather than rate-dependent changes in conduction (see Chapter 10).

Figure 5-T1.
TEST TRACINGS

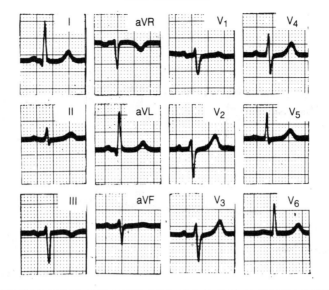

Is the heart position vertical or horizontal?	Horizontal.
What is the mean frontal plane QRS axis?	−20°
What is the PR interval?	0.14 s.
What is the QRS duration?	0-08 s.
Is the ECG normal or abnormal?	Normal

Figure 5-T2.
TEST TRACINGS

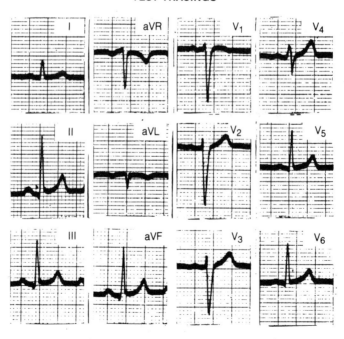

What is the mean frontal plane QRS axis?	+70°
What is the PR interval?	0.14 s.
What is the QRS duration?	0.08 s.
Is the heart position vertical or horizontal?	Vertical.
Is the ECG normal or abnormal?	Normal.

Figure 5-T3.
TEST TRACINGS

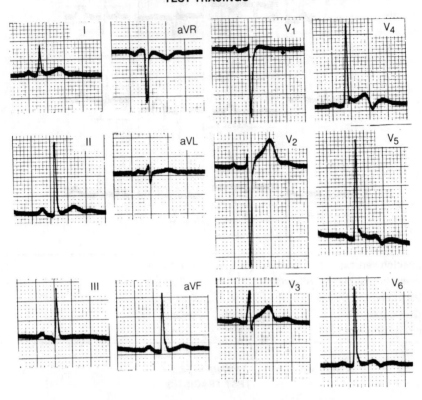

What is the mean frontal plane QRS axis?	$+60°$.	
What is the PR interval?	0.16 s.	
What is the QRS duration?	0.08 s.	
In which leads is a U wave apparent?	I, II, V_{2-4}.	
Describe the location of the J junction in lead V_2.	2 mm above the baseline.	
In which leads is the J junction elevated above the baseline?	I, V_{2-6}.	
Are the ST segments normal or abnormal?	Normal.	

This tracing represents a normal variant in a healthy 24-year-old black man. Despite the prominent precordial voltage (see Chapter 7), no clinical evidence of left ventricular hypertrophy was present.

Figure 5-T4.
TEST TRACINGS

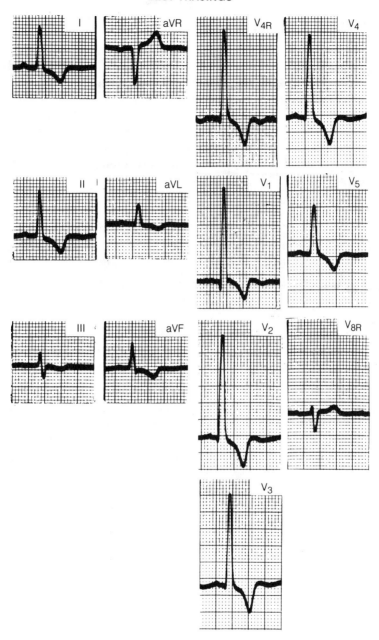

What is the mean frontal plane QRS axis?	+30°.
Identify the abnormalities in the ST segments and T waves and the leads in which they occur.	ST segment depression and T wave inversion are present in leads I, II, aVF, and V_{2-4}. T wave inversion is present in leads aVL, V_{4R}, V_1 and V_6.
Is the QRS voltage abnormally low or abnormally high? Which leads are involved?	Abnormally high voltage is present in leads V_{4R} through V_4.

This tracing represents anatomic rotation of the heart on its horizontal axis due to congenital dextroversion. Although the possibility of right ventricular hypertrophy is suggested by the tall right precordial voltage (see Chapter 7), the criteria are invalidated in the presence of dextroversion.

Figure 5-T5.
TEST TRACINGS

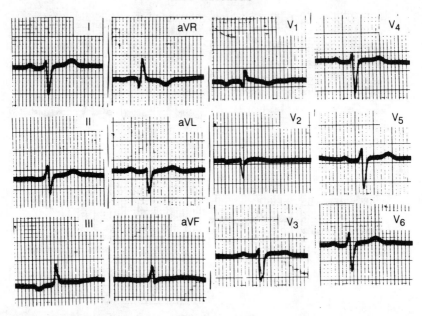

What is the mean frontal plane QRS axis?	+150°.
Describe the QRS morphology in lead V₁.	qR.
Describe the QRS morphology in lead V₆.	rS.
What is the PR interval?	0.2 s.

This tracing represents anatomic rotation of the heart on its horizontal axis due to congenital absence of the left pericardium. In this congenital abnormality the heart is displaced to the left and rotated in a true clockwise direction, resulting in the major QRS forces being directed rightward and posteriorly. This accounts for the QR pattern in V₁ and deep S waves persisting through V₆.

Figure 5–T6.
TEST TRACINGS

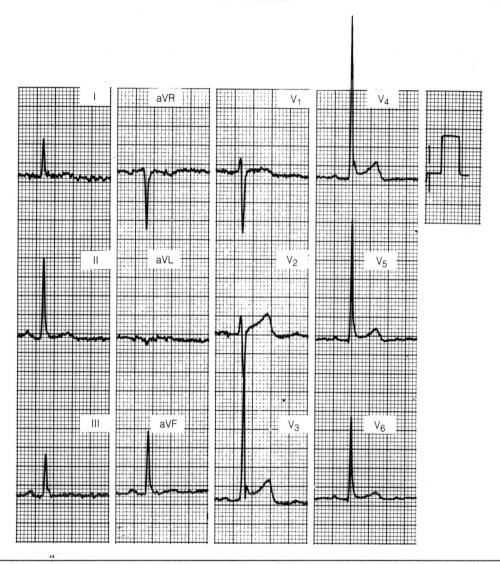

What is the mean frontal plane QRS axis?	Around +60°.
What is the QRS duration?	0.08 s.
Is the PR interval normal or abnormal?	Normal.
Describe the precordial voltage.	Prominent, suggesting, but not proving, left ventricular hypertrophy.
What is the amount (in millimeters) of J point elevation in leads V_3 and V_4?	4 and 4.5 mm, respectively.
Are the ST–T waves normal or abnormal?	Normal.
Is the ECG normal or abnormal?	A variant of normal.
What is the probable cause of the baseline artifact?	Muscle tremor; the patient was not relaxed.

This tracing was recorded from a 21-year-old healthy athlete.

6

P Wave Abnormalities

The normal P wave does not exceed 0.12 s in width and 2.5 mm in height. An increase in these values suggests the presence of atrial abnormality, which could be due to hypertrophy, dilatation, conduction delay within the atria, or a combination of these. Inasmuch as the ECG does not distinguish among these conditions, the term **atrial abnormality** is preferred to **atrial hypertrophy**. Where additional electrocardiographic evidence for the diagnosis of atrial hypertrophy exists (as, for example, when the pattern of ventricular hypertrophy is present) the diagnosis of actual atrial hypertrophy is more certain. Similarly, when electrocardiographic evidence of myocardial infarction or intraventricular conduction system disease is present, left atrial enlargement and interatrial conduction delay are more likely diagnoses, respectively, than is atrial hypertrophy. Thus, electrocardiographic evidence of a single clinical entity to explain the abnormalities in P wave configuration should be sought.

The sensitivity, specificity, and predictive accuracy of the electrocardiographic diagnosis of atrial hypertrophy, enlargement, or conduction delay for their actual existence will vary with the "gold standard" method applied to confirm the diagnosis, the particular diagnosis being made (eg, atrial hypertrophy or enlargement), and with the patient population being evaluated for the abnormality and the prevalence of the abnormality within that population (see Table 5-1).

Validation of the electrocardiographic criteria for atrial hypertrophy or dilatation has been obtained from cardiac catheterization studies with measurement of interatrial pressures; from M-mode and 2-dimensional echocardiographic studies, which provide knowledge of atrial size, wall thickness, and volume; and from postmortem studies, which provide direct measurement of size and wall thickness. The 2-dimensional echocardiogram is the superior clinical tool but is obviously more expensive and time-consuming than the 12-lead ECG. If the cause of the electrocardiographic abnormality cannot be inferred from the clinical picture, echocardiography can be used to evaluate if it is clinically warranted. None of these techniques directly measures interatrial conduction.

Left Atrial Abnormality

The criteria for left atrial abnormality are (1) a broad ($\geq$ 0.12 s), notched P wave usually best seen in leads I and II, and (2) a wide (1 mm $\times$ 0.04 s) terminal negative deflection in lead V_1. The broadened P wave results in an increased ratio of the P wave duration to the PR interval.

The early portion of the P wave represents right atrial depolarization, and the latter portion represents left atrial depolarization (Fig 6-1). Hypertrophy or enlargement of the left atrium results in an accentuation of the left atrial portion of the P wave, producing a broad, notched wave in the standard leads. Since the left atrium lies posterior

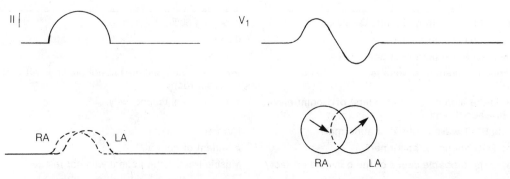

Figure 6-1. Diagram of atrial depolarization in relation to the P wave inscribed in leads II and V_1 of the surface ECG. The initial portion of the P wave results from right atrial depolarization, and the latter portion of the P wave results from left atrial depolarization. Enlargement or hypertrophy of either chamber will result in accentuation of that portion of the P wave to which it contributes most. In lead II, left atrial abnormality will result in a broad, notched P wave, and right atrial abnormality will result in a tall P wave. In precordial lead V_1, left atrial abnormality will result in a prominent terminal negative component of the P wave associated with a posteriorly directed depolarization, and right atrial abnormality will cause a tall, peaked initial portion of the P wave.

to the right atrium, depolarization of a hypertrophied or enlarged left atrium will produce the prominent negative component of the P wave in the right precordial leads (Fig. 6–2).

The sensitivity and specificity of the electrocardiographic pattern of left atrial abnormality are each about 66% when correlated with autopsy measurements; however, the electrocardiographic pattern almost always occurs in patients with underlying cardiac disease (often ventricular hypertrophy). Similarly, sensitivity and specificity of the electrocardiographic criteria (alone or in combination) for the diagnosis are about 57% and 65%, respectively, when using echocardiographic techniques to measure left atrial dimension.

Right Atrial Abnormality

The criteria for right atrial abnormality are (1) tall, peaked P waves in leads II, III, and aVF ($\geq$ 2.5 mm in height in lead II) (Fig 6–3), and (2) prominent peaked, diphasic, or markedly inverted P waves in lead V_1. The P wave duration is normal, and the mean P wave vector in the frontal plane is between +75 and +90°.

"Pseudo-P-Pulmonale"

This term denotes a prominent P wave in leads II, III, and aVF that is due to left, rather than right, atrial abnormality. The genesis of this wave is accentuation of that portion of the P wave which reflects left atrial depolarization, namely, the latter portion of the P wave (Fig 6–1). The initial portion of the P wave, reflecting right atrial depolarization, is normal. Depolarization of a severely diseased left atrium results in a tall terminal portion of the P wave. Involvement of the left atrium in production of the pseudo-P-pulmonale pattern is confirmed by identifying the deep, wide negative component of the P wave in lead V_1 (Fig 6–4).

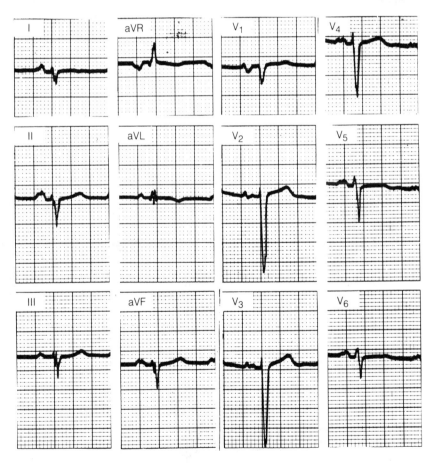

Figure 6-2. Left atrial abnormality characterized by broad, notched P waves best seen in leads II, aVF, and V_{2-5} and by a prominent (1 mm × 0.04 s) terminal negative deflection in lead V_1. The frontal plane QRS axis is −120°, and S waves are present in I, II, and III, suggesting right ventricular hypertrophy. In view of the possibility of right ventricular hypertrophy, a diagnosis of left atrial hypertrophy could be made. The patient had mitral stenosis.

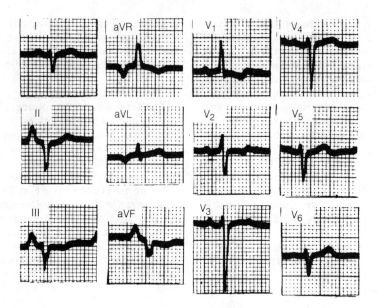

Figure 6-3. Right atrial and right ventricular hypertrophy. The P waves are abnormally tall in leads II, III, and aVF, indicating right atrial abnormality. The frontal plane QRS axis is oriented rightward (deep S in I) and superiorly (QS complexes in II, III, and aVF); the axis is −110°. A tall R wave is present in V_1. The rightward axis and tall R wave in V_1 indicate right ventricular hypertrophy. In the presence of right ventricular hypertrophy, QS complexes need not indicate myocardial infarction.

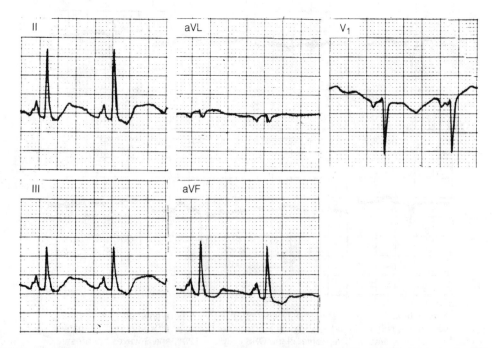

Figure 6-4. "Pseudo-P-pulmonale." The P waves appear markedly tall in leads II, III, and aVF. However, the initial (right atrial) portion of the P wave is normal; thus, the prominence is due to a left atrial abnormality, which is confirmed by the deep, wide negative P wave component in lead V_1.

Biatrial Abnormality

The criteria for biatrial abnormality are the presence of the independent criteria for both left and right atrial abnormality. The P waves will be notched and broad (≥ 0.12 s) in leads 1 and 11 and will have a prominent negative component (exceeding 1 mm $\times$ 0.04 s) in lead VI. In addition, the initial forces will be tall (≥ 2.5 mm) in lead II (Fig 6-5).

Transient P wave abnormalities, or reversible accentuation of existing P wave abnormalities, may accompany acute cardiac disease such as myocardial ischemia or infarction, or pulmonary edema (Fig 6-6), and are thought to reflect transient changes in atrial pressures, volumes, or both.

T_a Waves

T_a waves represent atrial repolarization. While a normal feature of some ECGs, these waves are accentuated in atrial hypertrophy or enlargement and in conditions that cause atrial injury, such as pericarditis or atrial infarction. A prominent T_a wave can mimic a Q wave of myocardial infarction by causing depression of the PR segment (Fig 6-7). If the T_a wave is of long duration, it can also mimic ST segment scooping or depression.

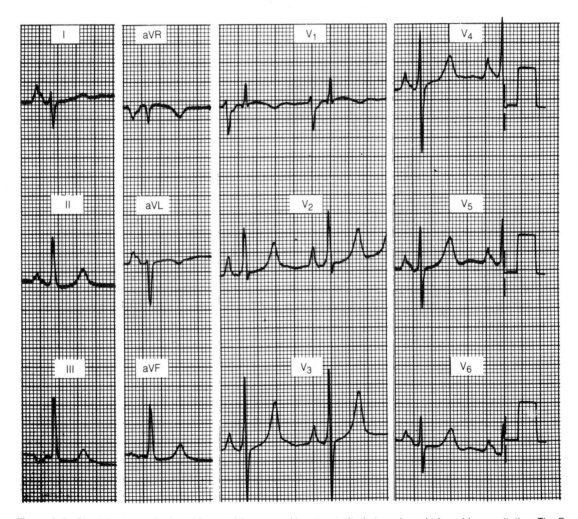

Figure 6-5. Biatrial abnormality in a 36-year-old woman with severe mitral stenosis and tricuspid regurgitation. The P wave is notched and has a duration of 0.16 s; the PR interval is 0.2 s. The P wave vector is oriented to the left and posteriorly. Note the markedly abnormal configuration in lead V_1 and the P wave height of 4.5 mm in lead V_2. Right ventricular hypertrophy is also present: the mean frontal plane QRS axis is about +125°, a qR is present in lead V_1 and a pure R wave in lead V_2. S waves persist in the precordial leads.

Figure 6-6. Transient P wave abnormalities recorded during (A) and after (B) an episode of chest pain in a patient with severe 3-vessel coronary artery disease. In (A), a pseudo-P-pulmonale pattern is recorded in lead II, and the P wave configuration in lead V_1 is entirely upright; a prominent negative component is not seen. In (B), after resolution of the chest pain, little change in lead II has occurred; however, the P wave configuration in V_1 now indicates biatrial abnormality, and a deep and wide negative component indicating left atrial abnormality is present. The alteration in P wave morphology during pain could represent acute atrial ischemia, interatrial conduction delay resulting from the ischemia, or an increase in intra-atrial pressure resulting from ischemia-related ventricular dysfunction. The diagnosis cannot be made from the ECG.

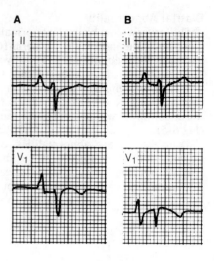

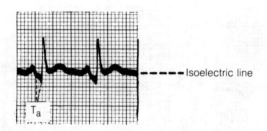

Figure 6-7. Prominent atrial repolarization (T_a) waves, producing pronounced PR segment depression.

REFERENCES

Chou TC, Helm RA: The pseudo P pulmonale. *Circulation* 1965;**32**:96.

DiBianco R et al: Left atrial overload: A hemodynamic, echocardiographic, electrocardiographic and vectorcardiographic study. *Am Heart J* 1979;**98**:478.

Josephson ME, Kastor JA, Morganroth J: Electrocardiographic left atrial enlargement: Electrophysiologic, electrocardiographic and hemodynamic correlates. *Am J Cardiol* 1977;**39**:967.

Surawicz B: Electrocardiographic diagnosis of chamber enlargement. *J Am Coll Cardiol* 1986;**8**:711.

Figure 6-T1.
TEST TRACINGS

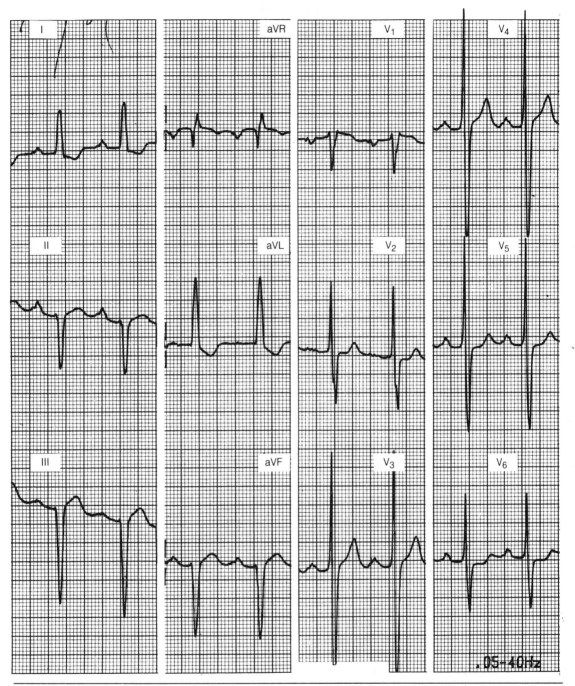

What is the P wave axis in the frontal plane?	+60°.
What is the P wave duration?	0.15 s. The P wave duration should be measured in those leads in which its onset is clearly defined. In this ECG, leads I and aVR show the P wave best.
What is the PR interval?	0.26 s.
Is right atrial abnormality present?	No. The initial forces of the P wave are normal.
Is left atrial abnormality present?	Yes. The P wave is abnormally broad, and there is an abnormal negative component in lead V₁. The maximum height of the P wave in lead II in this ECG is contributed to by the left, not the right, atrium.

Figure 6-T2.
TEST TRACINGS

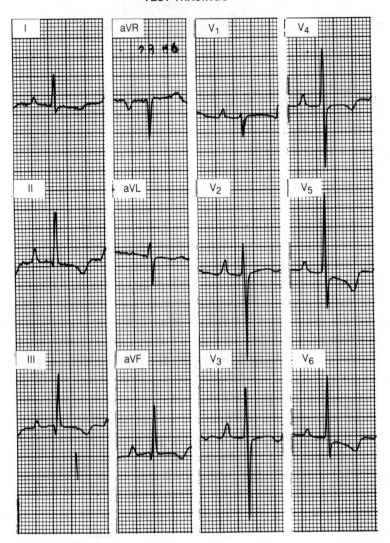

What is the mean frontal plane QRS axis?	+75°.
What is the P wave axis in the frontal plane?	+75°.
What is the height of the P wave in lead II?	3.5 mm.
Does this represent right or left atrial abnormality?	Right atrial abnormality since the initial P wave forces are abnormal in height.
Is an interatrial conduction delay present?	No. The P wave duration is 0.07 s.

This tracing was recorded from a patient with severe chronic obstructive pulmonary disease and clinical evidence of right ventricular hypertrophy. The lateral ST–T wave abnormalities are not explained by the right ventricular hypertrophy and are of uncertain significance.

Figure 6-T3.
TEST TRACINGS

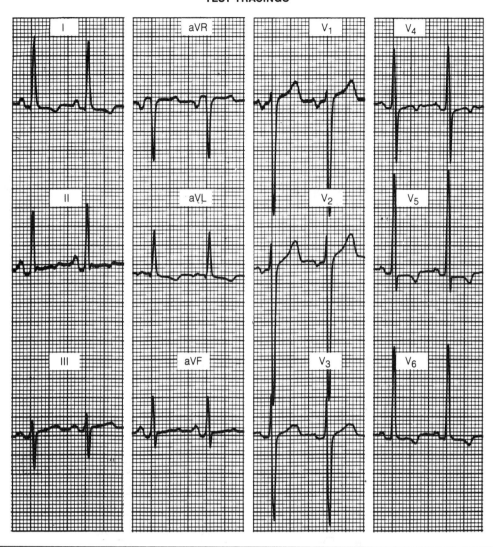

Is the P wave duration normal?	Yes, at about 0.09 s.
Is the mean frontal plane P wave axis normal?	Yes, at about +55°.
Is the PR interval normal?	Yes, at 0.16 s.
Are Q waves present in leads II and aVF?	No; the scooping prior to the onset of the QRS complexes is caused by a prominent T_a wave which depresses the PR segment.
In which leads is the T_a wave most prominent?	II, aVF, V_{4-6}.

This ECG was recorded in a patient with hypertension, as part of a routine yearly examination. There was no evidence of pericarditis.

Ventricular Hypertrophy

Ventricular hypertrophy develops as a result of pressure or volume load imposed upon the ventricles. A correlation exists between the thickness of ventricular muscle and the magnitude of its depolarization wave, although the underlying reasons for this are far from clear. A less good correlation is present between intracavitary blood volume and depolarization wave amplitude. In addition to, and in part because of, the increased muscle mass in ventricular hypertrophy, there is delay in conduction of impulses through the hypertrophied chamber, and often an alteration in the depolarization and repolarization pathways as well. Thus, the electrocardiographic features of ventricular hypertrophy are (1) an increase in the height of the depolarization wave representing the hypertrophied chamber, (2) prolongation of the QRS duration, (3) lengthening of the activation time (intrinsicoid deflection) over the hypertrophied ventricle to more than 0.05 s, (4) ST segment depression, and (5) T wave abnormalities consisting typically of asymmetric inversion, which may be shallow or deep (Fig 7–1). Those leads recording the electrical potentials from sites opposing the hypertrophied ventricle (eg, aVR or V_1 in left ventricular hypertrophy) will show (1) a deep S wave or QS complex, (2) an elevated ST segment, and (3) an upright T wave.

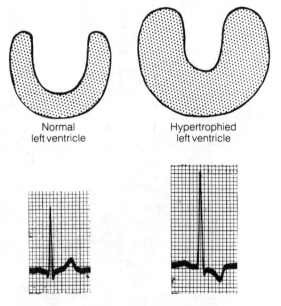

Figure 7–1. Diagram of a normal and a hypertrophied left ventricle and the associated QRS complexes recorded from overlying electrocardiographic leads. Compared to the normal QRS complex, the QRS complex recorded over the hypertrophied ventricle has greater height, prolonged intrinsicoid deflection (ventricular activation time), ST segment depression, and asymmetric T wave inversion.

Left Ventricular Hypertrophy

Left ventricular hypertrophy may result from a variety of conditions (Table 7–1). The electrocardiographic abnormalities may precede radiologic changes and thus may be the first clue to the diagnosis.

The mean frontal plane QRS axis may be deviated to the left, to between 0 and $-30°$, concomileftward axis deviation exceeds $-30°$, concomitant left anterior fascicular block may be present (see Chapter 8).

A left ventricular epicardial complex is recorded in lead aVL; therefore, a tall R wave with a depressed ST segment and an inverted T wave will be seen in this lead (Fig 7–2). An R wave equal to or exceeding 11 mm in lead aVL is highly specific for the diagnosis of left ventricular hypertrophy (although it is an insensitive criterion, occurring in only about 25% of cases), provided that the mean frontal plane QRS axis is not pathologically deviated to the left. In the presence of abnormal left axis deviation (superior to $-30°$), left ventricular hypertrophy is suggested (but not

proved) when the height of the R wave in lead aV_L exceeds 16 mm (Fig 7–3).

Tall R waves with depressed ST segments and inverted T waves will also be seen in precordial leads V_{4-6}. The QRS duration may exceed 0.11 s, and the ventricular activation time may be greater than 0.05 s. Deep S waves will be present in anterior precordial leads V_{1-2}, since these right precordial leads reflect the larger potential generated by the thick left ventricle compared to that of the

Table 7–1. Common causes of left ventricular hypertrophy.

(1)	Hypertension
(2)	Valvular aortic stenosis
(3)	Hypertrophic cardiomyopathy
	Concentric
	Asymmetric
(4)	Supravalvular aortic stenosis
(5)	Aortic regurgitation
(6)	Mitral regurgitation
(7)	Coarctation of the aorta
(8)	Patent ductus arteriosus
(9)	"Athletic heart" ("physiologic" hypertrophy)

right ventricle. As a general rule, left ventricular hypertrophy is present if the voltage of $SV_1 + RV_5$ or $SV_1 + RV_6$ exceeds 35 mm or if the R wave in V_5 or V_6 exceeds 27 mm. However, prominent precordial voltage alone (without concomitant ST and T wave abnormalities) is an *insufficient criterion* for the diagnosis of left ventricular hypertrophy, since large voltages may be recorded in normal young adults and thin-chested individuals. Voltage criteria alone have only about a 45% accuracy for the anatomic diagnosis of left ventricular hypertrophy as determined at autopsy.

In patients with marked anatomic left ventricular hypertrophy, and especially in those with septal hypertrophy, there can be a loss of anterior QRS forces (small or absent r waves in V_{1-3}), mimicking anterior wall myocardial infarction. Less commonly, abnormal Q or QS waves can be recorded in the inferior leads (II, III, and aVF) or lateral leads (I and V_6), simulating inferior or lateral wall myocardial infarction.

Some patients with left ventricular hypertrophy have hearts that are oriented vertically in the chest. The mean frontal plane QRS axis in such patients may be normal rather than leftward, and prominent voltage is present in leads II, III, and aVF (Fig 7–4). Precordial lead voltage criteria for left ventricular hypertrophy, along with the associated ST and T wave abnormalities, may be applied in making the correct diagnosis. Biventricular hypertrophy can also cause this pattern. Thus, clinical correlation is mandatory.

The QT interval may be prolonged due to abnormalities of, and delays in, ventricular repolari-

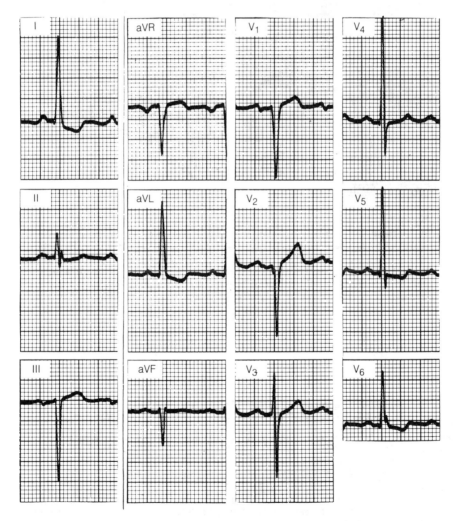

Figure 7-2. Left ventricular hypertrophy. The mean frontal plane QRS axis is −15°. The R wave exceeds 15 mm in aVL, and the sum of the S wave in V_1 and the R wave in V_5 exceeds 35 mm. ST segment depression is present in leads I and aVL, and T wave inversion is present in I, aVL, and V_{5-6}. The deep S waves in the right precordial leads reflect the large electrical force generated by the hypertrophied left ventricle. The ST segment elevation in V_{1-2} is consistent with left ventricular hypertrophy.

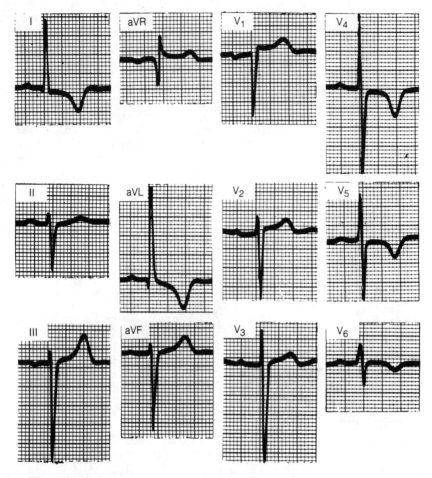

Figure 7-3. Left ventricular hypertrophy with left (superior) axis deviation. The mean frontal plane QRS axis is −45°, suggesting the possibility of coexisting left anterior fascicular block. The R wave of 24 mm in aVL, however, strongly suggests (but does not prove) the presence of left ventricular hypertrophy. ST segment depression and T wave inversion are present in aVL, and T wave inversion is present in V_{4-6}. Precordial lead voltage criteria for left ventricular hypertrophy are not met. This may be due to the superior axis, as a result of which the lead axes of V_{5-6} are far removed from the mean QRS vector. Left ventricular hypertrophy was confirmed at autopsy examination.

Table 7-2. Electrocardiographic criteria for left ventricular hypertrophy.

I. Precordial Leads:
  A. R waves in V_5 or V_6 > 27 mm. S in V_1 + R in V_5 or V_6 > 35 mm (over 35 years of age).
  B. Ventricular activation time > 0.05 s in V_{5-6}.
  C. QRS interval may be prolonged over 0.1 s.
  D. ST segment depression and T wave inversion in V_{5-6}.

II. Frontal Plane Leads:
  A. Horizontal Heart: R wave of 11 mm or more in aVL (except when frontal plane axis is superior to −30°; VAT, QRS interval, and ST-T changes as described for precordial leads. R_1 + S_3 > 26 mm; pattern in I similar to aVL.
  B. Vertical Heart: R wave of over 20 mm in aVF; VAT, QRS interval, and ST-T changes as described for precordial leads. Unless confirmed by precordial leads, this pattern in aVF is not diagnostic of left ventricular hypertrophy (since right ventricular hypertrophy can give a similar pattern in aVF).

Minimal Criteria
  R in aVL greater than 11 mm; or R in V_{5-6} greater than 27 mm; or S in V_1 + R in V_{5-6} greater than 35 mm.

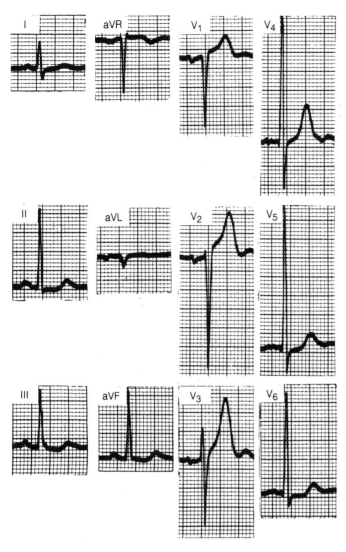

Figure 7-4. Left ventricular hypertrophy in a patient with a normal mean frontal plane QRS axis of +75°. There are tall R waves in II, III, and aVF. The sum of $SV_1 + RV_5 = 55$ mm, and ST depression is present in V_{5-6}. The P waves are notched in all leads, suggesting the possibility of left atrial hypertrophy. Prominent precordial voltage associated with a normal or rightward deviation of the mean frontal plane QRS axis should also raise the suspicion of biventricular hypertrophy.

zation. A prominent U wave may be present. In some patients with left ventricular hypertrophy due to hypertension, a negative U wave occurs. The electrocardiographic features of left ventricular hypertrophy are summarized in Table 7-2.

Sensitivity, Specificity, & Predictive Accuracy

As discussed in Chapter 6, the sensitivity, specificity, and predictive accuracy of the ECG for the anatomic diagnosis of left ventricular hypertrophy will vary with the prevalence of the condition in the population under study. ECG criteria for left ventricular hypertrophy in a patient with known aortic stenosis or essential hypertension almost always indicate true hypertrophy, whereas these same criteria in an otherwise normal individual do not necessarily indicate this diagnosis. Some causes of prominent precordial voltage in the absence of anatomic left ventricular hypertrophy are listed in Table 7-3.

Because of the suboptimal accuracy of the electrocardiographic diagnosis for left ventricular hypertrophy, the M-mode and 2-dimensional echocardiogram have been widely utilized in confirming the presence or absence of this diagnosis by measuring wall thickness and calculating left ventricular mass. Based on echocardiographic data, specific electrocardiographic variables (such as R wave height and mean frontal plane QRS axis), alone and in combination, have been analyzed in order to develop improved electrocardiographic criteria for the diagnosis. However, when specificity is maintained at about 90% in order to avoid a high false-positive incidence rate, little improvement in an overall sensitivity of about 50% has been achieved.

Table 7-3. Some causes of prominent voltage in subjects without anatomic left ventricular hypertrophy.

(1) Thin chest wall (closer proximity of the recording electrodes to the myocardial surface).
(2) Race (blacks tend to have higher voltages than whites).
(3) Sex.
(4) Age.
(5) Left anterior fascicular block (the superiorly directed mean frontal plane axis per se results in abnormally high voltages in I and aVL).
(6) Left-sided intraventricular conduction delay or left bundle branch block pattern (the abnormal depolarization sequence per se can produce abnormally high voltages).
(7) WPW conduction (abnormally tall voltages can be caused by the abnormal depolarization sequence per se).
(8) Acute myocardial ischemia (changes in voltage may be secondary to local intraventricular conduction delay).
(9) Left mastectomy (close proximity of the recording electrodes to the myocardial surface).

Right Ventricular Hypertrophy

Right ventricular hypertrophy may result from several common clinical conditions (Table 7-4). In right ventricular hypertrophy, the mean frontal plane QRS axis may be normal or deviated to the right. Axis deviation to the right of $+110°$ in an adult suggests the presence of right ventricular hypertrophy, provided that left posterior fascicular block (see Chapter 8) is not present. Tall R waves are seen in leads II, III, and aVR; in aVR, this may be a QR, qR, or R complex. The right precordial leads typically show tall R or qR waves with prolonged ventricular activation time. QR or qR waves in aVR or V_1 may reflect a delay in activation of the hypertrophied right ventricle (such that the early forces of left ventricular depolarization are recorded) and depolarization of a hypertrophied interventricular septum in a superior-inferior direction rather than a left-to-right direction (or both). QR or q waves in the right precordial leads may also reflect enlargement of the right atrium. Although the QRS duration in right ventricular hypertrophy may be slightly prolonged, it does not exceed 0.12 s. ST segment depression and T wave inversion are inscribed in the right precordial leads (Fig 7-5). Since prominent

Table 7-4. Common causes of right ventricular hypertrophy in the adult.

(1) Chronic obstructive pulmonary disease
(2) Pulmonary hypertension
    Primary
    Pulmonary emboli (acute, massive)
    Pulmonary emboli (chronic, recurrent)
    Mitral stenosis
    Mitral regurgitation
    Chronic left ventricular failure
(3) Tricuspid regurgitation
(4) Atrial septal defect

voltage in leads II, III, and aVF may be seen in patients with left ventricular hypertrophy and a vertically oriented heart, confirmation in the right precordial leads (V_{3-5}) must be sought to diagnose right ventricular hypertrophy with greater certainty.

In the absence of a conduction delay involving the right ventricle, tall R wave voltage in the right precordial leads is helpful in diagnosing right ventricular hypertrophy. A better criterion, however, is the R:S ratio in lead V_1. This ratio is normally less than 1 in the adult, but as the right ventricle hypertrophies some of the leftward forces normally recorded in the right precordial leads are canceled, resulting in an R:S ratio that approaches or exceeds 1. In addition to an abnormal R:S ratio in V_1, the R wave decrease in amplitude and the S wave increases in amplitude as the left precordial leads are recorded, reflecting prominent right ventricular forces. These features are summarized in Table 7-5.

Electrocardiographic Variations in Patients With Right Ventricular Hypertrophy

Not infrequently, the criteria for the diagnosis of right ventricular hypertrophy are not met in patients with clinical, echocardiographic, or hemodynamic evidence of this condition. Occasionally, a tall, peaked P wave in the inferior leads, which suggests right atrial abnormality (hypertrophy), may be indirect evidence of right ventricular hypertrophy (which must be inferred) (Fig 7-6). Some electrocardiographic findings correlate better with some specific disease states than with others, and may correlate better with some techniques of evaluation of that disease state (such as hemodynamic observations) than with others (such as echocardiographic data). For example, the electrocardiographic recognition of right ventricular hypertrophy is more commonly made in patients with significant pulmonary hypertension due to congenital heart disease, pulmonary vascular disease, and mitral stenosis. It is less commonly recognized in patients with chronic obstructive pulmonary disease.

Although the mean frontal plane QRS axis is deviated to the right in older patients with chronic lung disease and cor pulmonale, it may be directed posteriorly rather than anteriorly, resulting in normal, small, or even absent R waves in the right precordial leads (Fig 7-6). In these cases, anterior wall myocardial infarction may be mimicked. The T wave inversion in leads V_{1-3} that may also be seen can further mimic anterior wall myocardial ischemia or infarction. As a general rule, when the diagnosis of cor pulmonale due to chronic obstructive lung disease is known, the electrocardiographic diagnosis of myocardial infarction should not be made without clinical correlation.

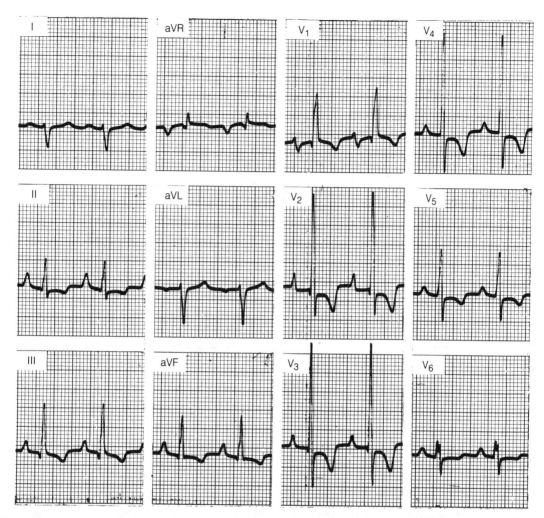

Figure 7-5. Right ventricular hypertrophy. The mean frontal plane QRS axis is deviated to the right at +120°. A QR complex is inscribed in aVR and V$_{1-3}$. The T waves are inverted in V$_{1-5}$. A deep S wave persists across the precordium as the R wave amplitude decreases. Right atrial hypertrophy is suggested by the tall, peaked P waves in II, III, aVF, and V$_1$.

Table 7-5. Electrocardiographic criteria for right ventricular hypertrophy.

I. Precordial Leads: These are the best leads for diagnosis.
   A. R wave of greater voltage than S wave in V$_1$ or V$_{3R}$ (R:S ≥ 1.0)
   B. qR pattern in V$_1$ or V$_{3R}$.
   C. Ventricular activation time > 0.03 s in V$_1$ or V$_{3R}$.
   D. Persistent S waves in V$_{5-6}$.
   E. ST segment depression and T wave inversion in V$_{1-3}$.

II. Frontal Plane Leads:
   A. Right axis deviation (greater than or equal to +110°); depressed ST segment and inverted T wave in II and III.
   B. Tall R in aVR (unless accompanied by the criteria in lead I, this alone is not indicative of right ventricular hypertrophy).
   C. Tall R with depressed ST segment and inverted T wave in aVF (unless confirmed by precordial leads, this pattern itself is not diagnostic of right ventricular hypertrophy).

Minimal Criteria
   Rs or qR complex in V$_1$ or V$_{3R}$ with VAT > 0.03 s.
   Right axis deviation.

Helpful (But Not Diagnostic) Criteria
   Abnormally tall or notched P waves; ST depression with T wave inversion in V$_{3R}$ and V$_{1-3}$ in the absence of a tall R in these leads; right intraventricular conduction delay.

Figure 7-6. Probable right ventricular hypertrophy in an older man with pulmonary emphysema. The frontal plane QRS axis is +115°. Tall, peaked P waves are present in II, III, and aVF, suggesting right atrial hypertrophy. QS complexes are present in V_{1-2}, and persistent S waves are seen in the left precordial leads. Old anterolateral wall myocardial infarction must be excluded on clinical grounds (see Chapter 9).

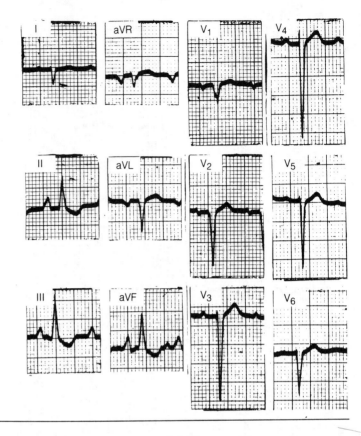

The ECGs of patients who have emphysema with hyperinflation of the lungs may show diffuse low voltage (due to the hyperinflated lung tissue), with no QRS complex exceeding 5 mm in height in the frontal leads and 10 mm in height in the precordial leads; terminal QRS forces in the frontal plane that are directed rightward (S wave in I) and superiorly (S waves in II, III, and aVF), or terminal QRS forces in the frontal plane that are directed leftward (R wave in I) and superiorly (S waves in II, III, and aVF), resulting in superior axis deviation (Fig 7-7). When the diagnosis of pulmonary emphysema is known, superior deviation of the mean frontal plane QRS axis does not connote disease in the intraventricular conduction system (left anterior fascicular block) but is, rather, a (poorly understood) feature of the lung disease.

The electrocardiogram is neither highly sensitive nor specific for the diagnosis of right ventricular hypertrophy compared to autopsy or echocardiographic data. Reported sensitivity of the ECG for the anatomic diagnosis is about 30% compared to 93% for the echocardiogram, and reported specificity is about 85% compared to 95%, respectively, for the ECG and echocardiogram.

Combined Right & Left Ventricular Hypertrophy

The electrocardiographic diagnosis of ventricular hypertrophy is not highly correlated with ven-

tricular weights as determined at autopsy; the correlation depends in part on the etiology of the hypertrophy. Whereas a correct electrocardiographic diagnosis of left ventricular hypertrophy can be made up to 85% of the time using all the criteria given above (Table 7-2), a false-positive diagnosis is still made 10-15% of the time. False-positive diagnoses are much more likely if voltage criteria alone (without concomitant ST segment and T wave abnormalities) are used. The correlation of the electrocardiographic diagnosis of right ventricular hypertrophy with autopsy findings is not as good as for left ventricular hypertrophy, ranging from as low as 23% to as high as 100% in patients with congenital heart disease. Correlation of the electrocardiographic diagnosis of combined ventricular hypertrophy with autopsy results is quite poor, with an accuracy of only 8-26%; thus, this diagnosis cannot be made reliably from the ECG. The poor correlation is better understood if one recognizes that in biventricular hypertrophy an increase in left ventricular forces counterbalances an increase in right ventricular forces (and vice versa); thus, the mean forces may be those of the left ventricle or neither ventricle, if left and right ventricular hypertrophy are "balanced."

The most reliable criteria for the electrocardiographic diagnosis of biventricular hypertrophy are the *combination* of right axis deviation (exceeding +90°) in the frontal plane and precordial lead

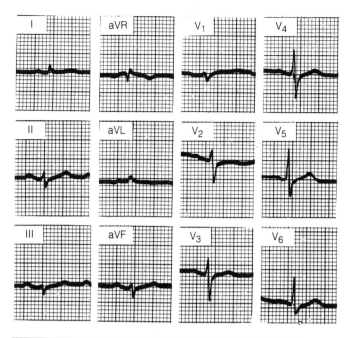

Figure 7-7. Possible right ventricular hypertrophy in a patient with pulmonary emphysema. The QRS complexes are of low voltage (none exceeds 5 mm in the standard leads). The mean frontal plane QRS axis is $-35°$, indicating a leftward and superior direction of depolarization. S waves are seen in V_{5-6} and may be due in part to the superior axis deviation.

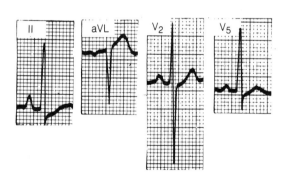

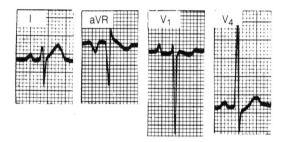

Figure 7-8. Combined right and left ventricular hypertrophy. The mean frontal plane QRS axis is $+105°$. ST segment depression is present in leads II, III, aVF, and V_6. $SV_1 + RV_5 = 39$ mm. The combination of right axis deviation and precordial lead voltage criteria for left ventricular hypertrophy is a reliable indicator of biventricular hypertrophy.

voltage criteria for left ventricular hypertrophy (Fig 7-8). The combination of precordial lead voltage for left ventricular hypertrophy with an R:S ratio in V_1 approaching or equaling 1 (reflecting the prominent anterior forces of the large right ventricle) is also helpful in making the diagnosis. The superior clinical tool for evaluation of left, right, or combined ventricular hypertrophy is echocardiography.

REFERENCES

Casale PN et al: Electrocardiographic detection of left ventricular hypertrophy: Development and prospective validation of improved criteria. *J Am Coll Cardiol* 1985;**6**:572.

Prakash R: Echocardiographic diagnosis of right ventricular hypertrophy: Correlation with ECG and necropsy findings in 248 patients. *Cathet Cardiovasc Diagn* 1981;**7**:179.

Selzer A: The Bayes theorem and clinical electrocardiography. *Am Heart J* 1981;**101**:360.

Surawicz B: Electrocardiographic diagnosis of chamber enlargement. *J Am Coll Cardiol* 1986;**8**:711.

Figure 7-T1.
TEST TRACINGS

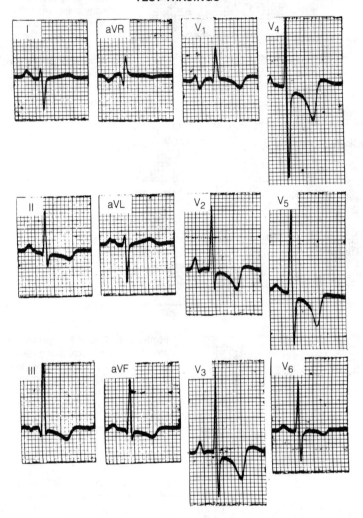

What is the mean frontal plan QRS axis?		+125°.
What is the PR interval?		0.18 s.
What is the QRS duration?		0.08 s.
List 3 abnormalities of the P waves.		Broad (leads I and aVL), notched (I and aVL), abnormal terminal negative component (exceeding 1 mm × 0.04 s) in lead V_1. The P waves are also tall in V_{1-3}.
What criteria for right ventricular hypertrophy are met in this tracing?		The right axis deviation, the qR in V_{1-2}, and the persistent S wave in V_6. The right atrial abnormality tends to confirm the diagnosis of right ventricular hypertrophy.

The patient had mitral stenosis, with biatrial and right ventricular enlargement and hypertrophy.

Figure 7-T2.
TEST TRACINGS

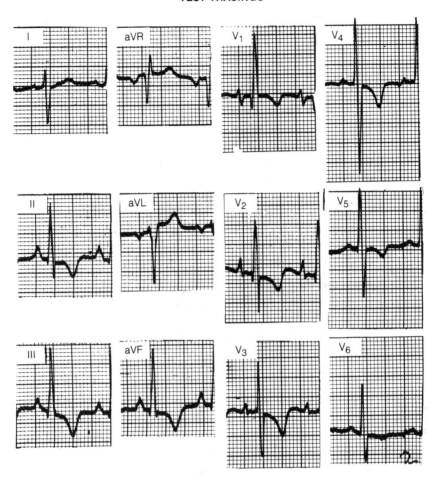

What is the PR interval?	0.16 s.
Is the QRS duration normal or abnormal?	Normal.
What is the mean frontal plane QRS axis?	+110°.
Is the P wave duration normal or abnormal?	Normal.
Is the P wave axis vertical or horizontal?	Vertical.
What abnormality do the P waves suggest?	Right atrial abnormality.
Which leads show ST segment depression?	II, III, aVF, and V_{1-5}.
What is the diagnosis?	Right ventricular hypertrophy, right atrial abnormality (probably hypertrophy).

The patient had schistosomiasis with pulmonary involvement and cor pulmonale. He had right atrial and right ventricular hypertrophy.

Figure 7-T3.
TEST TRACINGS

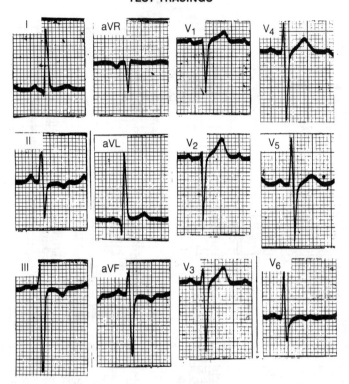

What is the mean frontal plane QRS axis?	−40°.
Are the P waves normal or abnormal?	Normal.
What is the PR interval?	0.14 s.
What is the height of the R wave in lead aVL?	17 mm.
Is the QRS duration normal or abnormal?	Normal.
Are precordial voltage criteria for ventricular hypertrophy met?	No.
What is the diagnosis?	Either left ventricular hypertrophy with concomitant left axis deviation or left

Figure 7-T4.
TEST TRACINGS

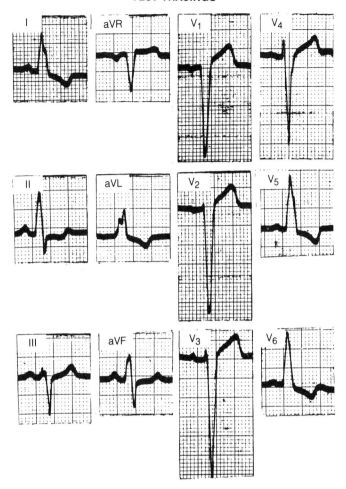

What is the mean frontal QRS axis?	0°.
Are the P waves normal or abnormal?	Normal.
Is the PR interval normal or abnormal?	Normal (0.16 s).
What is the QRS duration?	0.13 s.
Describe the QRS complexes in leads I and aVL, and in the precordial leads.	Notched R waves in leads I, aVL, and V_{5-6}; QS in lead V_1 and rS in V_{2-4}.
What is the pattern of intraventricular conduction?	Left bundle branch block (see Chapter 8). The accompanying ST–T wave abnormalities are secondary to the bundle branch block, and are termed "secondary" abnormalities.
Are precordial voltage criteria for left ventricular hypertrophy met?	Yes.
What is the impact of the intraventricular conduction delay on the electrocardiographic diagnosis of left ventricular hypertrophy?	In the presence of a left-sided conduction delay, voltage criteria cannot be accurately applied in the diagnosis of left ventricular hypertrophy.

Figure 7–T5.
TEST TRACINGS

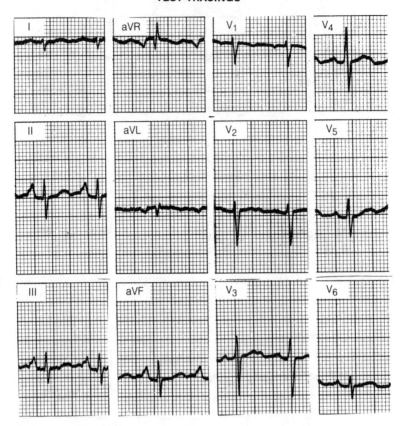

List the P wave abnormalities.	Tall and peaked in leads II, III, and aVF.
Describe the mean frontal plane QRS axis.	Initial forces are directed leftward (small r wave in lead I); terminal forces are directed rightward and superiorly (S wave in I, II, III, and aVF).
Describe the R:S progression in the precordial leads.	The R waves progress, and then regress; there are persistent precordial S waves.
What is a possible diagnosis?	Right ventricular hypertrophy due to chronic obstructive pulmonary disease.

Figure 7–T6.
TEST TRACINGS

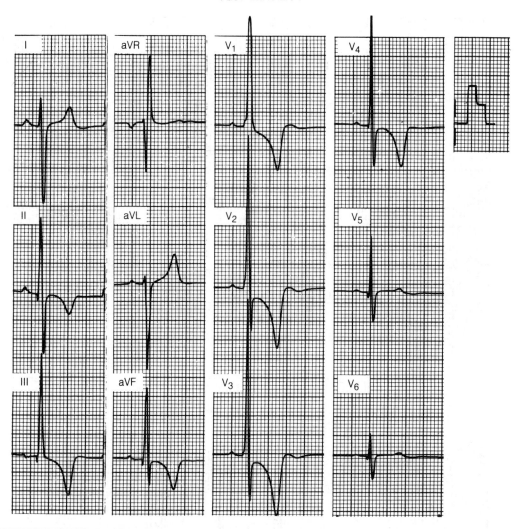

Are the P waves normal or abnormal?	Normal.
Is the mean frontal plane QRS axis normal, horizontal, or vertical?	Vertical.
Describe the QRS morphology in aVR.	rSR′
Describe the QRS morphology in lead V₁.	Notched R wave
Describe the R:S progression in the precordial leads.	The R waves progress, then regress; a persistent precordial S wave is present in the left precordial leads.
What are the criteria for combined ventricular hypertrophy? Are they met in this tracing?	Right axis deviation of the QRS complexes in the frontal plane and/or an abnormal R:S in V₁, combined with precordial voltage criteria for left ventricular hypertrophy. Voltage for left ventricular hypertrophy is present (note that the precordial leads are recorded at half-standard); thus, the diagnosis of combined ventricular hypertrophy can be made.

The patient is a 20 year old woman with a ventricular septal defect and pulmonary hypertension. Right atrial abnormality is not present, perhaps due to cancellation of forces by combined atrial abnormality.

Figure 7–T7.
TEST TRACINGS

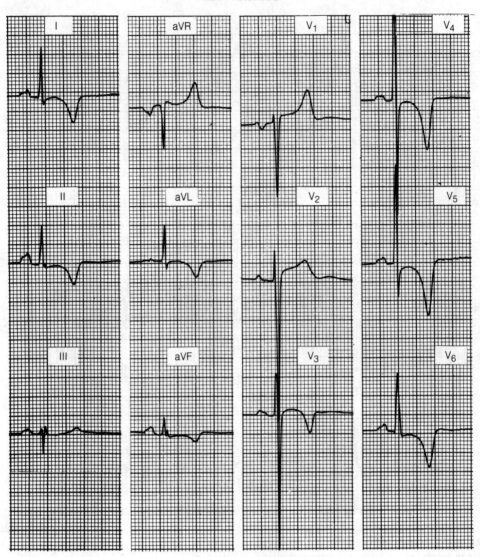

Is the mean frontal plane QRS axis normal or abnormal?	Normal.
What is the P wave axis in the frontal plane?	+60°.
What criteria for left atrial abnormality are met in this tracing?	The P waves are broad (0.12 s) and notched, and there is an abnormally wide and deep negative component (exceeding 1 mm × 0.04 s) in lead V_1.
Why is the P wave tall in lead II?	The second (not the first) component of the P wave is abnormally tall in lead II, reflecting left atrial abnormality. (The left atrium begins its depolarization after that of the right atrium.) The abnormality is termed "pseudo-P-pulmonale."

Intraventricular Conduction Delays 8

An intraventricular conduction delay is the result of **impaired impulse conduction** through one or more of the divisions of the intraventricular conduction system distal to (or within the lower portion of) the bundle of His (Fig 8–1). The conduction fibers that participate in the depolarization of ventricular tissue are the **right bundle branch,** the **common left bundle branch,** and the anterosuperior and inferoposterior radiations **(fascicles)** of the left bundle branch; there are also septal fibers originating from the left bundle branch, but because of their variability these do not constitute a true fascicle. Thus, the intraventricular conduction system of the heart is a **quadrifascicular** one (Fig 8–1).

Terminology

Intraventricular conduction delays are commonly referred to as "blocks" and have been classified as "incomplete" or "complete," indicating different degrees of conduction delay. "Incomplete bundle branch block" refers to a conduction delay within a portion of the intraventricular conduction system that does not result in abnormal prolongation of the QRS interval; "complete bundle branch block" refers to a conduction delay that does result in abnormal lengthening of the QRS interval. Neither of these terms is accurate, however, and are best avoided unless the term "pattern" is also used. "Block" in a conduction fiber should serve to indicate only that a conduction *delay* is present, not to indicate total inability of an impulse to be transmitted through that fiber. The differential diagnosis of conduction block and conduction delay cannot be determined from the ECG. Similarly, the terms "incomplete" and "complete" are misleading in that they refer only to lesser and greater *degrees* of conduction delay, rather than to the presence or absence of conduction. Thus, these terms have no anatomic or electrophysiologic counterpart and describe conduction *patterns* only.

As a result of conduction delay of an impulse in a fascicle, there is delay in, and abnormal spread of, excitation through the portion of ventricular muscle served by that fascicle. Therefore, the QRS duration may be prolonged to 0.12 s or longer; the QRS morphology becomes abnormal; the ventricular activation time (the time from onset of the QRS complex to the peak of the R wave) over the involved ventricle becomes prolonged; and the ST segments are depressed and the T

waves inverted in leads recording the abnormal depolarization. Lesser degrees of conduction delay produce less prolongation of the QRS duration and ventricular activation time but similar QRS–T morphology.

RIGHT BUNDLE BRANCH BLOCK PATTERN

The pattern of right bundle branch "block" is a common electrocardiographic finding; although it often occurs in the presence of heart disease of various causes, it is not diagnostic of cardiac disease and therefore does not predict its presence (Table 8–1).

Mechanism of Impulse Conduction

The spread of excitation from the SA node to the AV node and through the main portion of the bundle of His is normal (see Chapter 11). Activa-

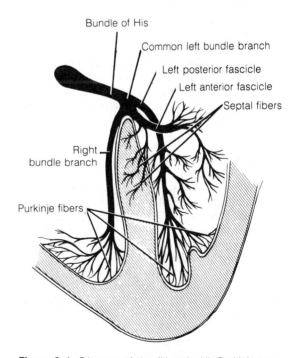

Figure 8-1. Diagram of the AV node–His-Purkinje conduction system. The intraventricular conduction system is a **quadrifascicular** one, consisting of the right, left anterior, and left posterior fascicles, and the septal fibers.

Table 8-1. Some causes of bundle branch block pattern in the adult ECG.[1]

(1) Clinically normal individual
(2) Lenegre's disease (idiopathic fibrosis of the conduction tissue)
(3) Lev's disease (calcification of the cardiac skeleton)
(4) Cardiomyopathy
Dilated
Hypertrophic (concentric or asymmetric)
Infiltrative
Tumor
Chagas' disease
Myxedema
Amyloidosis
(5) Ischemic heart disease
Acute myocardial infarction
Past myocardial infarction
Coronary artery disease without myocardial infarction
(6) Aortic stenosis (left bundle branch block)
(7) Infective endocarditis with abscess formation within the conduction system
(8) Trauma
(9) Hyperkalemia
(10) Ventricular hypertrophy
(11) Rate-dependency
(12) Massive pulmonary embolism (right bundle branch block)

[1]In most patients with bundle branch block, the prognosis is dependent not upon the conduction delay per se but on the underlying heart disease.

tion of the interventricular septum occurs in normal fashion, from left to right (Fig 8-2A).

Left ventricular depolarization occurs in a normal fashion. The initial 0.04–0.06 s of the QRS complex is normal. Because of the right intraventricular conduction delay (which could be located in the distal portion of the His bundle, the proximal portion of the right bundle branch, or the Purkinje fibers of the right ventricle), right ventricular depolarization is delayed (Fig 8-2B and C).

Electrocardiographic Pattern

The characteristic feature of right bundle branch block is a late, delayed electrical force of right ventricular depolarization oriented to the right and anteriorly (Fig 8-2). This late rightward vector produces a wide s wave in leads I and V_{4-6} and a wide R or R′ wave in aVR (Fig 8-3). The anterior vector of this late force produces the wide R′ waves in right precordial leads V_{3R}, V_1 and V_2. This late force may be directed either superiorly or inferiorly. If superiorly directed, it produces a wide s wave in aVF; if inferiorly directed, it produces a wide R′ in aVF. The ST segment and the T wave are opposite in direction to this late force of ventricular depolarization, resulting in *secondary* ST depression and T wave inversion in right precordial leads V_{1-3}. The QRS interval is 0.12 s or greater (Fig 8-3).

If a right bundle branch block pattern is present but the QRS interval is not prolonged beyond 0.12 s, a lesser degree of conduction delay is present (Fig 8-4); the phrase **"right intraventricular conduction delay"** is preferred to the older phrase "incomplete right bundle branch block." This pattern may be a variant of normal (Table 8-2).

The pattern of septal and left ventricular depolarization in right intraventricular conduction delay is normal. Thus, right bundle branch block does not itself alter the initial frontal plane QRS axis. The frontal plane QRS axis should be determined from the initial 0.04–0.06 s of ventricular activation rather than from the entire QRS complex; thus, the duration of the right-sided conduction delay, as measured from the broad s wave in lead I, should be disregarded when determining the frontal plane axis.

Right Bundle Branch Block With Left Ventricular Hypertrophy

Since right bundle branch "block" reflects delayed activation of the right ventricle, left ventricular events will be not obscured. Thus, the typical

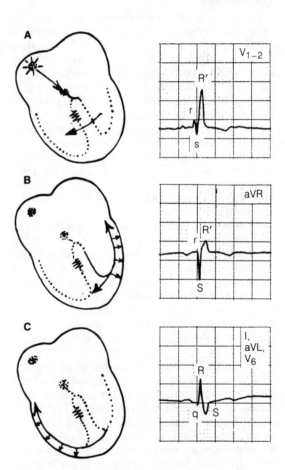

Figure 8-2. Right bundle branch block pattern. (〜〜, area of conduction delay.)

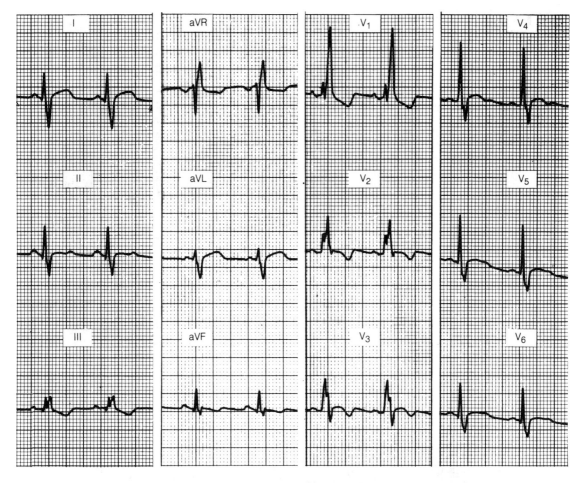

Figure 8-3. Right bundle branch block pattern. The mean frontal plane axis of the initial 0.04 s of the QRS complex (measured by subtracting the duration of the wide S wave in lead aVL) is $+40°$. The QRS interval is 0.13 s. The wide S waves in leads I, aVL, and V_{4-6} and the R′ waves in leads V_{1-2} are typical of right intraventricular conduction delay. ST–T abnormalities are recorded in the right precordial leads and are secondary to the abnormality of ventricular depolarization. Prominent U waves are seen in V_{4-5}.

electrocardiographic features of left ventricular hypertrophy in leads I, aVL, and V_{4-6} will usually be seen (Fig 8–5).

Right Bundle Branch Block With Right Ventricular Hypertrophy

Right ventricular hypertrophy can cause a conduction delay in the right ventricle, much as left ventricular hypertrophy can cause a left ventricular conduction delay. However, marked widening of the QRS complex is not usual with hypertrophy alone, and an abnormally rightward mean frontal plane QRS axis is not expected from the conduction delay alone. Determination of the initial 0.04 to 0.06 frontal plane QRS vector is therefore helpful. An abnormal rightward axis (greater than $+90°$) is consistent with right ventricular hypertrophy (or associated left posterior fascicular con-

Table 8-2. Some causes of "incomplete" bundle branch block patterns in the adult ECG.

Right intraventricular conduction delay
Variant of normal (late depolarization of the crista supraventricularis)
Atrial septal defect
Anomalous pulmonary venous drainage
Obstructive pulmonary disease
Pulmonary embolism (conduction delay is often transient)

Left intraventricular conduction delay
Left ventricular hypertrophy
  Hypertension
  Aortic valve disease
Ischemic heart disease
Cardiomyopathy
Hyperkalemia

Figure 8-4. Right intraventricular conduction delay. The pattern is similar to that of right bundle branch block, except that the QRS interval is 0.1 s. The right axis deviation (+110°) and the rR′ complex in V₂ indicate associated right ventricular hypertrophy, and the ST–T wave abnormalities in V₂₋₄ are consistent with this diagnosis. The P wave is 2.5 mm tall in lead II, suggesting right atrial abnormality and further substantiating the diagnosis of right ventricular hypertrophy.

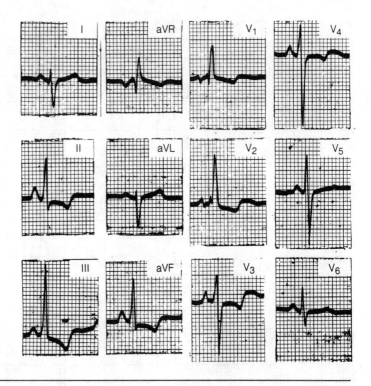

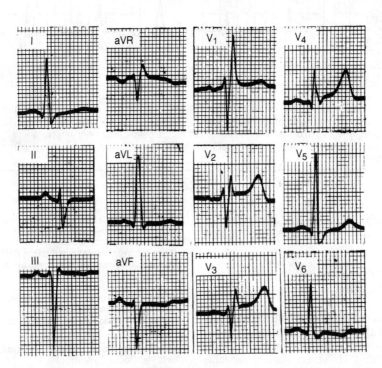

Figure 8-5. Right bundle branch block pattern and probable left ventricular hypertrophy. The precordial leads show the typical pattern of right bundle branch block. The R wave in aVL is 17 mm, suggesting left ventricular hypertrophy; the T wave is inverted in V₆, consistent with this diagnosis. The mean frontal plane QRS axis, determined from the first 0.06 s of the QRS complex, is superiorly directed at −50°, consistent with the left ventricular hypertrophy but also possibly reflecting a delay in conduction in the anterior fascicle of the left bundle branch. If the latter is true, then the diagnosis of left ventricular hypertrophy cannot be made with certainty.

duction delay) (Fig 8–4). In addition, the QRS configuration in lead V_1 is qR or pure R wave in right ventricular hypertrophy, but not in right bundle branch block. Finally, ventricular activation time over the right ventricle (time from onset of QRS complex to peak of the R′ wave) is not markedly delayed in right ventricular hypertrophy, whereas it usually exceeds 0.06 s in right ventricular conduction delay.

LEFT BUNDLE BRANCH BLOCK PATTERN

The pattern of left bundle branch "block" is more commonly associated with heart disease than is right bundle branch block, but it may also be seen in individuals without evidence of overt heart disease (Table 8–1).

Mechanism of Impulse Transmission

The spread of excitation from the SA node to the AV node and bundle of His occurs in a normal fashion (see Chapter 11). The impulse is then either not transmitted at all, or is transmitted with delay, in the left bundle branch or fascicles (or both) (Fig 8–1). Since in left bundle branch block the septal fibers do not participate in activation of the interventricular septum, the septum is depolarized from fibers arising in the distal portion of the right bundle branch. This results in a septal depolarization vector that is oriented to the left.

The right ventricle is depolarized in normal fashion. The left ventricle is depolarized in an abnormal manner (Fig 8–6). If antegrade conduction in the left bundle branch is totally blocked, the left ventricle is depolarized from impulses transmitted from the right bundle branch system across the interventricular septum and right ventricle into the left ventricle. If conduction is delayed in the left bundle branch, the left ventricle will be depolarized by the fibers of the left bundle branch but in a delayed and often abnormal sequence.

Electrocardiographic Pattern (Fig 8–6)

The abnormal septal depolarization from right to left results in an initial vector oriented to the left. Therefore, the normal septal q wave is not recorded in leads I and V_{5-6} (Fig 8–6A). If q (or Q) waves are recorded in these leads in the presence of left bundle branch block, the possibility of additional disease, such as myocardial infarction, is suggested. In this circumstance, the left ventricular conduction delay is distal to the common left bundle branch (peri-infarction block) (see Chapter 9).

Right ventricular depolarization occurs in a normal fashion, but because of the dominance of left ventricular forces there is little evidence of this in the conventional ECG. The abnormal left ventricular depolarization results in wide (0.12 s or greater), notched or slurred QRS complexes oriented to the left and posteriorly, typically recorded in leads I and V_{4-6} (Figs 8–6B and C and 8–7). The polarity of QRS complexes in leads II, III, and aVF will depend upon the mean frontal plane QRS axis. Since this axis usually lies between 0 and $-30°$, lead aVL will commonly show the pattern described above.

An abnormal superior axis (to the left of $-30°$) indicates additional conduction delay in the left anterior fascicle of the left bundle branch (Fig 8–8). An abnormal rightward axis (greater than

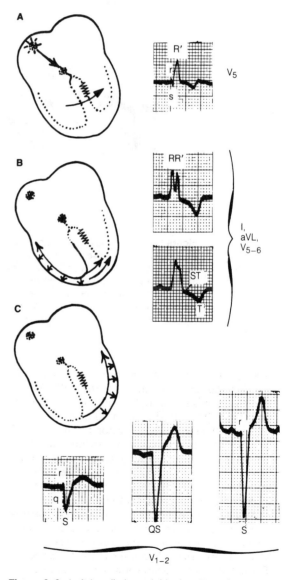

Figure 8–6. Left bundle branch block pattern. (〜〜, area of conduction delay.)

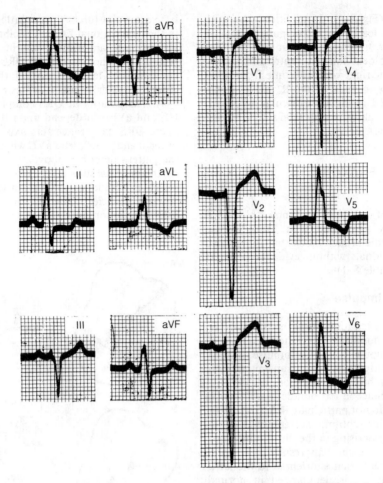

Figure 8-7. Left bundle branch block pattern. The mean frontal plane QRS axis is 0°. A wide, notched R wave with depressed ST segment and T wave inversion is seen in leads I, aVL, and V_{5-6}. A wide S wave is seen in precordial leads V_{1-4}; the ST segments are elevated in V_{1-3} and the T waves are upright. The QRS duration is prolonged to 0.12 s and the ventricular activation time is 0.1 s. Note the absence of Q waves in leads I, aVL, and V_{5-6} caused by right-to-left septal depolarization.

+90°) indicates additional conduction delay in the left posterior fascicle of the left bundle branch, or associated right ventricular hypertrophy (Fig 8-9); clinical correlation must be made.

The dominant posterior vector results in small or absent anterior forces in V_{1-3} (producing rS or QS complexes), mimicking anterior wall myocardial infarction. At times, Q waves are recorded in leads III and aVF, but these are *not diagnostic* of inferior wall myocardial infarction.

As a result of abnormal ventricular depolarization, ventricular repolarization is altered, resulting in *secondary* ST–T wave changes. The ST and T vectors are oriented opposite to the QRS vector. Thus, there is ST depression and asymmetric T wave inversion in leads I and V_{4-6} and elevated ST segments with upright T waves in leads V_{1-3} (Fig 8-7). The direction of the ST–T vectors in leads

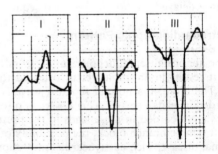

Figure 8-8. Left bundle branch block pattern with leftward axis deviation. The mean frontal plane QRS axis is −65°. The QRS complex in lead I is typical of left bundle branch block. The axis deviation is presumed to be due to additional conduction delay in the anterosuperior fascicle of the left bundle branch, resulting in early forces being oriented inferiorly and late forces superiorly.

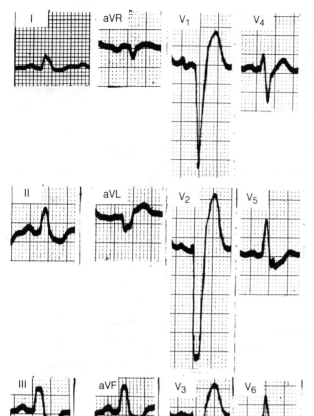

Figure 8-9. Left bundle branch block pattern with rightward axis deviation. The mean frontal plane QRS axis is +70°. The QRS morphology is otherwise typical of left intraventricular conduction delay. The rightward axis deviation is presumed to be due to disease in the inferoposterior fascicle of the left bundle branch, resulting in the early forces being oriented in an anterosuperior direction and the late forces in an inferoposterior direction.

III, aVF, and aVL will depend upon the mean frontal plane QRS axis and will be opposite to the direction of the QRS vectors.

If a left bundle branch block pattern is present but the QRS interval is not prolonged beyond 0.12 s, a lesser degree of conduction delay is present, and the phrase "**left intraventricular conduction delay**" is preferred to the older terminology "incomplete left bundle branch block" (Fig 8-10).

Differential Diagnosis of Left Bundle Branch Block & Left Ventricular Hypertrophy

The pattern of left bundle branch block may be seen in the same clinical conditions as those of left ventricular hypertrophy (Table 8-1). The major differential point between the 2 electrocardiographic patterns is the absence of a septal q wave in leads that record septal activity in the right-left axis (such as leads I and V_{5-6}). The presence of a q wave in these leads is evidence against the diagnosis of left bundle branch block, or it indicates associated myocardial infarction. In view of the abnormality of ventricular depolarization, voltage criteria for left ventricular hypertrophy are not valid in the presence of definite left bundle branch "block". However, echocardiographic studies suggest that extremely prominent voltage (SV_2 and $RV_6 \geq 45$ mm), together with a pattern of left atrial abnormality, do indicate the presence of left ventricular hypertrophy.

ST SEGMENTS & T WAVES IN INTRAVENTRICULAR CONDUCTION DELAY

In bundle branch block patterns, the ST segments are depressed and the T waves inverted in those leads reflecting the conduction delay; these abnormalities result from the conduction delay

Figure 8-10. Left intraventricular conduction delay ("incomplete" left bundle branch block pattern). The QRS duration is 0.1 s. Septal q waves are absent in leads I and V_{5-6}. The R wave is slurred in leads I, aVL, and V_{5-6} and notched in V_4. ST segment straightening is present in these leads. Precordial voltage criteria for left ventricular hypertrophy are met ($SV_1 + RV_5 = 38$ mm). In tracings such as this one, either the ventricular hypertrophy or the conduction delay is known or has to be assumed to be primary. If ventricular hypertrophy is known to be primary, the conduction delay is presumed to be due to the impulse having to travel through increased ventricular muscle thickness. If, however, the conduction delay is primary, voltage criteria for left ventricular hypertrophy cannot be applied.

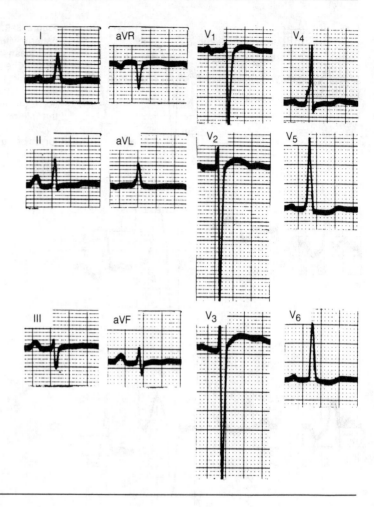

and are therefore described as *secondary* ST-T wave changes. Occasionally, the ST-T waves are upright, a finding termed *primary* ST-T wave changes, in contrast to the secondary ST-T abnormalities occurring as part of the conduction delay (Figs 8-11 and 8-12). Although primary ST-T wave changes are neither sensitive nor specific for acute myocardial ischemia or infarction, these diagnoses should be considered.

RATE-DEPENDENT (TACHYCARDIA-DEPENDENT) INTRAVENTRICULAR CONDUCTION DELAY

The right bundle branch usually has the longest refractory period of all the fascicles, followed by the left anterior fascicle of the left bundle branch and finally by the left posterior fascicle of the left bundle branch. Sinus impulses occurring at normal rates or, more commonly, premature supraventricular impulses, may therefore find various portions of the conduction system refractory when they reach them, producing a **rate-dependent conduction delay** (Figs 8-13 and 8-14). An increase in the atrial rate may also produce this form of intraventricular aberration (Fig 8-15). Rate-dependent intraventricular conduction delay is a function of the refractory period of conduction tissue, and its occurrence therefore does not imply the presence of heart disease. Following the return of normal intraventricular conduction after a period of conduction delay, the T waves of the normally conducted complexes may be abnormal; the precise mechanism of such T wave abnormalities is not clear, but their occurrence is not predictive of organic heart disease. (Similar T wave abnormalities can follow the appearance of spontaneous QRS rhythm in patients whose sequence of ventricular depolarization has been rendered abnormal by a cardiac pacemaker.) Occasionally, a QRS complex with a bundle branch block pattern will terminate a pause in QRS rhythm (**bradycardia-dependent** conduction delay).

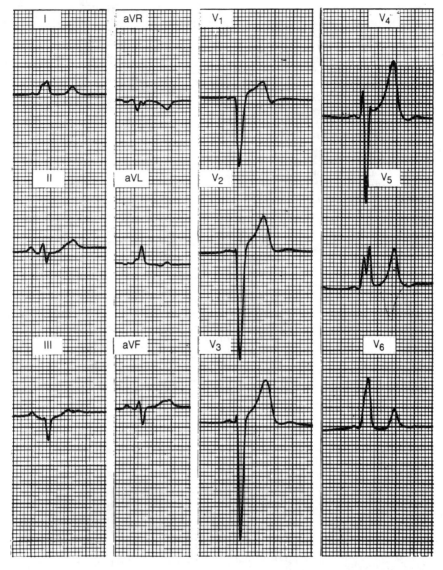

Figure 8-11. Left bundle branch block pattern with upright T waves in Leads I and V_{5-6}. Upright T waves in leads reflecting the intraventricular conduction delay are unexpected, and are termed *primary*, in contrast to the expected secondary ST-T wave abnormalities. Such T waves are not specific for a particular cardiac diagnosis, although their presence deserves mention. Despite the tented T waves in V_{5-6} suggesting hyperkalemia, the serum K^+ was normal.

FASCICULAR CONDUCTION DELAYS

The common left bundle branch divides into its fascicles: the anterior (anterosuperior) fascicle and the inferior (inferoposterior) fascicle (Fig 8-1). The septal fibers are not sufficiently organized to be termed a fascicle. The anterosuperior fascicle radiates out over the anterior and superior surfaces of the left ventricle, and the inferoposterior fascicle radiates out over the inferior and pos-

terior surfaces of the left ventricle. Peripherally, the fibers from both fascicles intertwine.

Normally, impulse transmission proceeds simultaneously down both left fascicles, resulting in a normally directed QRS vector in the frontal plane. However, if conduction delay is present in one of the fascicles, the spread of activation proceeds down the normal fascicle first, thus altering the direction of the mean QRS vector in the frontal plane. Since fascicular conduction is so rapid (10–20 ms), the conduction delay is not associated

Figure 8-12. Right bundle branch block pattern with upright T waves in V$_{2-3}$ and diphasic T waves in V$_1$. Deep, wide Q waves in leads II, III, and aVF indicate inferior wall myocardial infarction (old, suggested by the upright T waves in these leads); and the notched R wave in lead V, indicates posterior wall infarction. The upright T waves in the leads reflecting the right intraventricular conduction delay are not expected, and are termed *primary* T wave abnormalities. While primary T wave abnormalities are not specific for the diagnosis of ischemic heart disease, this should be considered. In this patient, the occurrence of the inferior wall myocardial infarction was associated with the change from the expected secondary ST depression and T wave inversion in V$_{1-3}$ to this primary pattern.

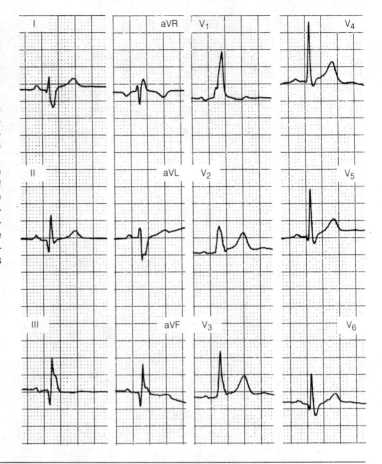

Figure 8-13. Rate-dependent right intraventricular conduction delay. *A:* During paroxysmal reciprocating supraventricular tachycardia (see Chapter 10) at a rate of 160/min, the QRS morphology shows a right bundle branch block pattern. (No P waves are visible.) *B:* Several minutes later, the rate has slowed to 135/min. QRS complexes having a right bundle branch block pattern alternate at regular intervals with QRS complexes having an RS configuration. *C:* Sinus rhythm, restored several minutes later. The QRS morphology of the sinus-conducted impulses has an RS configuration and is identical to the alternate QRS complexes in (B). Thus, in (B), normal sinus-conducted QRS complexes are alternating with right bundle branch block complexes, indicating 2:1 block in the right bundle branch; in (A), conduction in the right bundle branch did not occur or was delayed.

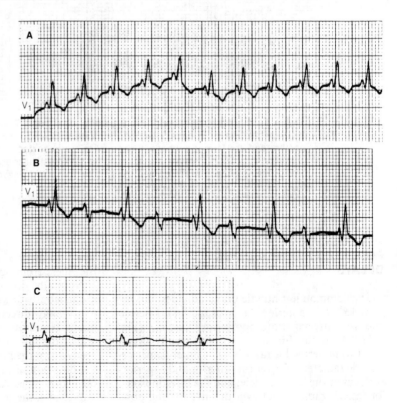

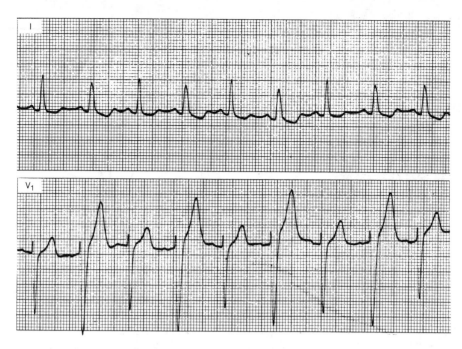

Figure 8-14. Rate-dependent left intraventricular conduction delay. Regular sinus rhythm at a rate of about 92/min is present. In lead V₁ the rS morphology of the QRS complexes alternates in 2:1 fashion between complexes of 0.08 s and 0.13 s durations, respectively, and have associated normal and tall T waves, respectively. The wider QRS complexes with tall T waves also have accompanying elevations of the ST segments. The septal q wave is not present in lead I. The rhythm strips indicate 2:1 conduction delay in the left bundle branch; the finding may presage the development of established left bundle branch "block," since it occurs during a normal sinus rate rather than during tachycardia.

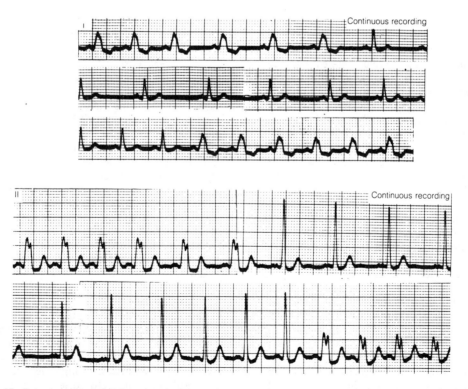

Figure 8-15. Rate-dependent left intraventricular conduction delay. At a critical sinus cycle length the left bundle branch is refractory, and the pattern of intraventricular conduction is that of left bundle branch block. Note the disappearance of the septal q wave in lead I (present in the normally conducted complexes) when the left bundle branch block pattern is present.

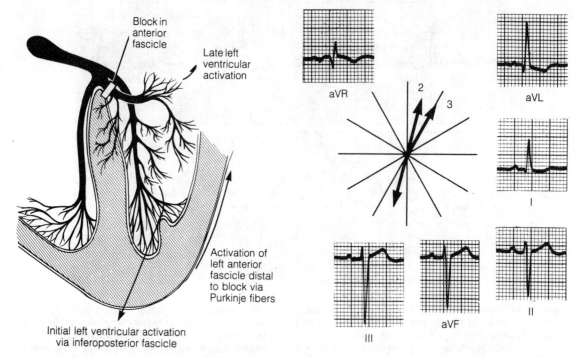

Figure 8-16. Left anterior fascicular conduction delay. The initial QRS (arrow 1) is oriented to the right (q in I) and inferiorly (r in II, III, and aVF). The terminal QRS (arrow 2) is oriented to the left (R in I) and superiorly (S in II, III, and aVF). The mean QRS frontal plane vector is −60° (arrow 3).

with measurable prolongation of the QRS complex duration in the conventional ECG.

Fascicular "blocks" are associated with the inscription of q waves (see below) that, although they might mimic those of myocardial infarction, are not sufficiently wide nor deep to indicate infarction. Should the pattern of preexistent q wave infarction be present, however, and fascicular conduction delay develops, the q waves of infarction may disappear, to be superceded by the depolarization sequence of remaining noninfarcted myocardium.

Conduction Delay in the Left Anterior Fascicle

Left anterior fascicular conduction delay ("block") results in an abnormal spread of activation through the left ventricular myocardium (Fig 8-16). Ventricular activation is initiated from the fibers of the inferoposterior fascicle of the left bundle branch, resulting in a vector oriented inferiorly (r wave in leads II, III, and aVF) and rightward (q wave in lead I and, occasionally, small q waves of brief (< 0.03 s) duration in V_{2-3}). Later activation of the ventricle occurs via the fibers of the anterior fascicle through interconnecting Purkinje fibers distal to the site of conduction delay, resulting in a late vector oriented to the left (R wave in lead I) and superiorly (S waves in leads

II, III, and aVF). The mean frontal plane QRS axis is superior to −30° (Fig 8-17), although any acute leftward axis shift may indicate some degree of conduction delay in the anterior fascicle. Since conduction time through the Purkinje system is so rapid, the 10–20 ms conduction delay caused by anterior fascicular "block" does not produce a measurable increase in the QRS interval.

Since the mean QRS vector is directed leftward and superiorly in the left anterior fascicular block, voltage criteria for left ventricular hypertrophy using lead aVL cannot be applied. Whether or not precordial lead voltage can be used to diagnose left ventricular hypertrophy has not been definitely established.

The development of the left anterior fascicular block will mask the q waves of inferior wall myocardial infarction.

Conduction Delay in the Left Posterior Fascicle

Left posterior fascicular conduction delay ("block") results in abnormal activation of the left ventricle (Fig 8-18). Left ventricular depolarization initially spreads through the anterior fascicle, resulting in a vector oriented to the left (r wave in lead I) and superiorly (q wave in leads II, III, and aVF). Later ventricular activation occurs via fibers from the posterior fascicle through in-

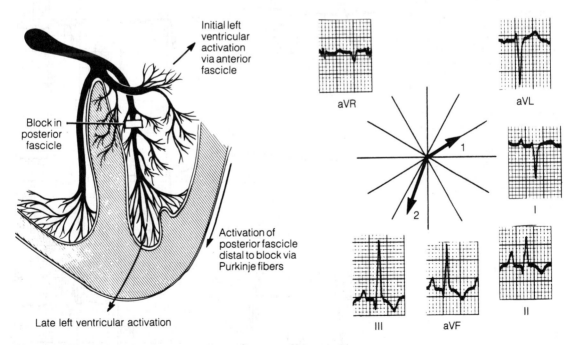

Figure 8-17. Left anterior fascicular conduction delay ("block"). The mean QRS axis is −50°. The QRS interval is 0.1 s. The R wave voltage in aVL is 14 mm. In the presence of left anterior fascicular "block," this voltage in aVL is not diagnostic of left ventricular hypertrophy. There is ST segment depression in I, aVL, and V_6. The small q waves in V_{1-3} are the result of early QRS forces directed inferiorly, rightward, and posteriorly. The s waves in V_{5-6} are the result of the superiorly directed late QRS forces.

Figure 8-18. Left posterior fascicular "block." The initial QRS (arrow 1) is oriented to the left (r in I) and superiorly (q in II, III, and aVF). The terminal QRS (arrow 2) is oriented rightward (S in I) and inferiorly (R in II, III, and aVF), resulting in a mean frontal plane QRS axis of +110°.

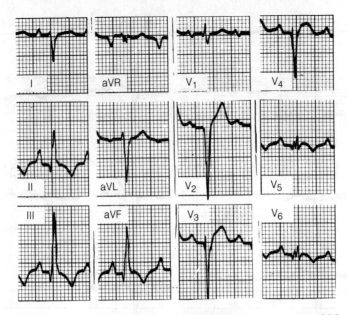

Figure 8-19. Left posterior fascicular "block." The mean frontal plane QRS axis is +110°. The QRS interval is 0.1 s. The P waves are tall in II and aVF. These findings are consistent with right atrial and right ventricular hypertrophy; however, cardiac catheterization revealed normal right heart pressures, emphasizing the need to exclude right ventricular hypertrophy before an electrocardiographic diagnosis of left posterior fascicular block is made. The precordial leads are indicative of anterior wall myocardial infarction (see Chapter 9).

Figure 8-20. ECGs taken 1 year apart in a 53-year-old man. *A:* The mean frontal plane QRS axis is −30°. The R wave voltage in lead aVL of 13 mm cannot be considered to indicate left ventricular hypertrophy in view of the leftward axis deviation. A broad Q wave is present lead aVL, and QS complexes are present in V_{2-3}, indicating prior anterior wall myocardial infarction. *B:* The interim development of left posterior fascicle block (right axis deviation of +100° and qR complexes in leads II, III, and aVF) has masked the Q wave in lead aVL. The precordial leads are unchanged. The q waves in leads III and aVF are too wide to indicate fascicular block alone; they represent inferior wall myocardial infarction.

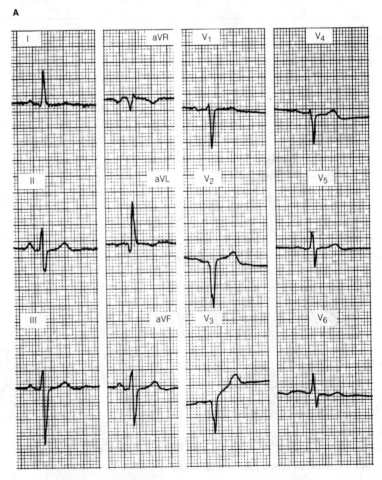

terconnecting Purkinje fibers distal to the site of conduction delay; this results in a vector oriented to the right (S wave in lead I), inferiorly (R wave in leads II, III, and aVF), and posteriorly (S wave in V_{1-2}) (Fig 8-19). The initial q waves in leads II, III, and aVF can suggest myocardial infarction, but they are usually of too brief a duration (< 0.03 s) to diagnose it. The mean frontal plane QRS axis equals or exceeds $+110°$, although any acute rightward shift in axis may indicate some degree of conduction delay in the posterior fascicle.

Left posterior fascicular block occurs only rarely as an isolated abnormality. The concomitant presence of a right bundle branch block pattern helps to confirm the diagnosis of left posterior fascicular block. Much more common causes of rightward axis deviation are a vertically oriented heart in a normal individual, right ventricular hypertrophy, and lateral wall myocardial infarction (see Chapter 9).

The development of left posterior fascicle block will mask the q waves of lateral wall myocardial infarction (Fig 8-20).

Conduction Delay in the Septal Fibers

Normal initial septal depolarization results from impulses transmitted by the septal fibers that arise from the proximal portion of the left bundle branch. The resulting vector is oriented to the right, producing small q waves in leads I and V_{5-6}. It might be anticipated that absence of septal q waves would suggest conduction delay in the septal fibers; however, up to 20% of normal individuals do not have septal q waves. This suggests that the interventricular septum may be oriented parallel to the frontal plane of the body. Thus, even though the septum is activated from its left to its right, the projection of this force is anterior but not rightward. Therefore, the diagnosis of "block" in the left septal fibers cannot be made from the ECG. Prominent anterior forces (abnormal R:S ratio in V_1) have been described as a manifestation of septal fiber block, but the specificity is poor.

Peri-infarction Conduction Delays

See Chapter 9.

B

Figure 8-20. (continued)

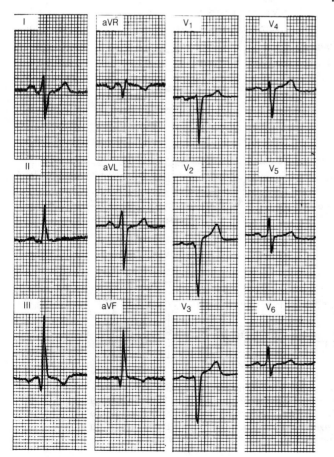

BIFASCICULAR CONDUCTION DELAYS

Bifascicular conduction delays ("block") indicate more diffuse involvement of the intraventricular conduction system by disease than does unifascicular block. They do not themselves predict the development of AV block (see Chapter 11), although the same disease processes that give rise to bifascicular conduction delays can also produce varying degrees of AV block. In acute myocardial infarction, however, the new development of bifascicular block is of ominous prognostic significance, since it implies extensive necrosis of the ventricular myocardium, including the interventricular septum.

Right Bundle Branch Block With Left Anterior Fascicular Block

This is one of the most common types of bifascicular bundle branch block. It is recognized by the combination of the criteria for each type of block: (1) delayed terminal QRS forces oriented to the right and anteriorly, producing wide S waves in I and V_{5-6} and wide R or R' waves in V_1 and V_2; plus (2) a mean 0.04 to 0.06 s QRS vector in the frontal plane superior to $-30°$ (Fig 8–21).

Right Bundle Branch Block With Left Posterior Fascicular Block

The electrocardiographic features that permit recognition of this type of bifascicular bundle branch block are (1) typical findings of right branch block, and (2) a mean 0.04 to 0.06 s frontal plane QRS axis of $+110°$ or greater (Fig 8–22). As in isolated left posterior fascicular block, right ventricular hypertrophy as the cause of the rightward axis must be excluded by clinical evaluation.

TRIFASCICULAR CONDUCTION DELAYS

Trifascicular conduction delay is suggested by the patterns of bifascicular conduction delay and a prolonged PR interval (Fig 8–23). However, the

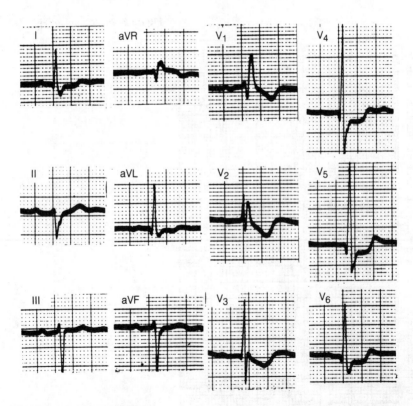

Figure 8–21. Bifascicular conduction delays involving the right bundle branch (terminal portion of the QRS oriented to the right and anteriorly, with wide S waves in leads I and V_{5-6} and wide R' waves in V_{1-2}) and the left anterior fascicle of the left bundle branch (mean frontal plane QRS axis of $-60°$). Since right bundle branch block is a terminal conduction delay, the mean forces of left ventricular activation are not obscured by its presence.

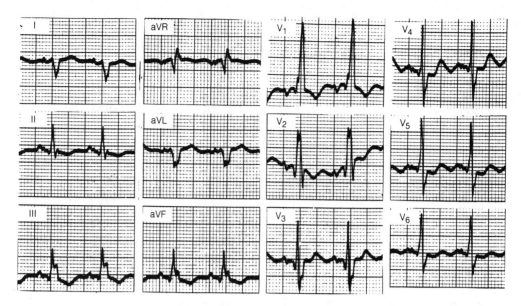

Figure 8-22. Bifascicular conduction delays involving the right bundle branch (delayed terminal portion of the QRS, with late orientation to the right and anteriorly, wide S waves in leads I and V_{5-6} and wide, notched R waves in V_{1-2}) and the posterior fascicle of the left bundle branch (mean frontal plane QRS axis +120°). The q waves in V_{1-3} indicate anterior wall myocardial infarction—old, as indicated by the upright T waves. Both right ventricular hypertrophy and lateral wall myocardial infarction as causes of the right axis deviation must be excluded on clinical grounds.

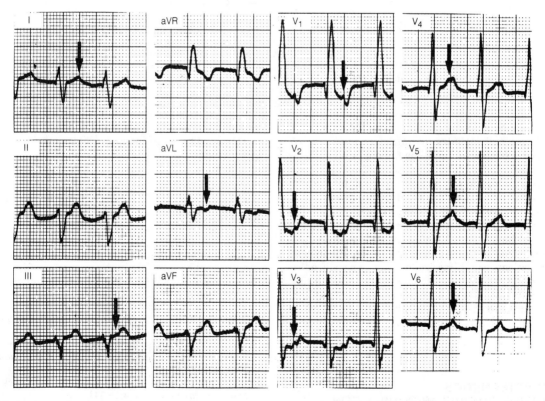

Figure 8-23. Possible trifascicular conduction system disease. The QRS duration is 0.13 s. The wide S waves in lead I and wide R' waves in V_{1-2} are indicative of conduction delay in the right bundle branch. The q waves in V_{2-3} are probably too wide to be due to the anterior fascicular block and likely represent past myocardial infarction. The PR interval is 0.35 s, indicating first-degree AV block; the visible portions of the P waves are indicated by arrows. The conduction delay resulting in the prolonged PR interval could be in the AV node or in the posterior fascicle of the left bundle branch; His bundle electrography is required for precise localization.

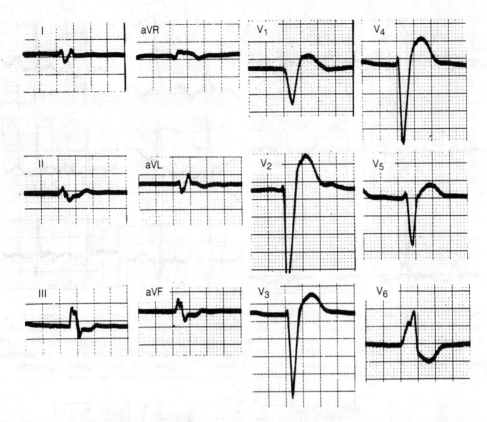

Figure 8-24. Indeterminate intraventricular conduction delay. The rhythm is atrial fibrillation. The QRS interval is 0.18 s. The pattern in the precordial leads is typical of left bundle branch block. A significant s wave is seen in lead I, indicating rightward forces. These findings could be the result of a greater degree of conduction delay in the left posterior fascicle than in the left anterior fascicle or could indicate associated right ventricular hypertrophy or myocardial infarction.

PR interval includes interatrial conduction, AV nodal conduction, and His bundle conduction in addition to fascicular conduction. Thus, PR interval prolongation in the presence of bifascicular conduction system disease does not always indicate disease in the remaining fascicle of the intraventricular conduction system; in fact, there is a 50% chance that AV nodal conduction delay is responsible for the prolongation of the PR interval in patients with bifascicular block. Specialized recording techniques that measure His-Purkinje conduction time (His bundle electrography) are required to make the definitive diagnosis of the location of conduction delay.

INDETERMINATE INTRAVENTRICULAR CONDUCTION DELAYS

At times, a bizarre intraventricular conduction defect will be seen that cannot be placed in any of the above categories. It is therefore called an indeterminate type of intraventricular conduction defect (Fig 8-24).

REFERENCES

Dhingra RC et al: Significance of chronic bifascicular block without apparent organic heart disease. *Circulation* 1979;**60**:33.

Fisch C, Zipes DP, McHenry PL: Rate-dependent aberrancy. *Circulation* 1973;**48**:714.

Flowers NC: Left bundle branch block: A continuously evolving concept. *J Am Coll Cardiol* 1987;**9**:684.

Massumi RA: Bradycardia-dependent bundle-branch block: A critique and proposed criteria. *Circulation* 1968;**38**:1066.

McAnulty JH, Rahimtoola SH: Bundle branch block. *Prog Cardiovasc Dis* 1984;**26**:333.

McAnulty JH et al: Natural history of "high-risk" bundle-branch block: Final report of a prospective study. *N Engl J Med* 1982;**307**:137.

Narula OS, Samet P: Right bundle branch block with normal, left or right axis deviation. *Am J Med* 1971;**51**:432.

Figure 8–T1.
TEST TRACINGS

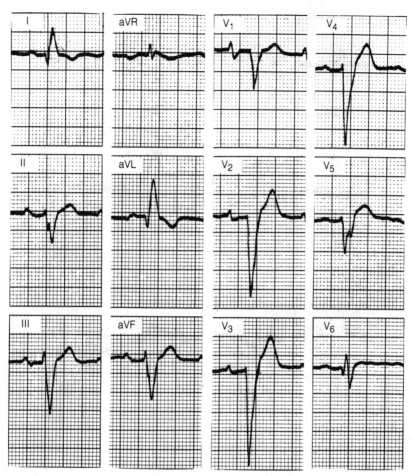

What is the PR interval?	0.23 s.
What is the QRS duration?	0.15 s.
What is the mean frontal plane QRS axis?	−60°.
Does this axis indicate left anterosuperior or left posteroinferior fascicle block?	Left anterosuperior fascicular block.
Is there a right intraventricular conduction delay?	No. Wide S waves are not present in I, aVL, and V_{5-6}, and R′ waves are not present in aVR and V_1.
Is there a left intraventricular conduction delay?	Yes. There is a delayed R wave in leads I, aVL, and V_6.
Is left ventricular hypertrophy present?	In view of the intraventricular conduction delay, this diagnosis cannot be made with certainty.
Explain the presence of the Q waves in leads I and aVL.	If left bundle branch "block" is present, septal Q waves should not be seen. The Q waves seen here are likely due to anterior wall myocardial infarction.
Are the ST and T wave abnormalities primary or secondary?	Secondary to the left intraventricular conduction delay.

Figure 8–T2.
TEST TRACINGS

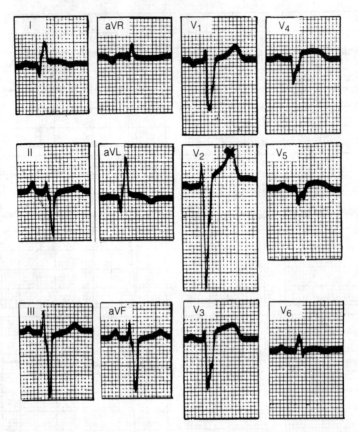

What is the mean frontal plane QRS axis?	−60°
What does this axis signify?	Left anterior fascicular conduction delay (block).
Are the Q waves in leads I, aVL, and V₄₋₅ part of the conduction delay? If not, what are they due to?	No. They are too wide. Q waves accompanying fascicular conduction delay do not exceed 0.03 s. These are Q waves of myocardial infarction.
What accounts for the QRS duration of 0.12 s?	Left intraventricular conduction delay, possibly due to the anterior wall myocardial infarction. Fascicular conduction delays do not prolong the QRS duration.

Figure 8–T3.
TEST TRACINGS

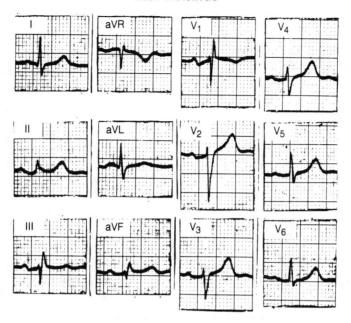

Is the QRS duration normal or abnormal?	Within normal limits.
What is the pattern of intraventricular conduction? How would you describe it?	Right-sided conduction delay, manifested by the S wave in leads I and aVL and V_6, and the R' in V_1.
Could this tracing be a variant of normal?	Yes.

Figure 8–T4.
TEST TRACINGS

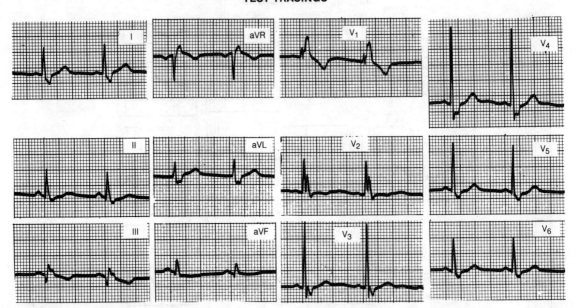

What is the heart rate?	75/min.
What is the mean frontal plane QRS axis?	+30°.
What is the P wave axis?	+60°.
What is the pattern of intraventricular conduction? Why?	Right bundle branch block, manifested by a deep, wide S wave in leads I, aVL, and V_{5-6}, and a wide R′ wave in V_1.
Is right ventricular hypertrophy present?	No. The QRS axis is normal, and neither a qR or pure R wave is present in lead V_1.
Describe the anterior forces.	They are prominent, with a tall R (not R′) wave in V_{2-3}.

Figure 8-T5.
TEST TRACINGS

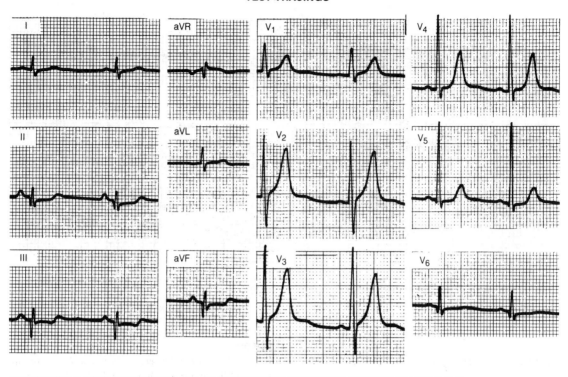

What is the mean frontal plane QRS axis?	0°
Explain why the initial QRS forces are directed superiorly.	There has been an inferior wall myocardial infarction (see Chapter 9), indicated by the Q waves in leads II, III, and aVF.
Is right bundle branch block present?	No. The QRS interval is normal, and wide deep S in leads I, aVL, and V_6, and an rR' in V_1 are not present.
Is right ventricular hypertrophy present?	No. The QRS axis is normal. The tall R wave in V_1 in this case, in which inferior Q waves are present, is due to posterior wall myocardial infarction (see Chapter 9).

Figure 8–T6.
TEST TRACINGS

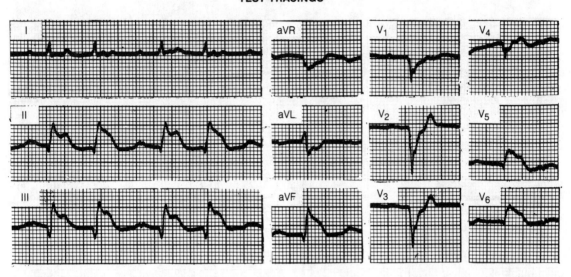

What is the mean frontal plane QRS axis?	+60°.
Is bundle branch block present?	No. The QRS complexes are of normal duration. Do not confuse the elevated ST segments (seen well in leads II, III, aVF, and V_{5-6}) with portions of the QRS complex.
Is left posterior fascicular block present?	No. The ST segment elevation indicates an acute inferolateral wall myocardial infarction; the q waves in leads II, III, and aVF are due to the infarction rather than to fascicular conduction delay.
In which leads is ST segment depression present?	aVL, and V_{2-3}.

The rhythm is sinus with type 1 (Wenckebach) second-degree AV block (see Chapter 11).

Figure 8-T7
TEST TRACINGS

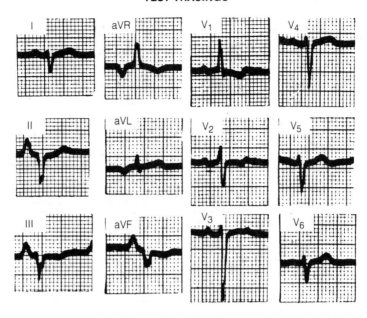

What is the P wave axis?	+80°.
Are the P waves normal?	No. They are abnormally tall in lead II, suggesting right atrial abnormality.
What is the frontal plane QRS axis?	Superior and rightward.
Is the QRS duration normal?	Yes, at 0.08 s.
Is a left-sided intraventricular conduction delay present?	No.
Is a right-sided conduction delay present?	No. The right axis deviation, pure R wave in V_1 and persistent S wave across the precordium indicate right ventricular hypertrophy.
Is right-sided conduction delay responsible for the mean QRS axis in this patient?	No. Right ventricular conduction delays *per se* do not cause deviation of the mean frontal plane QRS axis since they are terminal conduction delays.
Is inferior wall myocardial infarction present?	In this ECG which suggests an underlying diagnosis of obstructive pulmonary disease, QS complexes do not indicate myocardial infarction. The diagnosis cannot be made without clinical correlation.

Figure 8-T8.
TEST TRACINGS

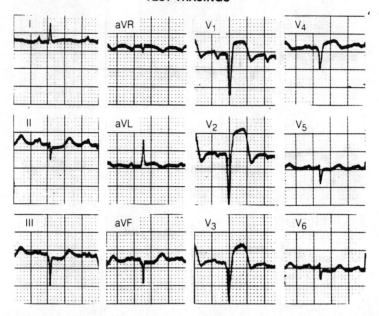

What is the mean frontal plane QRS axis?	−45°.
Is inferior wall myocardial infarction accounting for this axis?	No. The initial forces are directed inferiorly, yielding an rS pattern in leads II, III, and aVF. Moreover, the ST–T waves in these leads do not indicate inferior wall myocardial infarction.
Describe the ST segments in leads V_{1-4}.	They are elevated, compatible with acute anterior wall myocardial infarction.
Describe the ST segment in lead aVL.	It is elevated.
Describe the QRS morphology in the precordial leads.	QS complexes in V_{1-4}, rS complexes in V_{5-6}.
What is the diagnosis?	Acute anterior wall myocardial infarction with left anterior fascicular block.

Figure 8–T9.
TEST TRACINGS

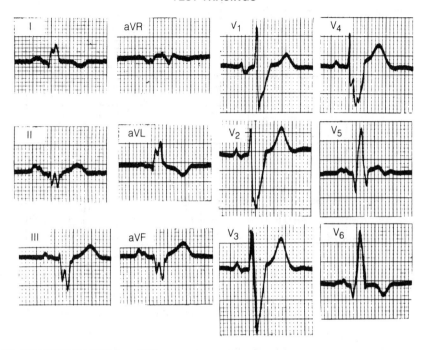

Is the conduction delay right- or left-sided?	Left-sided.
Explain the presence of the q waves in leads I and aVL.	Past anterior wall myocardial infarction is likely.
What is the P wave axis?	+60°.
Is right or left atrial abnormality present, and why?	Left atrial abnormality is present because the P waves are broad and notched and have a duration of 0.12 s as well as a prominent terminal negative component in V_1.

Figure 8-T10.

TEST TRACINGS

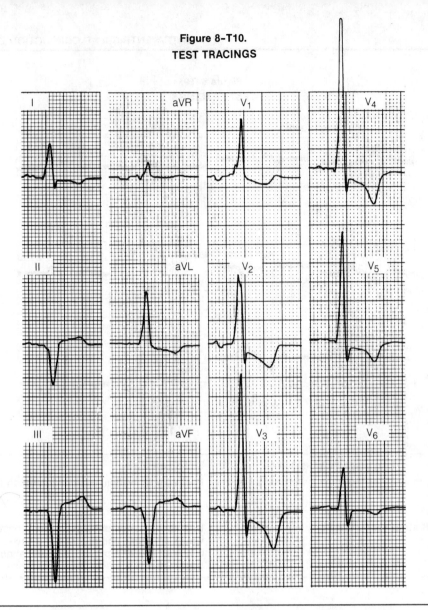

Describe the orientation of the mean frontal plane QRS axis?	Superior.
Is there a left-sided conduction delay?	Yes. The activation time is prolonged over the left ventricular leads.
Is there a right-sided conduction delay?	Yes. There is a broad terminal r' in aVR and V_1.
Is left ventricular hypertrophy present?	If the left-sided conduction delay is known to be primary, the diagnosis of left ventricular hypertrophy cannot be known with certainty, since the sequence of left ventricular depolarization is abnormal. If, however, left ventricular hypertrophy is known to be primary, the left-sided conduction delay may well be secondary to it.
Is inferior wall myocardial infarction present?	Because of the left-sided intraventricular conduction delay, this diagnosis cannot be made with certainty. Left anterior fascicular block may account for the superior axis deviation.
Is there an atrial abnormality? Which and why?	Left atrial abnormality, indicated by the broad, notched P waves and the wide terminal negative component in V_1.
Do the ST–T wave abnormalities indicate ischemia?	Because of the abnormal sequence of ventricular depolarization, the diagnosis of ischemia cannot be made with certainty; clinical correlation is required.

Figure 8-T11.
TEST TRACINGS

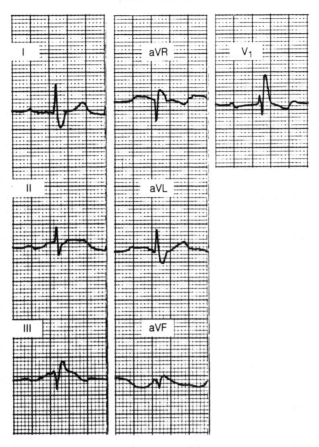

What is the pattern of intraventricular conduction?	Right bundle branch block with left axis due to mild conduction delay in the left anterior fascicle (mean frontal plane QRS axis −30°).
What is the PR interval?	0.32 s.
What comprises the PR interval?	Intraatrial conduction, intra-AV nodal conduction, and His-Purkinje conduction.
Does this tracing represent trifascicular conduction system disease?	Possibly, but since the PR interval comprises several areas of conduction, it cannot be known with certainty that its prolongation is due to conduction disease in the left posterior fascicle.

9   Myocardial Ischemia & Infarction

MYOCARDIAL ISCHEMIA

Myocardial ischemia occurs when coronary artery blood flow is insufficient to meet myocardial metabolic requirements. By definition, it is a transient and reversible phenomenon. The electrocardiographic findings are usually limited to ST segment and T wave abnormalities, although transient Q waves sometimes occur if the ischemia is of sufficient severity. Since the underlying process is transient, so are the electrocardiographic features; thus, a single ECG is *never* diagnostic of myocardial ischemia, since the transient, reversible nature of the abnormalities cannot be demonstrated in a single tracing. Similarly, separate ECGs recorded weeks, months, or years apart that show identical ST and T wave abnormalities are extremely unlikely to be reflecting myocardial ischemia, since ischemia is a dynamic process not expected to remain the same over time. The diagnosis of myocardial ischemia, therefore, depends upon the clinical evaluation of the patient and the electrocardiographic changes *during and after* spontaneous angina pectoris, whether it occurs at rest or during exercise. Many conditions unrelated to myocardial ischemia can produce ST and T wave abnormalities similar to those of ischemia, including hypokalemia, left ventricular hypertrophy, drugs, pericarditis, and myocarditis. Most commonly, however, the ST and T wave abnormalities have no clear cause and are thus idiopathic. Unless the diagnosis of myocardial ischemia is proved, the ST-T wave changes must be considered to be *nonspecific* or *nondiagnostic,* and interpreted as such.

MECHANISM OF ELECTROCARDIOGRAPHIC PATTERNS IN MYOCARDIAL ISCHEMIA

Cellular Basis of Ischemic Electrocardiographic Changes

Recent studies of transmembrane action potentials and epicardial electrograms recorded simultaneously from the surface of the ventricle have shown the following events during ischemia: (1) decrease in resting membrane potential, producing depression of the QT segment of the surface electrogram; and (2) decrease in the action potential duration, amplitude, and rate of change of voltage, producing ST segment elevation in the surface electrogram and prolongation of the activation time over the involved tissue (Fig 9-1). The deterioration of the action potential can render it incapable of propagating an impulse, and complete inability to excite the tissue may occur. Depending on the duration of ischemia, these changes may be transient or permanent.

The intracellular compartment of ischemic cells is positive with respect to that of nonischemic cells, resulting in a current flow from ischemic to normal cells, and an opposite current flow in the extracellular compartment. Depending upon whether the ischemia is transmural or nontransmural, current flows are established from endocardium to epicardium, in which epicardial electrograms show QT and ST changes that are reciprocal to endocardial events. T wave alterations reflect differences in repolarization of ischemic and normal myocardium. If repolarization lasts longer in ischemic tissue than in nonischemic tissue, the extracellularly recorded T wave will be negative, whereas it will be positive if repolarization in ischemic cells does not outlast that in nonischemic cells.

Injury Current of Rest

In contrast to the intracellular space, injured muscle tissue is electrically negative in relation to

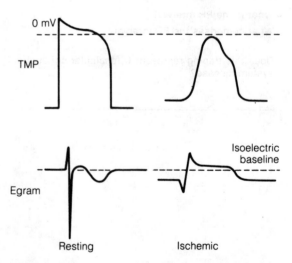

Figure 9-1. Schema of events during acute ischemia, recorded simultaneously from an intracellular electrode (TMP, transmembrane action potential) and the surface of the ventricle (local electrogram, Egram). (Adapted from Janse MJ: *Can J Cardiol* 1986;**46A(Suppl A)**)

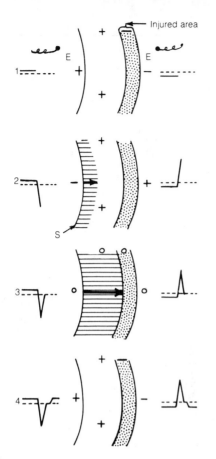

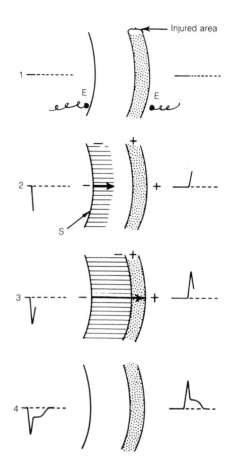

Figure 9-2. Injury current of rest. (The dotted lines indicate the isoelectric baseline.) The injured area is negative relative to the rest of the muscle. (1) An electrode (E) overlying the injured muscle will record a depression relative to the baseline, and an electrode overlying the noninjured muscle will record an elevation relative to the baseline. When the muscle is stimulated (S) (2), an advancing negative charge (in front of which is a positive charge) exists, producing an upward deflection recorded by the electrode overlying the injured area and a downward deflection recorded by the electrode overlying the noninjured area. When there ceases to be a potential difference between the injured and uninjured areas of the muscle, the deflections return to the baseline (3). When the muscle returns to its resting state, the deflections recorded from the 2 electrodes return to their original positions (4); the electrode overlying the injured area records ST segment elevation, and the electrode overlying the noninjured area records ST segment depression.

Figure 9-3. Injury current of activity.

When an electrode overlies an uninjured area of the muscle, the reverse occurs. Since the electrode overlies a positively charged area, the deflection it produces is elevated relative to the baseline (Fig 9-2). When the muscle is stimulated, a negative charge results, producing a downward deflection. When a potential difference between the uninjured and the injured areas of the muscle is not present, the deflection returns to the baseline. Since the original deflection recorded over the uninjured area was elevated relative to the baseline, the inscribed deflection gives the appearance of ST segment depression. When the muscle returns to its resting state, the deflection returns to its resting position above the baseline (Fig 9-2).

Injury Current of Activity

Experimental evidence suggests that when injured muscle is stimulated, it does not become as electrically negative as normal muscle. Thus, stimulated injured muscle will have less of a negative charge and therefore a relatively larger positive charge than normal stimulated muscle. An electrode overlying the injured portion of a muscle will face this positive charge, resulting in elevation of the ST segment (Fig 9-3). An electrode overlying the uninjured portion of the muscle will face a negative charge, resulting in depression of the

normal resting muscle (Fig 9-2). Thus, a potential difference between these areas exists, producing a flow of current. An electrode overlying the injured area of muscle will record a depression relative to the baseline. When the muscle is stimulated, an advancing negative charge (in front of which is a positive charge) is initiated, and the overlying electrode records a positive deflection. When a potential difference no longer exists between the advancing stimulus and the injured area, the recorded deflection returns to the baseline.

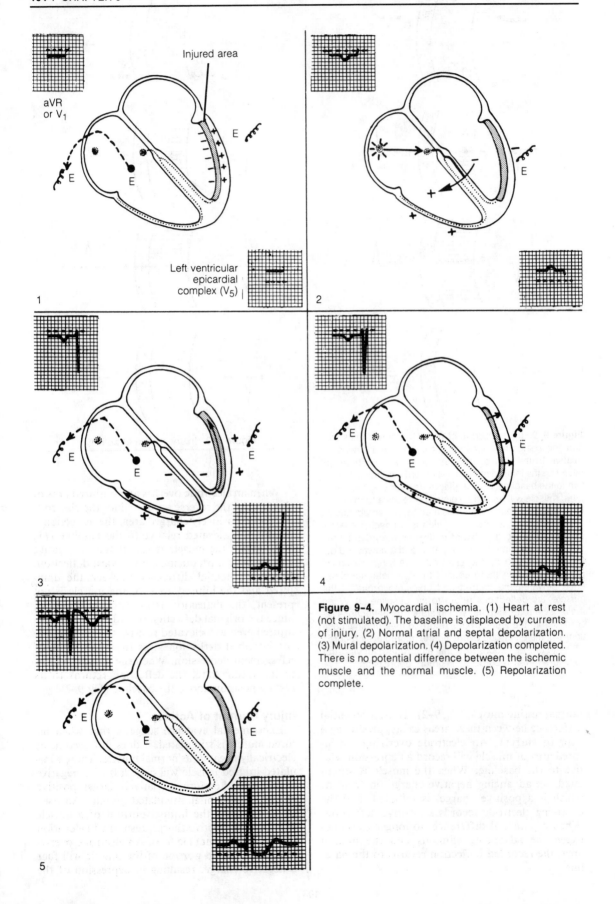

aVR
or V₁

Injured area

E

E

E

Left ventricular
epicardial
complex (V₅)

1

2

3

4

E

E

E

E

E

E

5

Figure 9-4. Myocardial ischemia. (1) Heart at rest
(not stimulated). The baseline is displaced by currents
of injury. (2) Normal atrial and septal depolarization.
(3) Mural depolarization. (4) Depolarization completed.
There is no potential difference between the ischemic
muscle and the normal muscle. (5) Repolarization
complete.

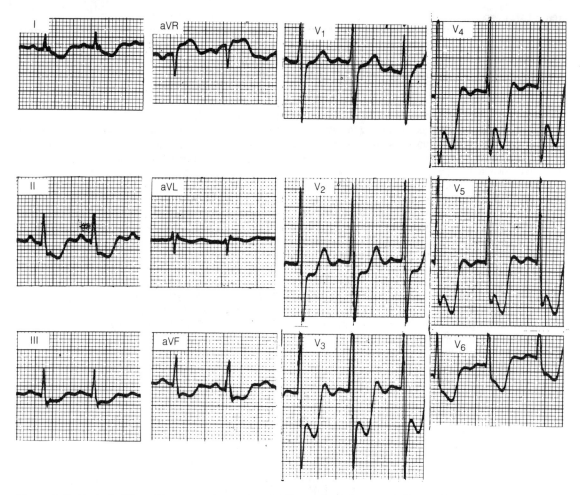

Figure 9-5. Marked, diffuse ST segment depression with T wave inversion recorded in a patient with 3-vessel coronary artery disease during an episode of anginal pain. Tracings before and after the pain were entirely normal. ST segment depression is most prominent in II, III, aVF, and V$_{2-6}$; in leads V$_{3-5}$ the ST depression is 10 mm.

ST segment. As a practical rule, an electrocardiographic tracing recorded directly over injured muscle records ST segment elevation. If normal muscle lies between injured muscle and the recording electrode, ST segment depression results (Fig 9–4).

T Wave Changes

As a result of the ST segment depression, the T wave may be "dragged" downward, producing the appearance of T wave inversion; however, true T wave inversion can also occur in leads showing ST segment depression (Fig 9–5). The T wave vector points away from an area of ischemia and toward an area of normal myocardium.

ELECTROCARDIOGRAPHIC PATTERNS RESULTING FROM MYOCARDIAL ISCHEMIA

ST-T Abnormalities

ST Segment Depression. ST segment depression is considered to reflect **nontransmural myocardial ischemia.** It often involves the subendocardial areas of the heart, which are the most vulnerable to ischemic injury due both to their bearing the brunt of systolic pressure developed by the ventricle and their smaller total blood supply which results in part from the transmyocardial coronary artery perfusion pressure gradient. The typical electrocardiographic pattern is ST segment depression with T wave inversion in left ventricular epicardial leads (Fig 9–5) and ST segment elevation (often not discernible) in leads facing the nonischemic portion of ventricular tissue.

Pseudonormalization. The T waves may be abnormal in a baseline tracing recorded in a patient with coronary artery disease, but during acute ischemic pain, they may become upright or less abnormal in some ECG leads ("normalization"). This phenomenon is termed **pseudonormalization** of baseline abnormal T waves and, in the presence of acute cardiac pain, indicates myocardial ischemia (Fig 9–6). However, since normalization of T waves which are abnormal at baseline may occur in conditions other than acute ischemia, this diagnosis requires clinical correlation.

ST Segment Elevation. ST segment elevation (Fig 9–7) reflects **transmural myocardial ischemia** and therefore indicates a more severe degree of ischemia than that responsible for the pattern of ST segment depression. Transient reversible transmural myocardial ischemia occurring at rest is frequently observed in patients with coronary vasospasm, with or without underlying fixed obstructive coronary artery disease. If ST segment elevation develops during exercise, it may reflect vasospasm or a critical degree of coronary artery luminal obstruction, provided that Q waves of prior myocardial infarction are not present. If Q waves are present, ST segment elevation during exercise reflects underlying wall motion abnormality rather than ischemia.

ST segment depression is often observed in leads opposite to those recording the ST segment elevation. This ST segment depression may be reciprocal to the ST elevation (Fig 9–7) or may indicate additional ischemia in areas remote from those showing ST elevation; the ECG does not differentiate between the two.

ST Segment Alternans. Rarely, during an episode of acute severe reversible transmural ische-mia, alternation in the amplitude, duration, and even polarity of the ST segment occurs, sometimes accompanied by alterations in the amplitude and duration of the QRS complexes themselves (Fig 9–8). While the cellular basis for this abnormality is not entirely clear, it is accompanied by alternation in cellular action potential amplitudes and durations, probably resulting from the interactions between the fast inward current of sodium and the slow inward current of calcium which are depressed during conditions of ischemia (see Chapter 2). ST segment alternans is an insensitive but highly specific marker for acute transmural ischemia, and may predict the development of ischemia-related ventricular arrhythmias.

PSEUDODEPRESSION & PSEUDOELEVATION OF THE ST SEGMENT VERSUS ISCHEMIC DEPRESSION & ELEVATION

Some normal individuals show apparent ST segment depression or elevation either at rest or during exercise. This phenomenon is usually associ-

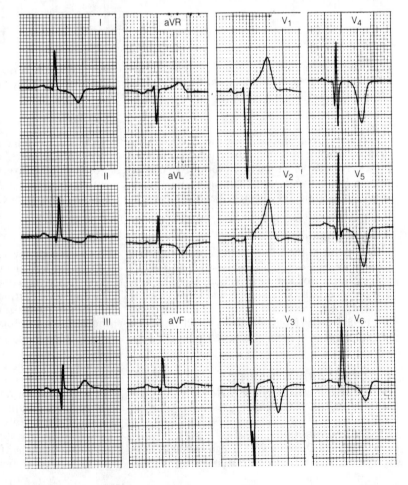

Figure 9–6. Pseudonormalization of T waves in a hypertensive patient with severe 3-vessel coronary artery disease and a 95% stenosis of the left main coronary artery. *A:* Baseline recording. T wave inversion is present in leads I, aVL, and V$_{3-6}$. J point elevation is present in V$_{1-2}$ and ST segment elevation in V$_3$. Q waves are present in leads II, III, aVF, and V$_{4-6}$ indicating past infarction of the inferior and anterior walls. *B:* Tracing recorded during severe anginal pain at rest. The T waves are less deeply inverted in leads I, aVL, and V$_{4-5}$, and are now upright in V$_3$. These changes reverted to the more abnormal ones recorded at baseline, when the chest pain had been relieved. Unless accompanied by an acute clinical event, the normalization of T waves is not specific for myocardial ischemia.

ated with tachycardia or anxiety and is explained by the presence of a **prominent atrial repolarization (T_a) wave.** In pseudodepression, the T_a wave continues through ventricular depolarization and is still evident after the inscription of the QRS complex. This pattern can be distinguished from ischemic ST segment depression by (1) the contour of the ST segment, which in pseudodepression displays a continuous ascent with upward concavity; and (2) associated downsloping of the PR segment. In ischemic ST segment depression, the J point is depressed and the ST segment is horizontal or downsloping (or very slowly upsloping). In pseudoelevation, the T_a wave may appear to represent isoelectricity, and the subsequent ST segment may therefore appear to be elevated (Fig 9–9).

Superimposition of atrial flutter waves upon the terminal portions of the QRS complexes can also cause pseudodepression and pseudoelevation, in addition to T_a waves.

INVERTED U WAVES

Occasionally, inversion of the U wave may be seen on a resting ECG (Fig 9–10) although it is more commonly seen after exercise. It may occur transiently during anginal pain. This finding is considered to represent severe obstructive coronary artery disease involving the left anterior descending coronary artery; it is an insensitive marker for this condition, however, and its specificity is not known. An inverted U wave may also be seen in left ventricular hypertrophy of any etiology and during periods of blood pressure elevation in hyertensive patients.

MYOCARDIAL INFARCTION TERMINOLOGY

Myocardial infarction occurs when insufficient coronary artery blood flow over a critical length

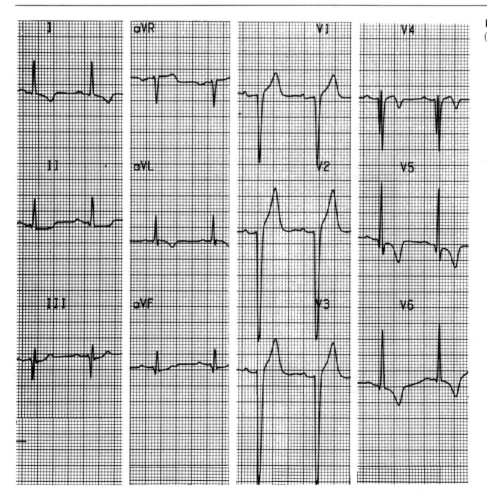

Figure 9–6.
(*continued*)

Figure 9-7. Spontaneous angina with ST elevation, indicating transmural myocardial ischemia. *A:* Tracing taken during an episode of anginal pain that occurred while the patient was at bed rest in the hospital. There is marked ST elevation in leads V₂₋₅ with ST depression in aVF. *B:* Tracing taken 30 min after (A) when the patient was pain-free and asymptomatic. The ST segments are isoelectric, and the ECG is normal. Subsequent evaluation, including serial ECGs and enzyme determinations, revealed no evidence of acute myocardial infarction. Although tracing (A) is quite typical of early infarction, the rapid disappearance of the ST elevation and the absence of clinical and electrocardiographic evidence of infarction on subsequent examinations indicate that tracing (A) represents severe acute but reversible ischemia.

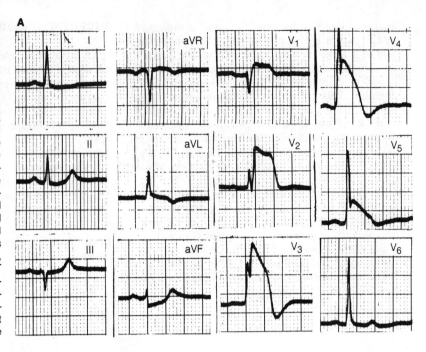

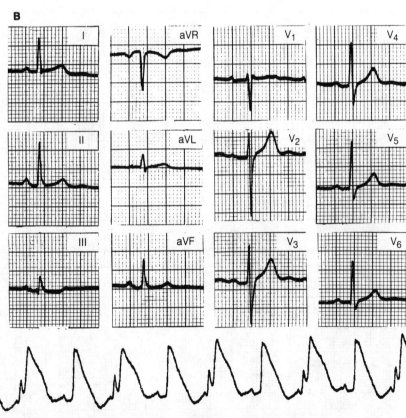

Figure 9-8. ST segment alternans recorded from a 24-hour ambulatory electrocardiographic examination in a patient with episodic pulmonary edema. Prior to the onset of the alternans, the rhythm was sinus with junctional bigeminy (see Chapter 10), in which the premature QRST complexes resembled identically the sinus generated complexes. In this rhythm strip, there is alternation in the amplitude of the R wave, QRST duration, and ST segment.

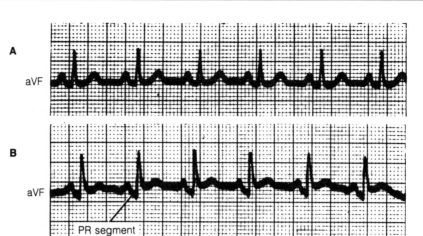

Figure 9-9. Pseudo-ST elevation. *A:* Normal tracing. *B:* Although the ST segment appears to be elevated, it is in fact isoelectric and on the same level as the TP segment. The downsloping PR segment, caused by a prominent T_a wave, causes the apparent ST segment elevation.

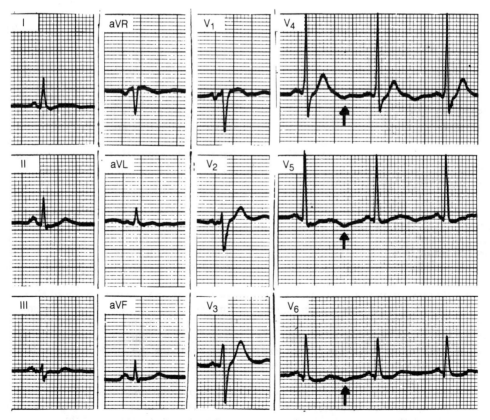

Figure 9-10. Inverted U waves (arrows) in a patient with aortic regurgitation and chest pain. Mild ST depression is present in I, II, aVL, and V_{4-6}. Inverted U waves are best seen in V_{4-6}.

of time causes death of myocardial tissue. This may result from atherosclerotic obstruction in the coronary arteries, thrombotic or embolic occlusion of a coronary artery, or spasm in an artery. The left ventricle is involved in virtually all instances of myocardial infarction; isolated right ventricular myocardial infarction is extremely rare. A single ECG recorded during acute myocardial infarction may be normal, may show nondiagnostic ST and T wave abnormalities only, or may reflect transmural ischemia and loss of ventricular forces. **Serial ECGs** and clinical correlation are mandatory in making the correct diagnosis.

It has recently become clear that the description of myocardial infarction as "nontransmural" ("subendocardial") and "transmural" is an oversimplification and therefore not correct. Electrocardiographic patterns of myocardial infarction that do not show Q waves (the classic criteria for transmural myocardial infarction) are often shown at autopsy to have been associated with necrosis of the entire ventricular myocardium from endocardium to epicardium. Conversely, ECGs that do show Q waves suggesting transmural infarction may be found at autopsy to have been limited to one or more layers of myocardium. Thus, the electrocardiographic distinction between transmural and nontransmural infarction based on the presence of Q waves is misleading. In recognition of this lack of specificity of the ECG for the anatomic situation, myocardial infarction will be described in this section as "Q-wave" and "non-Q-wave" infarction.

TRANSMURAL MYOCARDIAL INFARCTION

MECHANISM OF THE ELECTROCARDIOGRAPHIC PATTERNS

The Abnormal Q Wave & QS Complex in Transmural Myocardial Infarction

Since infarcted cardiac tissue is necrotic, and necrotic tissue is inexcitable and incapable of generating an action potential, it is electrically silent. The most diagnostic electrocardiographic finding for myocardial infarction is therefore the inscription of an abnormally wide (0.04 s) and deep (25% of the height of the R wave in a given lead) q wave or QS complex. Small, nonpathologic q waves that do not meet these criteria for width and depth are seen in normal individuals, where they are commonly recorded in leads I, aVF, and V_{4-6} and represent left-to-right depolarization of the interventricular septum. These **nonpathologic**

q waves should not exceed 0.03 s or 25% of the height of the R wave.

There are 3 exceptions to these criteria for the diagnosis of a pathologic Q wave: (1) If the Q wave is confined to lead III, it has no special significance. Q waves 0.04 s in duration and 25% of the height of the R wave may be recorded in normal individuals whose mean frontal plane QRS axis lies between +30 and 0°; lead aVF will not record a q wave. Thus, the diagnosis of myocardial infarction based on the presence of Q waves isolated to lead III should not be made. (2) If the q wave is confined to lead aVL alone and there are no other abnormalities in the ECG, it has no special significance. Q waves 0.04 s in duration and 25% of the height of the R wave may be recorded in normal persons whose mean frontal plane QRS axis is vertical (between +60 and +90°). (3) A small q wave (but not a QR or QS complex) may be present in lead V_2. While any q wave in this lead is often an abnormal finding, it may indicate conditions other than myocardial infarction (such as left bundle branch block, left anterior fascicular block, left ventricular hypertrophy, or chronic obstructive pulmonary disease) and thus is not helpful in establishing the diagnosis of infarction. The sensitivity and specificity of the ECG for the diagnosis of myocardial infarction and the causes of diagnostic error are given in Table 9–1.

Genesis of the Q Wave

The genesis of the Q wave is the redirection of electrical forces due to loss of forces that resulted from cell death. An electrocardiographic recording at a given moment in time represents the mean of electrical forces going in many directions in space. Ninety percent of such forces are canceled, leaving only about 10% that are recorded. When a myocardial infarction of significant size occurs, the depolarization forces in that area are lost, resulting in a change of direction of mean forces away from the area of infarction (Fig 9–11). The redirection of forces occurs most significantly during the initial 0.04–0.05 s of ventricular depolarization, resulting in a q wave (or QR or QS complex) in leads overlying the infarction zone. A small infarction, in which only a small amount of tissue is lost, may be insufficient to alter the mean forces so as to produce a q wave but may merely reduce the magnitude of the normal mean force, resulting in a reduction in R wave voltage in the leads overlying the infarction zone. It should be emphasized that a *reduction* in R wave voltage across the precordium (rather than lack of the expected *progression* of R wave voltage) may be an indicator of infarction, provided that other confirmatory electrocardiographic abnormalities (such as ST and T wave changes) are also present.

Table 9-1. Sensitivity and specificity of the ECG for the diagnosis of myocardial infarction (correlation with autopsy findings).

Sensitivity = 55-61%

Causes of false-negative diagnoses (Infarction present; ECG does not meet criteria for the diagnosis)
- (1) Cancellation of forces by second infarction
- (2) Left ventricular hypertrophy
- (3) Nonspecificity of ST-T abnormalities in the absence of Q waves
- (4) Lateral wall myocardial infarction
- (5) Posterior wall myocardial infarction
- (6) WPW conduction (see Chapter 15)

Specificity = 70-90%

Causes of false-positive diagnoses: (Infarction absent; ECG meets criteria for the diagnosis)

Q waves present when infarction is not present:
- (1) Left ventricular hypertrophy
- (2) WPW conduction
- (3) Chronic obstructive pulmonary disease
- (4) Fascicular conduction delays
- (5) Infiltrative heart disease (amyloid, hemochromatosis, myxedema)

Q waves absent
- (1) Right ventricular hypertrophy
- (2) Drug and electrolyte abnormalities
- (3) Secondary ST-T wave abnormalities in the presence of bundle branch block
- (4) Nondiagnostic ST-T wave abnormalities
- (5) Chronic obstructive pulmonary disease
- (6) Acute pulmonary embolism
- (7) Hyperventilation
- (8) Myocarditis

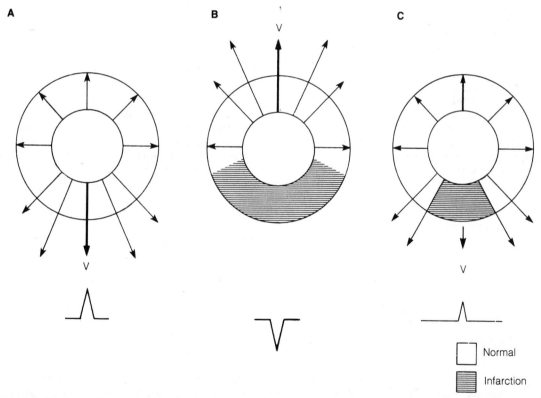

Figure 9-11. Cross section of the ventricle, showing arrows directed from the endocardium to the epicardium, representing the first 0.04 s of ventricular depolarization. *A:* Normal myocardium, in which there are greater forces directed downward, resulting in a mean force in that direction (heavy arrow) and an upright complex recorded by an electrode overlying that area. *B:* Loss of large forces because of myocardial necrosis, resulting in the mean force now being oriented in an opposite direction (heavy arrow). The electrode overlying the area of necrosis records a negative deflection (Q wave). *C:* Loss of some forces because of a small amount of myocardial necrosis, resulting in a reduction of mean force directed downward. The electrode overlying this area may not record a q wave but only a small R wave.

Table 9-2. Electrocardiographic diagnosis of acute myocardial infarction in patients with left bundle branch block.

Electrocardiographic findings in order of decreasing sensitivity*
(1) Serial changes in QRST complexes
(2) ST segment elevation
(3) Q waves in leads I, aVL, or V_{5-6}
(4) Q wave in V_6 and increased R wave in V_1
(5) Notch in ascending limb of S wave in anterior precordial leads

*Correlative data obtained from perfusion imaging using thallium-201.

Q waves can occur in conditions unassociated with myocardial infarction (Table 9–2). They are often transient, and clinically the differential diagnosis is generally not problematic.

ST Segment Changes in Transmural Infarction

Frequently, the first electrocardiographic finding in myocardial infarction is ST segment elevation in a lead overlying the area of infarction. The ST segment characteristically has a convex upward curvature.

Leads that are placed approximately 180° from the area of infarction show reciprocal ST segment depression. These changes are analogous to those described for injury currents in the isolated muscle strip. ST segment depression might also reflect additional ischemia in the area of myocardium recorded by those electrocardiographic leads; thus, the differential diagnosis between *reciprocal* ST segment depression and ischemia remote from the area of infarction must be made by independent means such as perfusion scintigraphy.

Because completely dead muscle is electrically silent, the occurrence of ST segment changes early in the course of infarction indicates the presence of some viable muscle in the epicardial region.

T Wave Changes in Transmural Infarction

Within the first few hours of infarction, "giant" upright T waves may be seen in leads overlying the infarct. The exact cause is not known but may be leakage of intracellular potassium from the damaged muscle cells into the extracellular spaces, producing a local hyperkalemia (Fig 9–12).

After a period of hours or days (up to 2 weeks), the ST segment returns to the isoelectric line and T wave changes occur. The T wave changes may begin to develop while the ST segments are still deviated. The T waves begin to invert in those leads that showed ST segment elevation.

The typical infarction T wave is symmetrically inverted; that is, its peak is midway between its beginning and the end. The inverted T wave may have an isoelectric ST segment but show an up-ward convexity ("coronary" T wave), or it may have an elevated ST segment and an upward convexity ("cove-plane" T wave) (Figs 9–13 and 9–14).

In transmural infarction, the abnormal Q waves may appear within hours of infarction or later in its evolution. They may occur while the ST segment changes are present or appear after they have become isoelectric. Q waves usually appear before marked T wave changes have occurred. With the expanding use of thrombolytic therapy in the early stages of myocardial infarction, the evolutionary electrocardiographic patterns become telescoped in time to minutes to hours rather than days to weeks.

LOCALIZATION OF TRANSMURAL INFARCTION BY ELECTROCARDIOGRAPHIC PATTERNS

By observing the infarction pattern in specific electrocardiographic leads, the anatomic site of infarction can often be localized. The *functional extent* of the infarction is *not assessable* from the ECG.

Coronary Artery Blood Supply to The Heart

The blood supply to the heart is derived from the left and right coronary arteries, which arise from the left and right aortic sinuses, respectively. The left coronary artery divides shortly after its origin into the **left anterior descending** and the **left circumflex** arteries (Fig 9–15). The former supplies the anterior surface of the left ventricle, the medial portion of the anterior surface of the right ventricle, and the lower third of the posterior surface of the right ventricle. The remainder of the right ventricle is supplied by the **right coronary artery.** The circumflex artery supplies the lateral wall and the lower (apical) half of the posterior wall of the left ventricle. The upper (basal) half of the posterior wall and the inferior wall of the left ventricle are supplied by the right coronary artery. Anatomic variations exist, depending upon the "dominance" of the right and left coronary systems. In atherosclerotic and vasospastic coronary disease, the blood supply to different areas of the myocardium will vary, depending upon the site and magnitude of the arterial obstruction and the presence and integrity of the collateral circulation.

The site of myocardial infarction can be determined by applying the electrocardiographic criteria for the diagnosis of myocardial infarction to specific leads; erroneous interpretations are not rare, however, and will be influenced by prior infarctions and coronary artery anatomy.

Site of Infarction	Electrocardiographic Leads Reflecting the Infarction
Anterior	V_{2-6}
Inferior	II and aVF (and III)
Lateral	I, aVL, and V_6
Posterior	V_{1-2}
Right ventricle	V_{2-4R}, occasionally V_{1-3}

ANTERIOR WALL MYOCARDIAL INFARCTION

Anterior wall myocardial infarction is best reflected in the precordial leads. Leads I and aVL may show the infarction pattern if lateral wall myocardial infarction is also present. The characteristic findings in the evolution of a Q-wave ante-

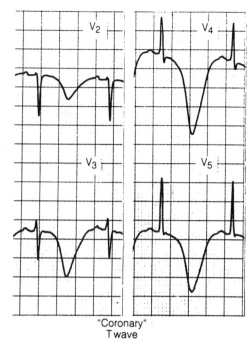

"Coronary" T wave

Figure 9-13. Markedly deep symmetric T wave inversion in the precordial leads in a patient with acute myocardial infarction. Serum electrolytes were normal, no drug therapy had been administered, and neurologic examination was normal. (Such T wave abnormalities are not infrequently seen with intracranial hemorrhage without myocardial necrosis.) Q waves did not evolve. Deep T wave inversion of this magnitude is most unusual.

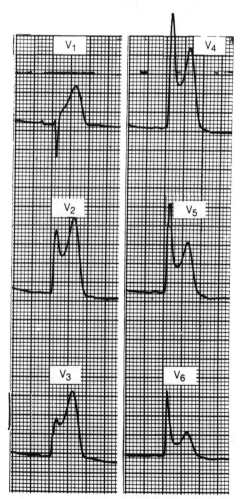

Figure 9-12. Giant upright T waves exceeding the QRS amplitude in a patient with acute anterior wall myocardial infarction. Accompanying the giant T waves is marked ST segment elevation. Q waves are not yet present.

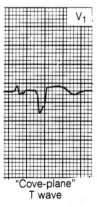

"Cove-plane" T wave

Figure 9-14. T wave abnormalities in acute myocardial infarction.

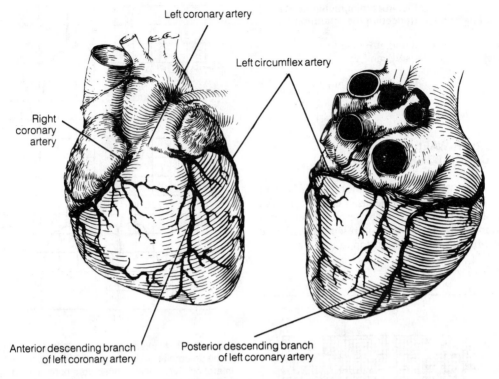

Figure 9-15. Coronary circulation.

rior wall myocardial infarction are summarized as follows (Fig 9-16):

Frontal plane: ST segment elevation occurs in leads I and aVL, reflecting transmural injury, followed by the inscription of a Q wave, reflecting loss of myocardium, and, finally, T wave inversion. Leads II and III may show ST segment depression, which is either reciprocal to the ST elevation or reflective of additional ischemia remote from the area of infarction.

Precordial leads: Depending upon the extent of the infarction and the position of the heart within the chest, several of the precordial leads will show the infarction pattern.

Vector analysis: The initial 0.04-s vector is directed posteriorly, away from the infarction zone, resulting in a q or QS wave in the precordial leads. If this initial vector is also oriented rightward, an abnormal q wave will be inscribed in lead I. In the early stages of myocardial infarction, the ST vector is oriented anteriorly and to the left, resulting in ST segment elevation in lead I and the left precordial leads. Within the first few hours of infarction, tall ("giant"), tented T waves may be recorded in the leads overlying the infarcted area. The tented T waves are thought to reflect local hyperkalemia due to potassium efflux from necrotic tissue. In later stages, the T vector is oriented posteriorly and to the right, away from the infarcted area, producing inverted T waves in these leads.

When a pattern of infarction involving the *inferior* leads occurs *in association with* an *anterior* wall myocardial infarction, it is likely that there is only a single infarction, involving both the anterior wall and the apical-inferior area of the heart. Leads II and aVF (and sometimes also III) may therefore show the infarction pattern, as they reflect events occurring at the cardiac apex. However, the possibility does exist that both anterior and inferior wall myocardial infarction may occur at the same time (Fig 9-17).

INFERIOR WALL MYOCARDIAL INFARCTION

Since this area of myocardium overlies the left diaphragm, the infarction pattern will be recorded in leads II, III, and aVF. The characteristic findings of Q-wave infarction in this area are summarized as follows (Fig 9-18):

Frontal plane: The infarct pattern will be seen in leads II, III, and aVF. At the time of ST segment elevation in these leads, reciprocal ST segment depression may be seen in leads I and aVL. Later, when the T waves become inverted in the inferior leads, the T waves in leads I and aVL will become tall.

Precordial leads: The precordial leads often show no abnormality. At times, however, depending upon the extent of infarction, abnormalities

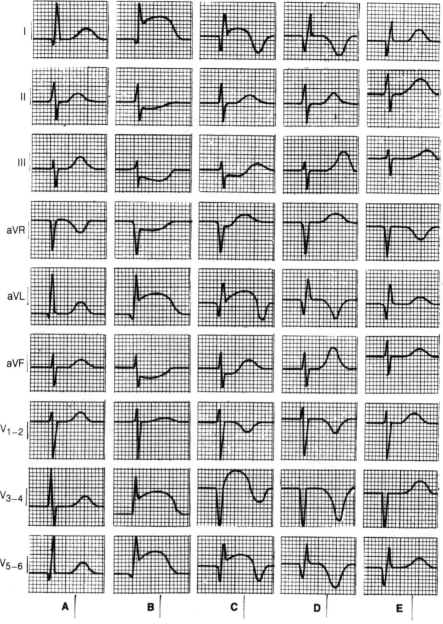

Figure 9-16. Diagrammatic illustration of serial electrocardiographic patterns in anterior wall myocardial infarction. *A:* Normal tracing. *B:* Early pattern. There is ST segment elevation in I, aVL, and V_{3-6} and ST depression in II, III, and aVF (the ST depression might reflect inferior wall ischemia or reciprocal depression). *C:* Later pattern (hours to days). Q waves are present in I, aVL, and V_{5-6}. QS complexes are present in V_{3-4}, indicating that the major area of infarction underlies the area recorded by V_{3-4}. ST segment changes persist but to a lesser degree, and the T waves are beginning to invert in those leads in which ST segment elevation is present. *D:* Late (established) pattern (days to weeks). The Q waves and QS complexes persist. The ST segments are isoelectric. The T waves are deeply and symmetrically inverted in the leads that showed ST elevation and tall in the leads that showed ST depression. This pattern may persist for the remainder of the patient's life. *E:* Very late pattern (months to years). The abnormal Q waves and QS complexes persist, but the T waves have returned to normal. Without the benefit of serial ECGs, it is not possible to determine when myocardial infarction occurred. Therefore, no conclusions should be drawn as to the age of the process on the basis of a single ECG. Patterns A through D may evolve much more rapidly (hours to days) if thrombolytic agents are used in the very early stages of infarction.

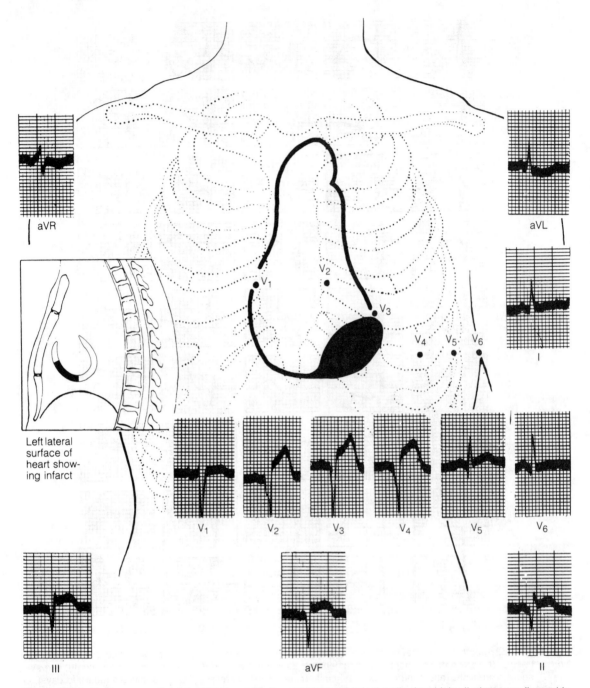

Figure 9–17. Single myocardial infarction involving the anterior and apical walls, in which all electrocardiographic changes occur over the same period of time. There are deep, wide Q waves with elevated ST segments in leads II and III. Lead aVF shows a Q wave and ST elevation. This pattern indicates inferior wall myocardial infarction. The precordial leads show loss of R wave voltage between V_1 and V_2, QS complexes in V_{3-4} and a qR complex in V_5. There is ST segment elevation in V_{2-5}, reflecting anterior wall myocardial infarction. The abnormalities in the inferior leads reflect infarction of the cardiac apex, which overlies the diaphragm in some patients. Since both anterior and inferior wall myocardial infarctions might have occurred at different times in this patient, clinical correlation is most important in correct interpretation of the site of infarction.

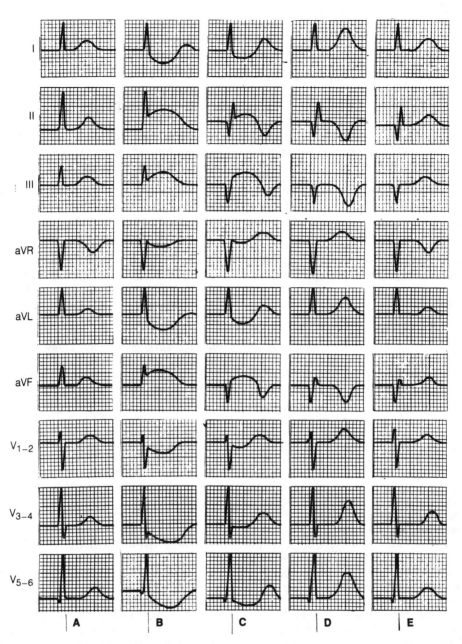

Figure 9–18. Diagrammatic illustration of serial electrocardiographic patterns in inferior myocardial infarction. *A:* Normal tracing. *B:* Very early pattern (hours after infarction). There is ST segment elevation in II, III, and aVF and ST segment depression in I, aVL, and aVR as well as in the precordial leads. *C:* Later pattern (hours to days). Abnormal Q waves have appeared in the inferior leads. There is less ST elevation in these leads and less ST depression in the anterior leads. The T waves are becoming inverted in II, III, and aVF. *D:* Late (established) pattern (days to weeks). The ST segments are isoelectric. Deep, symmetrically inverted T waves are seen in II, III, and aVF. The T waves are abnormally tall and symmetric in I, aVL, and the precordial leads. This pattern may persist for the remainder of the patient's life. *E:* Very late (months to years) pattern. The abnormal Q waves persist, but the T waves have become normal. As with anterior wall infarction, if thrombolytic therapy is used, the evolutionary changes may occur over a much shorter period of time.

will be recorded in the area of the interventricular septum (V_{2-3}) or in the area of the lateral wall (V_6). Not infrequently, ST segment depression, which is either reciprocal to the ST segment elevation or indicative of anterior wall ischemia, is recorded in V_{1-3}.

Vector analysis: The initial 0.04-s vector is directed superiorly because of the loss of inferior forces. Thus, abnormal Q waves are inscribed in leads II, III, and aVF, and the mean frontal plane QRS axis is directed leftward and superiorly. It is important to recognize that the superior axis deviation that results from inferior wall myocardial infarction is due *not* to conduction system disease involving the left anterior fasicle of the left bundle branch (see Chapter 8) but to loss of muscle. In the early stage of infarction, the ST vector is directed inferiorly, producing ST segment elevation in these leads. In the later stages, the T vector is oriented superiorly, resulting in inverted T waves in II, III, and aVF.

POSTERIOR WALL MYOCARDIAL INFARCTION

Myocardial infarction confined to the posterior wall of the heart is unusual; posterior wall infarction is almost always accompanied by inferior or lateral wall myocardial infarction (or both). In addition to the electrocardiographic pattern of inferior wall infarction, therefore, that of posterior wall infarction is added. As a result of posterior wall infarction, the initial 0.04 s of the QRS complex will be directed *anteriorly,* because of loss of the forces normally generated by the posterior portion of the ventricle (Fig 9–19). This condition will result in abnormally tall R waves in precordial leads V_{1-2} and an abnormal R:S ratio. Q waves may be recorded over the posterior surface of the heart by esophageal electrodes. ST segment depression in V_{1-2} is seen early in posterior wall myocardial infarction, which might be reciprocal to posterior wall ST elevation or might reflect additional anterior wall myocardial ischemia. Terminally upright T waves suggest the former, and inverted T waves may suggest the latter. Later, tall, symmetric T waves will be present.

Inferoposterolateral Wall Myocardial Infarction

The pattern of infarction will be recorded in the inferior leads, the anterior precordial leads, and the lateral leads. The inferior infarction will be manifested by abnormal Q waves and T wave inversion in leads II, III, and aVF. The posterior wall infarction will be manifested by abnormally tall R waves with upright T waves in V_{1-2}. The lat-

eral wall infarction will be manifested by abnormal Q waves and inverted T waves in V_{5-7} (Fig 9–20 on page 120).

NONTRANSMURAL MYOCARDIAL INFARCTION

As mentioned previously, although the ECG was used for many years to distinguish transmural from nontransmural myocardial infarction, it is now recognized that this differentiation cannot be made from the ECG alone. It had been considered that the subendocardial portion of the myocardium was electrically "silent" and that depolarization in this area would not be associated with an abnormal Q wave. However, correlations of electrocardiographic patterns with autopsy findings have documented the unreliability of the ECG in establishing an accurate differential *anatomic* diagnosis. Although many anatomic transmural infarctions are manifested by Q waves on the ECG, a significant number are not (Fig 9–21 on page 121); conversely, many anatomic nontransmural infarctions will demonstrate Q waves. When Q waves are not present, the electrocardiographic diagnosis of acute myocardial infarction depends upon *evolutionary* changes in *serial* records and clinical correlation. The differential diagnosis of non-Q-wave infarction from myocardial ischemia likewise depends upon the *serial* demonstration of evolutionary changes in the former and *reversibility* to normal (or baseline) in the latter; a single ECG is insufficient for the correct diagnosis.

MULTIPLE INFARCTIONS

If the ECG reverts to normal after an initial infarction, a second infarct will produce a pattern as would be expected with initial infarction. However, abnormal Q waves that persist following the initial infarct may not be altered by a second infarct involving the opposite wall. ST segment elevations that occur with the second infarct will cause ST segment depression in the area of the initial infarct. The development of inverted T waves as a result of the second infarct can cause the inverted T waves resulting from the initial infarct to become upright (Figs 9–22 and 9–23 on pages 122 and 123).

VENTRICULAR ANEURYSM (Akinesis & Dyskinesis)

An aneurysm of the left ventricle, in which a portion of the ventricular wall is fibrotic and thinned and does not contract (or even expands)

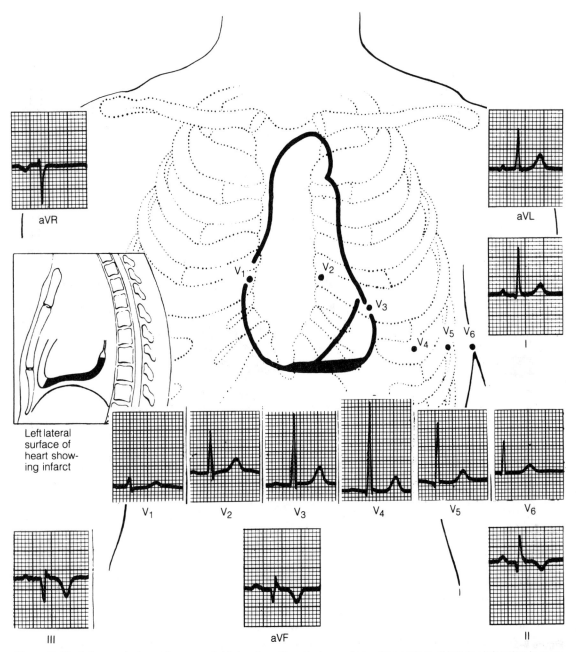

Figure 9-19. Inferoposterior wall myocardial infarction. The electrocardiographic pattern of inferior infarction is seen in leads II, III, and aVF. The posterior wall infarction is manifested by an abnormally tall R wave in V_{1-2}, indicating loss of posterior forces with consequent prominent anterior forces. The T waves are upright in V_{1-2}, indicating an anteriorly directed T wave vector, pointing away from the area of ischemic injury. The tall R waves in leads V_{1-2} might be due to right ventricular hypertrophy (see Chapter 7), but right axis deviation, tall, peaked P waves, and T wave inversion in V_{1-2} are all absent, whereas criteria for inferior infarction are present. Thus, the diagnosis of right ventricular hypertrophy is unlikely.

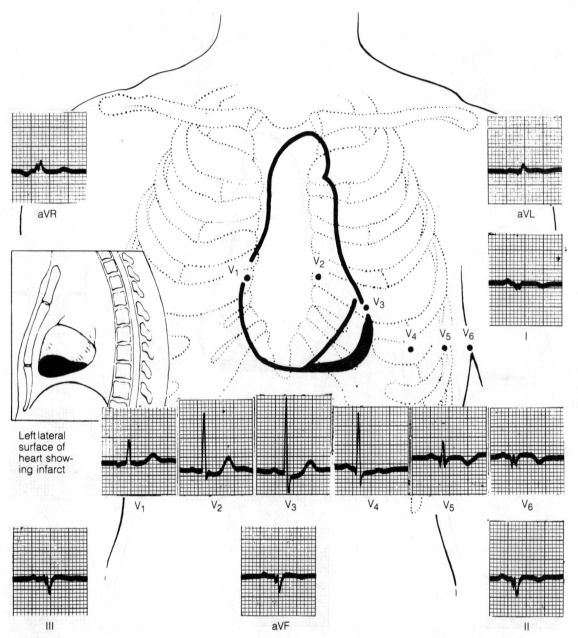

Figure 9-20. Inferoposterolateral wall myocardial infarction. Q waves and T wave inversion are present in the inferior leads, abnormally tall R waves with upright T waves are present in precordial leads V_{1-2}, and Q waves with T wave inversion are present in lateral leads V_{5-6}. The mean frontal plane QRS axis is directed rightward because of loss of left lateral forces. In view of the infarction patterns present in this tracing, the rightward axis deviation does not reflect increased muscle mass of the right ventricle (right ventricular hypertrophy).

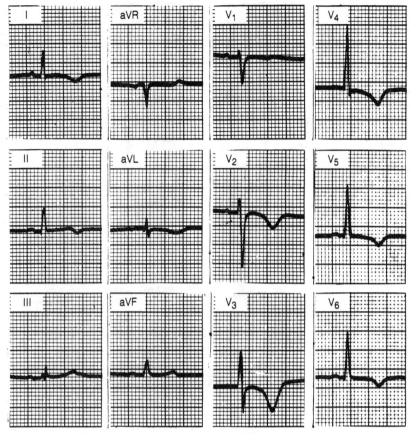

Figure 9-21. Non-Q wave myocardial infarction, documented at autopsy to be transmural. The T waves are symmetrically inverted in I, II, aVL, and V$_{2-6}$. Q waves are not present, despite the through-and-through infarction process.

during ventricular systole, may follow myocardial infarction. "Aneurysm" is a pathologic term, however, and describes the morphologic characteristics of the scarred muscle. The functional counterparts of aneurysmal tissue are **akinesis** (lack of motion), and **dyskinesis** (paradoxic bulging motion during ventricular systole). The most consistent electrocardiographic finding in these major wall motion disorders of the ventricle following myocardial infarction is the persistence of ST segment elevation in the epicardial leads reflecting the area of infarction (Figs 9–24 and 9–25 on page 124). The ST segments may remain elevated for months to years. Since this pattern is seen in only about half of autopsy-proved or surgically-proved cases (sensitivity about 50%), the absence of ST elevation does not indicate absence of significant ventricular wall motion disorders.

DIFFERENTIAL ELECTROCARDIOGRAPHIC DIAGNOSIS OF MYOCARDIAL INFARCTION (Table 9-1)

Normal Electrocardiogram

The criteria for an abnormal Q wave are a duration of at least 0.04 s or a Q:R ratio equal to or exceeding 25% (or both). These criteria are not valid for the diagnosis of myocardial infarction if they are present in lead III alone, since up to 35% of normal persons may have this finding. The additional finding of T wave inversion in this lead is also of no diagnostic value (Fig 9–26 on page 125). Recording lead III during deep inspiration and expiration has been recommended as a means of identifying the inconstancy of Q waves in this

Figure 9-22. Multiple myocardial infarctions. *A:* Acute anterior wall myocardial infarction. Deep Q waves are present in leads V_{1-3} with ST segment elevation in leads V_{1-5} and T wave inversion in leads I, aVL, and V_{1-5}. *B:* Ten months later, the ECG has reverted to normal. *C:* Second acute myocardial infarction, occurring 8 months after the tracing in (B) was recorded. New Q waves with ST segment elevation are present in leads I, II, III, aVF, and V_{5-6}. Abnormally tall R waves are present in V_{1-2}, with ST segment depression in these leads. This second myocardial infarction is inferoposterolateral in location.

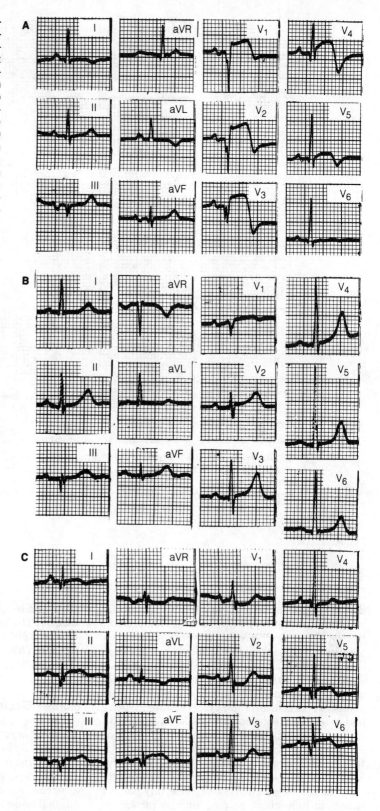

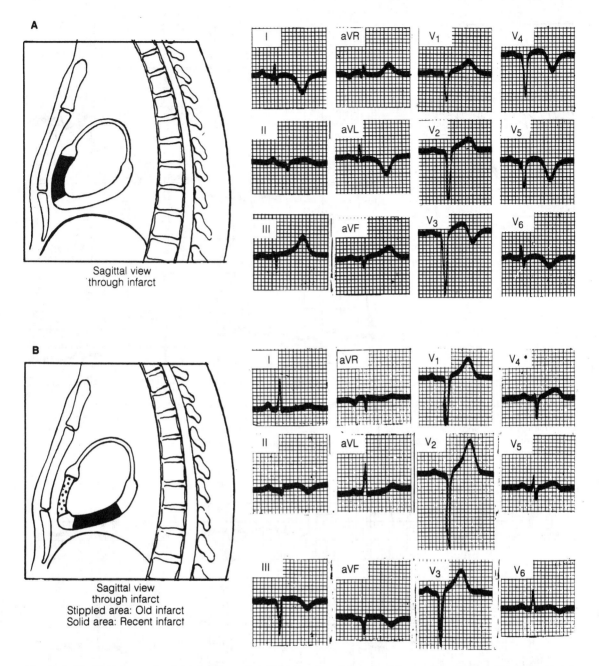

Figure 9–23. Multiple myocardial infarctions. *A:* Initial infarction. There are QS complexes in V_{1-5}. The T waves are inverted in I, aVL, and V_{3-6}. The pattern indicates anterior wall myocardial infarction, and the pattern was stable for several months. *B:* Second infarction. A deep Q wave with inverted T wave is now present in aVF, indicating inferior wall infarction. As a result, the T waves that were previously inverted in the precordial leads have now become upright.

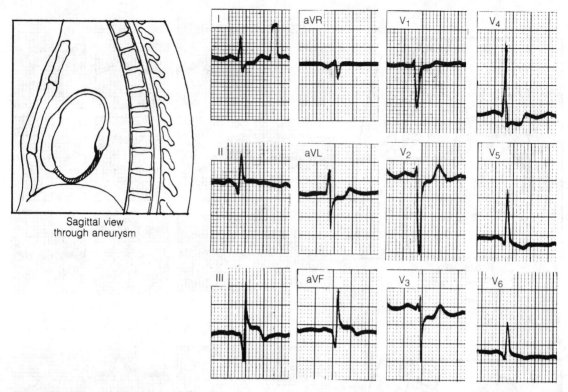

Sagittal view
through aneurysm

Figure 9-24. Ventricular aneurysm involving the inferior wall. Deep, wide Q waves with ST segment elevation and T wave inversion are present in II, III, and aVF, indicating inferior wall myocardial infarction. There is ST segment depression in leads I, aVL, and V$_{1-4}$. Although the ECG might suggest recent inferior wall infarction, this had been a stable pattern over 1 year, and the inferior wall ventricular aneurysm was confirmed by cineangiography and at surgery.

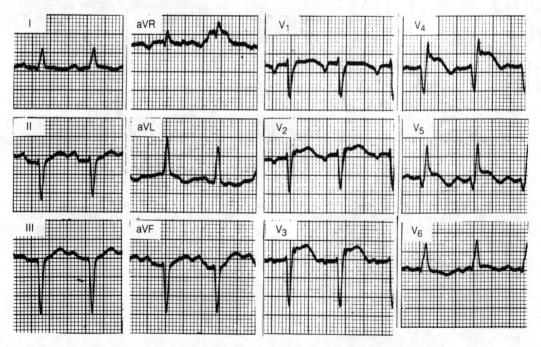

Figure 9-25. Anterior ventricular aneurysm. The frontal plane axis is −60°, indicating left anterior fascicular block. There is a diminutive r wave in V$_3$ and V$_4$ and wide Q waves in V$_{5-6}$. The ST segments are elevated in V$_{3-5}$. Although this is consistent with acute anterior wall infarction, clinically, the infarction had occurred 1 year before, and serial ECGs had shown no change. A large anterior ventricular aneurysm was documented by left ventricular angiography.

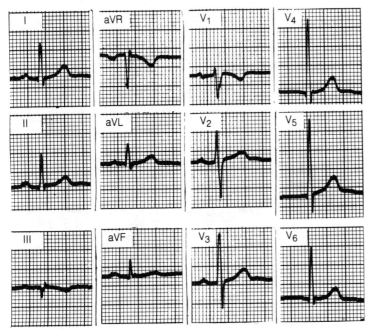

Figure 9-26. Normal ECG. There is a Q wave in lead III, and the T wave is inverted in this lead; no other abnormalities (specifically, in leads I and aVF) are present. Such a tracing should not be interpreted as showing inferior wall myocardial infarction.

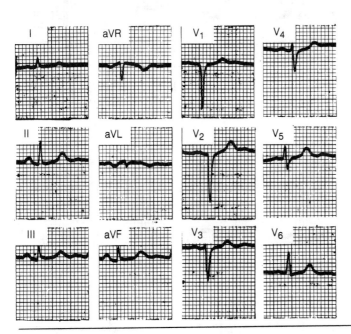

Figure 9-27. Normal electrocardiographic pattern with QS complexes in V_{1-2}. The R waves progressively increase in height, and the R:S ratio changes appropriately from V_{3-6}. There are no ST–T abnormalities. Although old anteroseptal myocardial infarction could have occurred, this sort of tracing is best interpreted as being within normal limits, depending upon the clinical circumstances.

lead, but neither its sensitivity nor its specificity for the absence of myocardial infarction is known.

QS complexes may occasionally be seen in V_2 in normal individuals (Fig 9-27).

Left Ventricular Hypertrophy

In hypertrophy of the left ventricle, the left ventricular forces are directed leftward, inferiorly, and posteriorly. Thus, QS complexes may be inscribed in V_{1-2} and are occasionally present through V_4. Anterior wall myocardial infarction cannot be diagnosed from the ECG with certainty, although it *cannot be excluded* as having occurred (Fig 9-28). In addition, the ST segment depression in I, aVL, and V_{5-6} and the ST segment elevation in V_{1-3} associated with left ventricular hypertrophy may further mimic myocardial ischemia or infarction, but they cannot be interpreted as such.

In patients with marked hypertrophy of the interventricular septum, abnormal Q waves can be recorded in several electrocardiographic leads,

Figure 9-28. Left ventricular hypertrophy in a patient with aortic regurgitation. The R wave in aVL is 13 mm, and Sv_1 + RV_6 is 47 mm. Associated ST elevation is present in leads V_{1-3} and ST depression in I, aVL, and V_{5-6}. QS complexes are present in V_{1-4}. In the presence of left ventricular hypertrophy, criteria for myocardial infarction cannot be accurately applied.

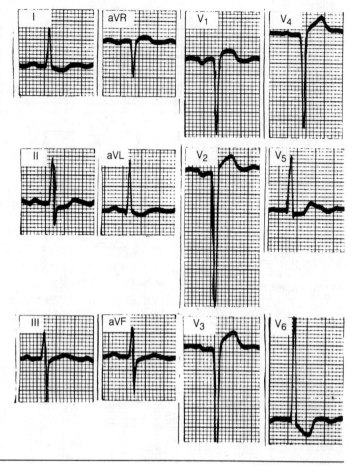

Figure 9-29. Right ventricular hypertrophy in a patient with severe chronic obstructive pulmonary disease. QS complexes are present in leads V_{1-3}, representing recordings made over a greatly dilated right ventricle. The progression of R waves over the precordium is poor for the same reason. The P waves are tall and peaked in leads II, III, and aVF, and there is marked rightward deviation of the mean frontal plane QRS axis. This ECG could represent extensive anterolateral wall myocardial infarction (old, because of the upright T waves); the correct diagnosis depends upon clinical correlation.

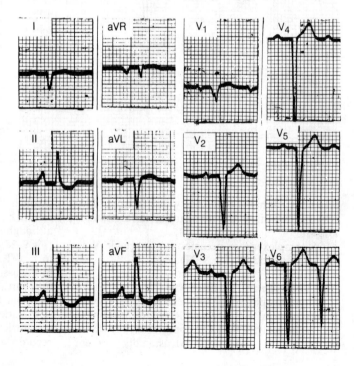

simulating anterior, inferior, lateral, or posterior wall myocardial infarction. Since the normal q wave is due in part to septal depolarization, septal hypertrophy will accentuate this initial force. In addition, the distorted anatomy of the myocardial fibers can contribute to abnormal and delayed impulse conduction through septal tissue. Coronary arteriographic and autopsy data have proved the absence of myocardial infarction in such patients with abnormal q waves.

Chronic Obstructive Pulmonary Disease With Right Ventricular Hypertrophy

The presence of chronic lung disease, with associated hyperinflation of the lungs, can produce changes in the ECG that mimic myocardial infarction. A marked reduction or even total absence of anterior QRS forces is most commonly observed, resulting in small r waves or QS complexes in precordial leads V_{1-4} (Fig 9–29). If there is additional right ventricular hypertrophy or acute right ventricular overload, the T waves may be inverted in these leads, further mimicking anterior wall myocardial infarction (Fig 9–30).

For reasons that are not quite clear, pulmonary emphysema may distort the mean frontal plane QRS axis, resulting in an abnormally leftward and superior axis (Fig 9–31). This should *not* be confused with left anterior fascicular conduction delay, since it is not involvement of the intraventricular conduction system that is causing the left axis deviation but alteration of the QRS vector in the frontal plane caused by the lung disease. In addition, abnormal Q waves or QS complexes can be recorded in leads aVF or I, thus mimicking inferior wall or lateral wall myocardial infarction. If the diagnosis of obstructive pulmonary disease is known, any ECG showing these features should not be interpreted as showing myocardial infarction unless there is clinical correlation.

Left Anterior Fascicular Conduction Delay

If there is a delay in conduction in the left anterior fascicle of the left bundle branch, the inferoposterior surface of the heart is depolarized in advance of the anterosuperior surface. This initial inferoposterior force may result in inscription of a q wave in leads I and aVL, which does not indicate myocardial infarction but occurs as a result of the fascicular conduction delay. In addition,

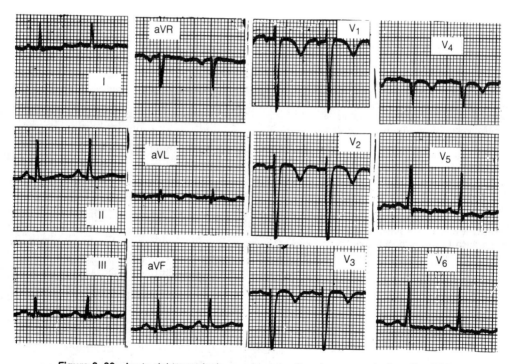

Figure 9-30. Acute right ventricular overload due to pulmonary embolism. The ECG shows deep symmetric T wave inversion in leads V_{1-4}. This electrocardiographic pattern is compatible with acute myocardial ischemia or infarction, but serial tracings failed to show evolution or resolution of the abnormalities, and a lung scan documented a large perfusion defect. Acute pulmonary embolism may be unassociated with rightward axis shift or a change in P wave morphology, with anterior precordial T wave abnormalities the only clue as to its occurrence (as in this case).

Figure 9-31. Right ventricular hypertrophy in a patient with severe chronic obstructive lung disease. The QRS complexes are of low voltage in the frontal plane, likely due to hyperinflation of the lungs. Q waves are present in the inferior leads, resulting in superior axis deviation. The P waves are peaked in II, III, and aVF. Inferior wall myocardial infarction was not present at autopsy.

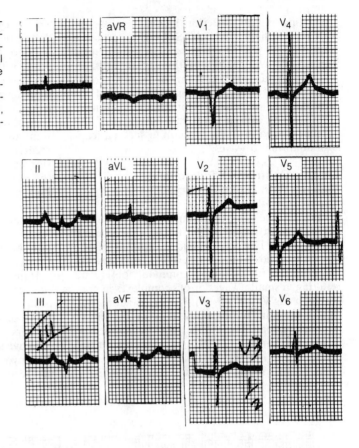

Figure 9-32. Left anterior fascicular and right bundle branch block patterns. Anterior wall myocardial infarction is simulated by the small q waves in V_{1-3}. These q waves are not due to loss of anterior force resulting from myocardial necrosis but to abnormal septal depolarization caused by conduction delay in the anterosuperior fascicle of the left bundle branch. Left anterior fascicular block is not expected to cause deep, wide Q waves in the precordial leads; when such Q waves occur, they most likely represent myocardial infarction.

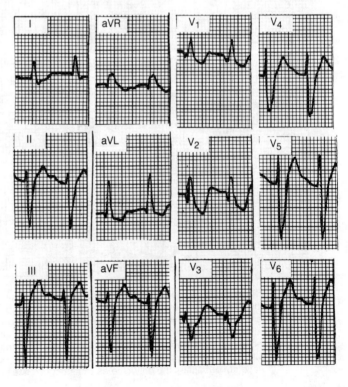

small (but not wide) q waves may be seen in V_{1-2} as a result of loss of the normal depolarization sequence of the anterior portion of the interventricular septum (Fig 9–32).

MYOCARDIAL INFARCTION WITH CONCOMITANT BUNDLE BRANCH BLOCK PATTERNS

In general, a right bundle branch block pattern does not obscure the patterns of myocardial infarction, whereas a left bundle branch block pattern does. The most diagnostic feature of myocardial infarction is the abnormal direction of the initial 0.04-s QRS vector (the Q wave). Since this portion of the QRS complex remains normal in *right-sided* intraventricular conduction delay, myocardial infarction can be detected when it occurs. However, the initial 0.04-s vector is *itself* abnormal in left bundle branch block; thus, the infarction pattern is obscured, and the expected abnormal Q wave will not be inscribed.

Right Bundle Branch Block Pattern & Myocardial Infarction

The concomitant occurrence of right bundle branch block pattern and anterior wall myocardial infarction indicates infarction of the interventricular septum and thus connotes an extensive degree of myocardial necrosis. As a result of the infarction, the initial r wave of the rSR' complex in right bundle branch block will disappear in right ventricular epicardial leads, resulting in QR complexes (Fig 9–33).

The occurrence of right bundle branch block and inferior wall myocardial infarction suggests that the proximal portion of the right bundle branch, which is supplied by branches of the right coronary artery, is itself ischemic or infarcted. The pattern of inferior wall myocardial infarction is not obscured by the right bundle branch block.

The occurrence of posterior wall myocardial infarction in association with right bundle branch block alters the QRS complexes in the right precordial leads. Conduction delay in the right bundle branch alters the late forces of ventricular depolarization, and posterior wall infarction alters the initial forces of ventricular depolarization. The initial forces of ventricular depolarization are oriented in an abnormally anterior direction in posterior myocardial infarction. The late forces (the R') reflecting the right bundle branch conduction delay are also oriented anteriorly. Thus, an abnormally tall, wide R or rR' wave will be inscribed in the right precordial leads (Fig 9–34). A similar pattern may be seen in patients with right ventricular hypertrophy and right intraventricular conduction delay and also in patients with right bundle branch block alone; thus, confirmatory evidence of myocardial infarction (usually involvement of the inferior wall) must be sought.

The development of right bundle branch block with left anterior or posterior fascicular block will result in the changes described above with the addition of a leftward or rightward shift, respectively, of the mean frontal plane QRS axis (Fig 9–35 on page 130; see Chapter 8). Infarction Q waves already present may be masked by the fascicular conduction delay.

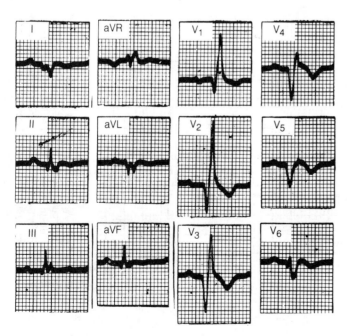

Figure 9–33. Anterior wall myocardial infarction associated with right bundle branch block. The QRS duration is 0.14 s and the VAT in V_{1-2} is 0.1 s. The initial r waves of an uncomplicated right bundle branch block pattern that are normally seen in right precordial leads are not present. Instead, deep, wide Q waves indicative of anterior wall myocardial infarction are recorded.

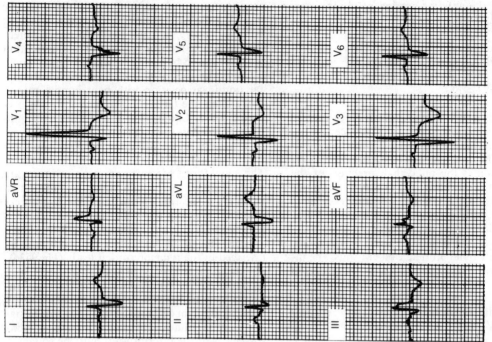

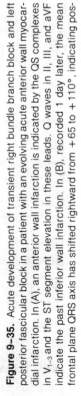

Figure 9–35. Acute development of transient right bundle branch block and left posterior fascicular block in a patient with an evolving acute anterior wall myocardial infarction. In (A), an anterior wall infarction is indicated by the QS complexes in V$_{1-3}$ and the ST segment elevation in these leads. Q waves in II, III, and aVF indicate the past inferior wall infarction. In (B), recorded 1 day later, the mean frontal plane QRS axis has shifted rightward from +65 to +110°, indicating posterior fascicular conduction delay. A delayed R' wave is present in V$_{1-3}$, and a deep wide S wave is present in I, aVL, and V$_{5-6}$, indicating right bundle branch block. The anterior and inferior Q waves are unchanged. Although the rightward shift in frontal plane QRS axis could suggest lateral wall myocardial infarction, the absence of associated ST–T wave changes together with evidence of conduction delay makes this diagnosis most unlikely.

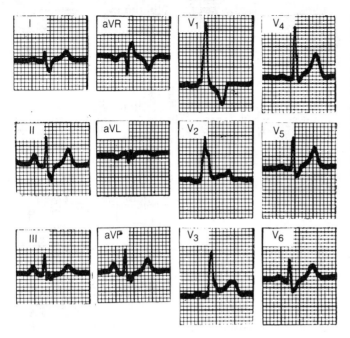

Figure 9-34. Posterior wall myocardial infarction and right bundle branch block. The QRS interval is 0.12 s. The wide s waves in leads I, II, III, aVF, and V_{5-6} and the late portion of the R waves in V_{1-3} are indicative of right bundle branch block. The initial tall R deflection in V_{1-3} is consistent with associated posterior wall infarction but not diagnostic of it, since the same pattern can occur in right ventricular hypertrophy or right intraventricular conduction delay. Clinical correlation is required.

Left Bundle Branch Block Pattern & Myocardial Infarction

The concomitant occurrence of left intraventricular conduction delay and acute myocardial infarction of either the anterior or inferior wall connotes extensive damage to the interventricular septum. Whether the left bundle branch block pattern is new or old, however, the diagnosis of acute myocardial infarction can be made only infrequently from the ECG. In the presence of left bundle branch block, 3 electrocardiographic findings suggest the diagnosis of acute infarction, which must nevertheless be confirmed by independent means: serial electrocardiographic changes, marked ST segment elevation (Fig 9-36), and the inscription of a new q wave where it is not expected (Fig 9-36) (Table 9-2). Q waves in association with a left bundle branch block pattern are

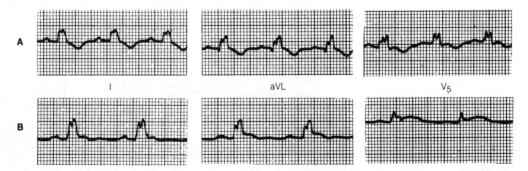

Figure 9-36. Myocardial infarction in the presence of left bundle branch block pattern. *A:* Prior to acute infarction. A left bundle branch block pattern is present; note the q wave in lead aVL, which suggests anterior infarction or a component of peri-infarction conduction delay. *B:* Recorded during an episode of severe chest pain. ST segment elevation is present in leads I, aVL, and V_5. Independent confirmation of myocardial infarction is required. (In this patient, infarction was confirmed by diagnostic elevations of serum creatine kinase MB fractions.)

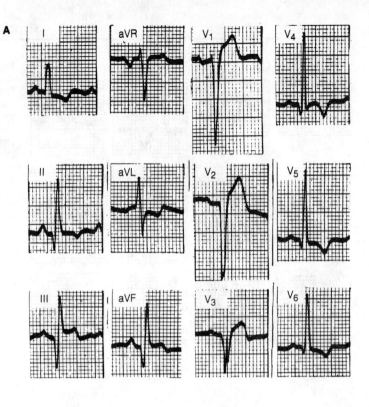

Figure 9-37. Infarction associated with left bundle branch block. *A:* The deep, wide Q waves with ST–T changes in II, III, and aVF are indicative of inferior wall infarction. The QS complexes in V_{2-3} and abnormal Q waves with T inversion in V_{4-6} are indicative of anterior wall infarction. The prominent precordial voltage is compatible with left ventricular hypertrophy. *B:* This ECG now demonstrates a left bundle branch block; the previous signs of infarction are no longer seen.

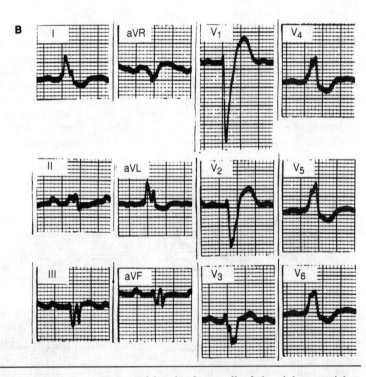

considered to be due to infarction of the anterior wall, as a result of which a conduction delay distal to the common left bundle occurs (peri-infarction block). An alternative mechanism of the inscription of a q wave in left bundle branch block is extensive infarction of the septum with loss of septal forces; the q wave then represents the forces generated by the free wall of the right ventricle.

The development of left bundle branch block in a patient with prior infarction obscures the electrocardiographic pattern of the infarction, which can then no longer be read (Fig 9–37). Similarly, myocardial ischemia cannot be diagnosed from the ECG (Fig 9–38).

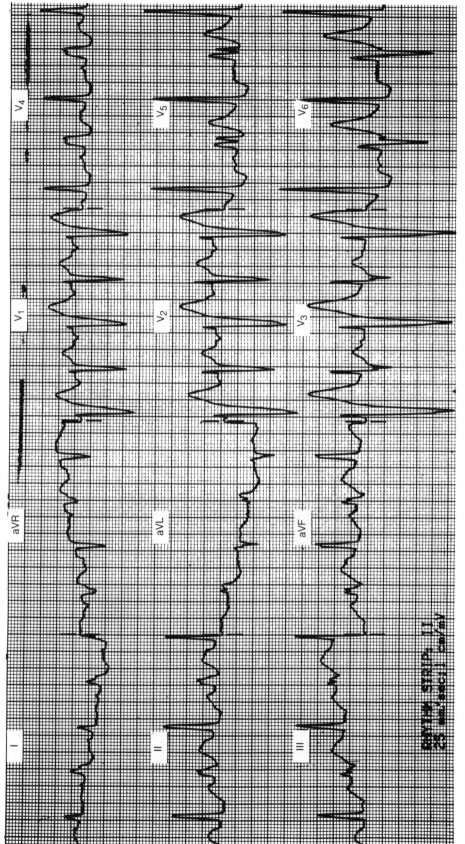

Figure 9-38. Development of 2:1 block in the left bundle branch in a patient with documented severe coronary artery disease and ischemic chest pain, in whom myocardial infarction was excluded by serial creatine kinase MB determinations. ST segment depression suggesting myocardial ischemia is present in those QRST complexes not showing the conduction delay (N = normal), in leads II, III, aVF, and V₄₋₆. These changes are obliterated in the QRST complexes showing the left bundle branch block pattern (B = block). The QRST complexes showing the intraventricular conduction delay, in contrast, display marked ST segment elevation in V₁₋₃. The tracing illustrates the fallacy of attempting to interpret ventricular morphologic events if depolarization and repolarization of the left ventricle is abnormal. (Tracing reduced by 12%.)

133

TRANSIENT Q WAVES

Although abnormal Q waves are often diagnostic of myocardial infarction, they occasionally appear only transiently (Fig 9–39). The conditions in which transient Q waves may be observed include coronary artery spasm and shock states (Table 9–3). The reason for the appearance and disappearance of the abnormal Q wave is not understood, but it is possible that transient, reversible, severe myocardial ischemia is the unifying underlying cause.

PSEUDOINFARCTION DUE TO INCORRECT LEAD PLACEMENT

The interchange of RA, LA, and LL electrodes can result in marked changes in the frontal plane leads, mimicking myocardial infarction (Figs 9–40 and 9–41). Lead misplacement will not alter the P–QRS–T configurations in the precordial leads, because the indifferent electrode is the sum of the potentials of RA + LA + LL, irrespective of the individual locations on the extremities.

Figure 9–39. Transient abnormal Q waves. *A:* The rhythm is sinus. The PR interval is 0.24 s, indicating first-degree AV block. The notched P waves in the frontal plane leads and the diphasic P with a wide negative deflection in V₁ are consistent with left atrial abnormality. The QRS interval is 0.15 s, and there is a wide S in I and wide, notched R' waves in V₁₋₂, indicating right bundle branch block pattern. Wide Q waves are seen in II, III, and aVF and are consistent with inferior wall infarction. *B:* Taken 1 day after (A). The QRS interval is reduced to 0.12 s, but the right bundle branch block persists. Q waves are no longer present in I and aVF. Clinical data: The patient had mitral stenosis. At the time of tracing (A), he was in shock as a result of thromboembolism of the abdominal aorta. At the time of tracing (B), his blood pressure and peripheral perfusion had been temporarily improved. It is concluded that the Q waves seen in (A) resulted from severe myocardial ischemia, which subsided at the time of record (B). Autopsy findings: Mitral stenosis with left atrial and right ventricular hypertrophy; extensive thrombosis of abdominal aorta; no myocardial infarction; no pulmonary embolization.

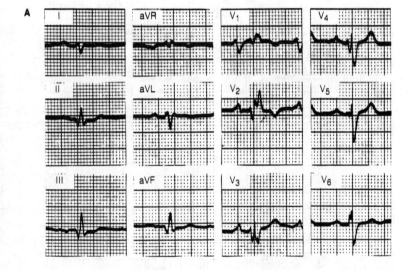

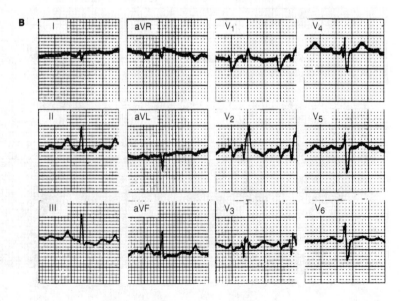

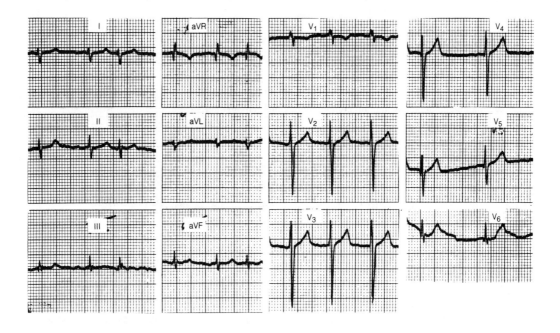

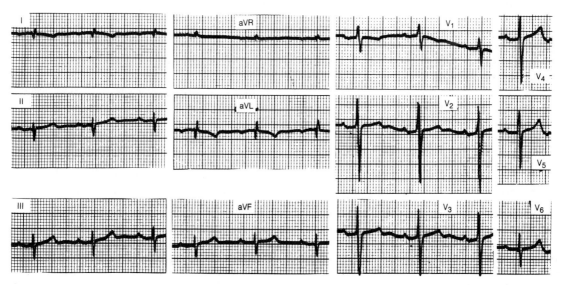

Figure 9-40. Right ventricular hypertrophy due to mitral stenosis. *A:* The rhythm is atrial fibrillation. The mean frontal plane QRS axis is +120°. There is a prominent R wave in V$_1$ with an R:S ratio approaching 1. *B:* ECG recorded after mitral valve replacement and direct current cardioversion. Sinus rhythm is present. A new Q wave with inverted T wave is present in lead I, suggesting lateral wall myocardial infarction. However, the P wave is also inverted in lead I and aVL, providing a clue to the diagnosis of lead misplacement. Leads II-III and aVR-aVL are reversed as a result of accidental interchange of the RA and LA electrodes.

A

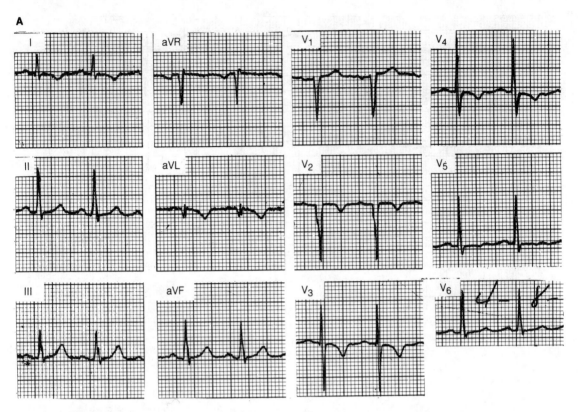

Figure 9-41. Electrode misplacement as a cause of pseudoinfarction pattern. *A:* Anterior wall myocardial infarction (QS complex in V_2, qRS complex in V_3, and T wave inversion in V_{2-4}) known to have occurred 3 years earlier. *B:* (at right) As a result of accidental interchange of the LA and LL electrodes, a pseudoinfarction pattern is present in the inferior leads. The diagram illustrates the resultant effect of LA-LL lead reversal.

PERIPHERAL CONDUCTION DELAYS IN ASSOCIATION WITH MYOCARDIAL INFARCTION (Peri-infarction Block)

Infarction of the myocardium can involve fibers from the anterior and posterior fascicles of

Table 9-3. Causes of transient q waves.

Acute reversible transmural ischemia
Pancreatitis
Intracerebral hemorrhage
Hyperkalemia
Transient fascicular conduction delay
Anaphylactic shock
Adrenal insufficiency

the left bundle branch as they radiate over the anterosuperior and inferoposterior surfaces of the ventricle, respectively, as well as the more distal Purkinje fibers. Conduction delay that is limited to the area surrounding the infarction zone is termed **peri-infarction block.** The QRS complexes that show the infarction pattern will therefore appear to be more prolonged than the QRS complexes recorded from areas remote from the infarction; notching may be present (Fig 9-42). Peri-infarction block should not be misinterpreted as fascicular block, which involves the fascicles of the left-sided conduction system. Fascicular block will produce axis deviation in the frontal plane and does not itself prolong the QRS duration, whereas in peri-infarction block the frontal plane QRS axis is not altered and the QRS duration appears lengthened over the leads that show q waves.

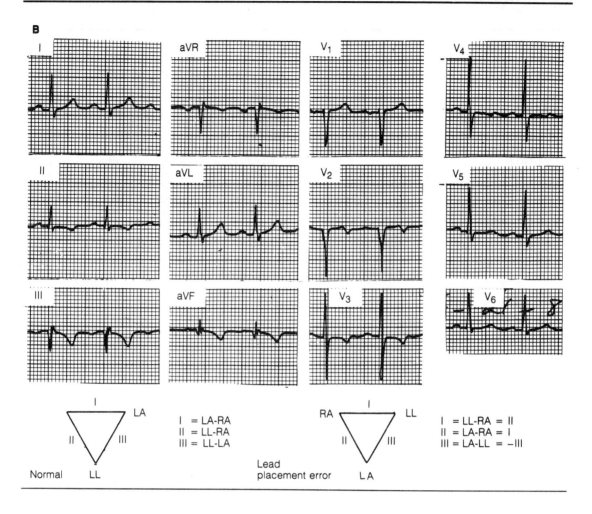

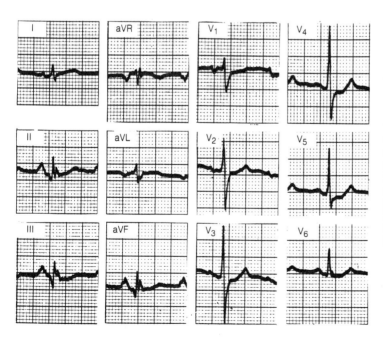

Figure 9-42. Peri-infarction block recorded in the inferior leads, occurring as a result of inferior wall myocardial infarction. The QRS duration in the inferior leads is 0.12 s, and the complexes are notched. There are Q waves in II, III, and aVF, and the terminal QRS forces are oriented inferiorly (notched R waves in II, III, and aVF) and slightly rightward (small s wave in I). Although the mean frontal plane QRS axis of +60° suggests the possibility of left posterior fascicular block, the prolongation of the QRS interval makes peri-infarction block a more likely diagnosis.

REFERENCES

Bateman TM et al: Transient pathologic Q waves during acute ischemic events: An electrocardiographic correlate of stunned but viable myocardium. *Am Heart J* 1983;**106**:1421.

DeGuzman M, Rahimtoola SH: What is the role of pacemakers in patients with coronary artery disease and conduction abnormalities? *Cardiovasc Clin* 1983;**13**:191.

Hassett MA, Williams RR, Wagner GS: Transient QRS changes simulating acute myocardial infarction. *Circulation* 1980;**62**:975.

Hindman MC et al: The clinical significance of bundle branch block complicating acute myocardial infarction. (2 parts.) *Circulation* 1978;**58**:679, 689.

Hnads ME et al: Electrocardiographic diagnosis of myocardial infarction in the presence of complete left bundle branch block. *Am Heart J* 1988;**116**:23.

Savage RM et al: Correlation of postmorten anatomic findings with electrocardiographic changes in patients with myocardial infarction: Retrospective study of patients with typical anterior and posterior infarcts. *Circulation* 1977;**55**:279.

Scheinman MM, Abbott JA: Clinical significance of transmural versus nontransmural electrocardiographic changes in patients with acute myocardial infarction. *Am J Med* 1973;**55**:602.

Shugoll GI: Transient QRS changes simulating myocardial infarction associated with shock and severe metabolic stress. *Am Heart J* 1967;**74**:402.

Wackers FJ et al: Assessment of the value of electrocardiographic signs for myocardial infarction in left bundle branch block. In: Wellens HJJ, Kulbertus HE (editors). *What's New in Electrocardiography*. Martinus Nijhoff, 1981.

Figure 9-T1.
TEST TRACINGS

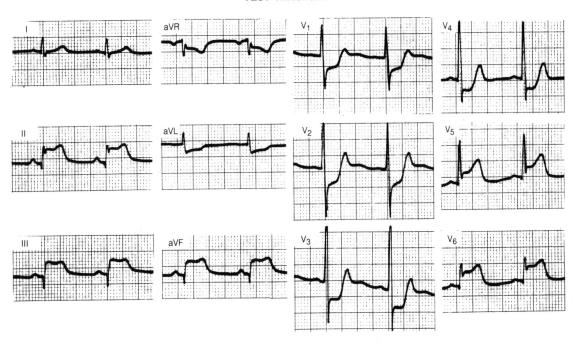

Which walls are involved in the ischemic process?	Inferior, posterior, and possibly anterior, although the ST segment depression in these leads could represent reciprocal changes.
Account for the tall R wave in lead V_1.	Loss of posterior forces leads to abnormally prominent anterior forces, registered in the horizontal axis as a tall R wave in leads V_{2-3}.
Does this tracing represent ischemia or infarction?	Cannot tell on the basis of a single ECG. Severe transmural ischemia can cause this tracing, as well as the early stages of transmural infarction.

Figure 9–T2.
TEST TRACINGS

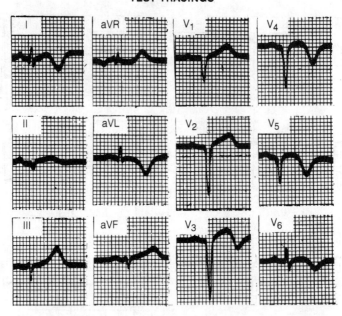

Which wall is involved in the infarction process?

Anterior. QS complexes are present in V_{1-6}, with coveplane ST elevation and T wave inversion. The ST segment is also elevated in I, and the T waves inverted in leads I and aVL.

What is the mean frontal plane QRS axis? Account for the axis.

$-40°$. It is probably due to left anterior fascicular block rather than to inferior wall infarction.

What is the age of the infarction (acute, recent, or old)?

Cannot tell. This pattern may be seen in the early evolution of the infarction, or may persist for years thereafter.

Figure 9-T3.
TEST TRACINGS

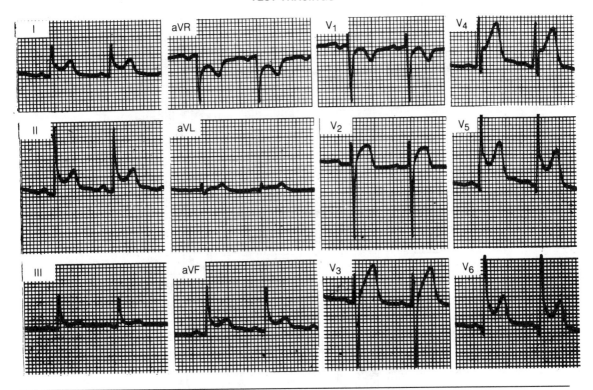

Which leads show ST segment elevation?

I, II, III, aVF, V₂₋₆.

Account for the widespread nature of the ST elevation.

Either extensive anterior wall myocardial infarction with involvement of the apical area, or another process.

The patient had acute pericarditis due to staphylococcus endocarditis. Clinical correlation and serial ECGs are required to arrive at the precise diagnosis.

Figure 9–T4.
TEST TRACINGS

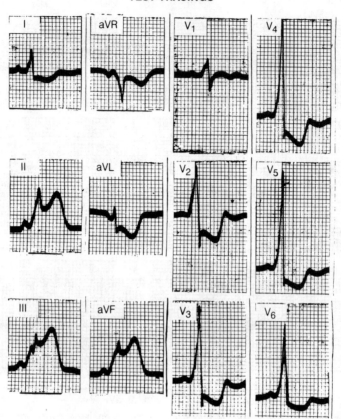

What is the pattern of intraventricular conduction?	WPW (see Chapter 15), indicated by the short PR interval and the delta wave.
What is the PR interval?	0.12 s.
Account for the prominent wide initial R wave in lead V_1.	This is the delta wave, not the R wave of posterior infarction.
Do the ST segment depressions in V_{2-6} indicate myocardial ischemia?	In the presence of abnormal ventricular depolarization, such as in WPW conduction, the ST segment and T wave changes are secondary to the conduction abnormality, and cannot be interpreted for the presence of ischemia.
Do the ST segment elevations in leads II, III, and aVF indicate ischemia or infarction?	Yes, since ST segment elevation is unexpected in WPW conduction.

Figure 9-T5.
TEST TRACINGS

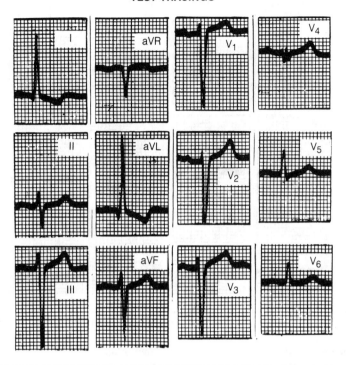

What is the PR interval?	0.16 s.
What is the QRS duration?	0.08 s.
What is the mean frontal plane QRS axis?	−30°.
What is the R wave voltage in lead aVL?	20 mm.
Is left ventricular hypertrophy present?	Probably, since the R wave height in aVL exceeds 17 mm and the QRS axis is only borderline at −30°.
Account for the lack of voltage criteria for left ventricular hypertrophy in the horizontal plane.	Since the vector is directed leftward, inferiorly, and posteriorly, poor R wave may be recorded in the precordial leads.
Account for the prominent q wave in leads I and aVL.	This is contributed to both by the ventricular hypertrophy with associated hypertrophy of the interventricular septum, and by the leftward axis.

Figure 9-T6.
TEST TRACINGS

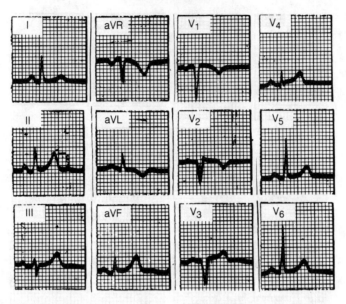

What is the diagnosis?	Anterior wall myocardial infarction. QS complexes are present in V_{1-3}; the QS complex is notched in V_2.
What is the age of the process?	Cannot tell.

Figure 9-T7.
TEST TRACINGS

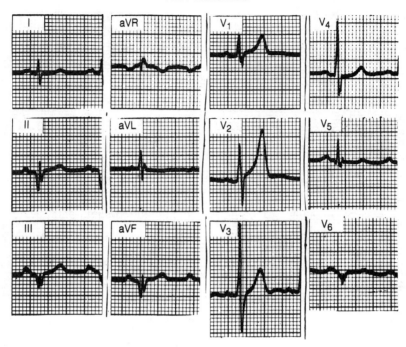

What is the diagnosis? Describe the relevant QRS morphology.	Inferoposterior wall myocardial infarction. Deep wide Q waves are present in II, III, aVF and V_6, and a tall R wave is present in V_1 (R:S ratio 4:1). The T waves are upright and tall in V_{1-3}.
What is the orientation of initial QRS vector? Why?	Superior, due to loss of inferior forces resulting from the myocardial infarction. Left anterior fascicular block does not account for the superior axis since the criteria for its presence are not met.
What is the age of the infarction?	Probably old, in view of the upright T waves in the inferior leads.

Figure 9-T8.
TEST TRACINGS

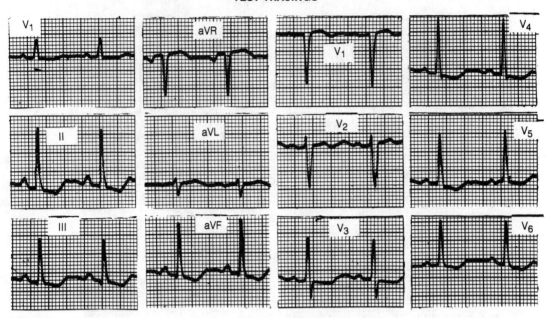

What is the PR interval?	0.18 s.
What is the QRS duration?	0.08 s.
What is the QT interval?	0.32 s.
What is the QTU interval?	About 0.52 s.
Describe the U waves.	They are abnormally prominent in V_{2-4}.
Describe the ST segment abnormalities.	There is ST segment depression in II, III, aVF, and V_{3-6}.
Does this ECG represent myocardial ischemia?	The ST–T wave abnormalities are nondiagnostic without a clinical correlation. The prolonged QTU interval suggests an electrolyte disorder or use of medication (see Chapter 16).

The ECG was recorded in a patient taking phenothiazines.

Figure 9-T9.
TEST TRACINGS

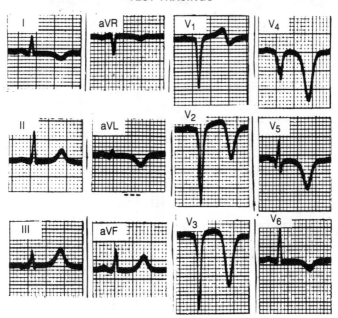

What is the diagnosis?

Anterior wall myocardial infarction.

Is the process acute, in evolution, or old?

Cannot tell.

If the infarction is old, what accounts for the ST segment elevations in leads I, aVL, and V_{2-6}.

Wall motion disorder (akinesis of dyskinesis) due to the infarction.

Figure 9-T10.
TEST TRACINGS

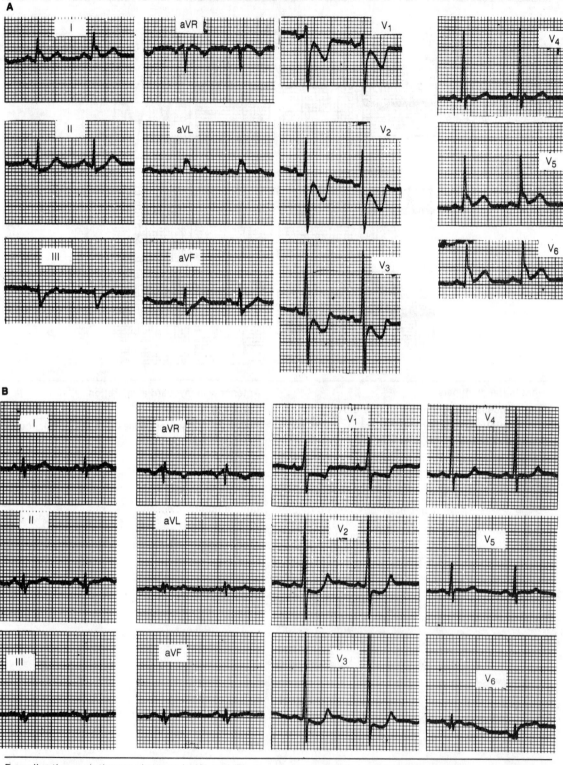

Describe the evolutionary changes in (A) and (B), recorded 24 hours apart.

An acute inferoposterolateral wall myocardial infarction is present. In (A) marked ST segment depression is present in V_{1-3} and ST segment elevation is present in V_{5-6}. In (B) Q waves are present in II, III, aVF and V_6, and tall R waves are present in V_{1-2}.

What accounts for the notching of the terminal portion of the R wave in leads I and V_{5-6} in tracing (A)?

This represents a conduction delay which overlies the area of infarction; it is not present in other leads. It thus suggests a peri-infarction conduction delay.

Figure 9-T11.
TEST TRACINGS

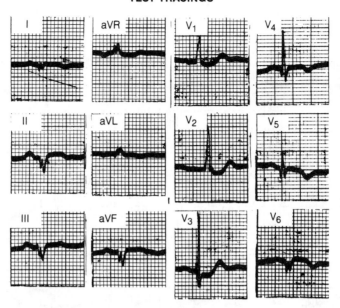

What is the mean frontal plane QRS axis?	−100°.
How do you account for this axis?	Loss of inferior forces due to inferior wall myocardial infarction.
Account for the tall R wave in V_{1-3}.	Posterior wall myocardial infarction.
Account for the notched QS wave in lead I and for the q waves in V_{4-6}.	Accompanying lateral wall myocardial infarction.
What is the diagnosis?	Inferoposterolateral wall myocardial infarction.

Figure 9–T12.
TEST TRACINGS

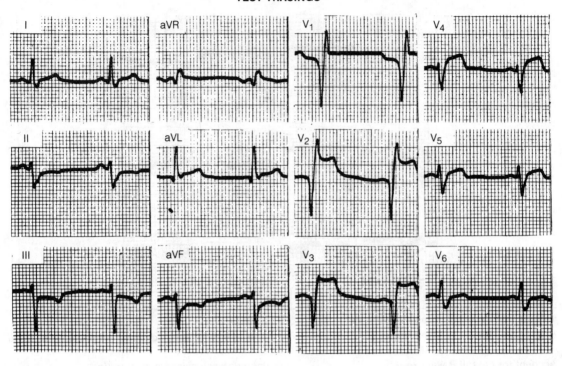

Where is the infarction?

Anterior wall. Deep wide Q waves are present in V_{1-3}, and ST segment elevation in V_{1-4}.

What is the QRS duration?

0.12 s.

What is the mean frontal plane QRS axis?

$-45°$.

What is the pattern of intraventricular conduction?

Right bundle branch block, with superior axis deviation resulting from left anterior fascicular conduction delay.

Account for the ST segment depression in leads II, III, and aVF.

These represent either reciprocal changes, or ischemia of the inferior wall.

Figure 9-T13.
TEST TRACINGS

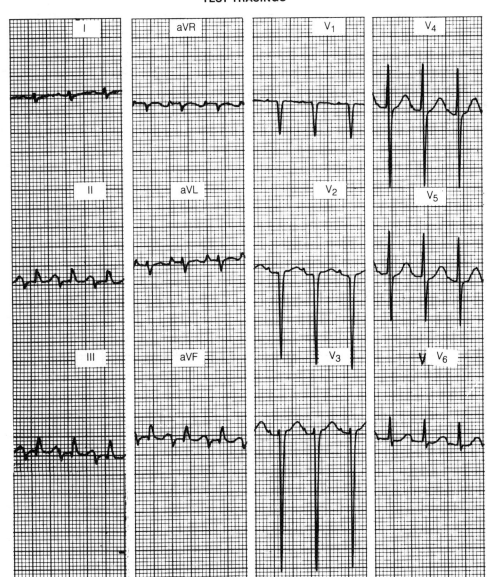

What is the mean frontal plane QRS axis?	+90°.
What is the heart rate?	About 150/min.
Are the P waves normal or abnormal?	Abnormal. They have a superiorly directed axis, and may be ectopic in origin (see Chapter 10).
Is anterior wall myocardial infarction present?	QS complexes are present in V_{1-2}. The T waves are upright. The differential diagnosis includes old myocardial infarction.

The tracing was recorded in a patient with chronic obstructive pulmonary disease with acute exacerbation. Myocardial infarction was not present. Clinical correlation is required for proper diagnosis.

Figure 9–T14.
TEST TRACINGS

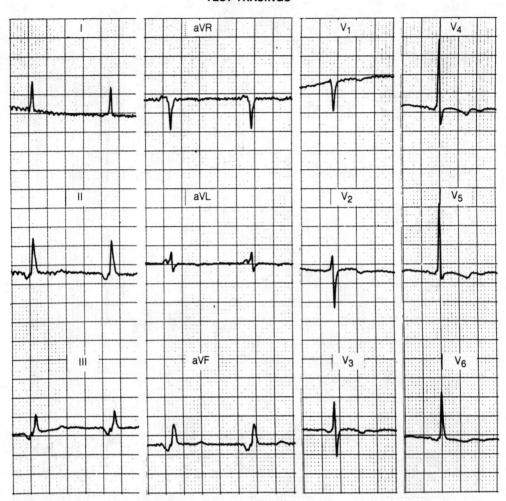

What is the mean frontal plane QRS axis?	+60°.
Describe the QRS complexes in leads II, III, and aVF.	Pure R wave. The negative deflection which precedes the R wave is not a Q wave but an inverted P wave (best seen in the second panel).
What is the significance of the ST-T wave abnormalities?	They are nondiagnostic of myocardial ischemia.

The patient has an ectopic atrial rhythm (see Chapter 10) and the P waves inscribe a pseudo–Q wave in the inferior leads. Myocardial infarction was not present.

Normal Cardiac Rhythm & the Supraventricular Arrhythmias

10

ELECTROPHYSIOLOGY OF CARDIAC RHYTHM

Activation of heart muscle results from spontaneous impulse formation occurring in a pacemaker cell and conduction of this impulse from cell to cell. Disturbances of cardiac rhythm are related to the basic processes of **automaticity, conduction**, and **triggering**.

Automaticity

Cells that are capable of pacing the heart have the property of automaticity, the basis for which is the *spontaneous depolarization* of the cell during phase 4 (see Chapter 2). Normally, the sinus node serves as the pacemaker for the heart, since its phase 4 depolarization is the most rapid and thus its automatic rate is the fastest. However, should the firing rate of the sinus node slow below that of other, *subsidiary* pacemaker cells, these *escape* pacemakers will take over the pacing function of the heart. Pacing tissue is present within the specialized conduction system of the heart—portions of atrial tissue, areas in the AV junction, the common bundle of His, the bundle branches, and the peripheral Purkinje system.

The rate at which pacemaker cells discharge depends on the following: (1) the membrane potential present at the end of repolarization, (2) the slope (rate) of phase 4 diastolic depolarization, and (3) the threshold potential at which the cell is able to be depolarized. Lowering the membrane potential away from the threshold potential, slowing the slope of phase 4, or raising the threshold potential toward zero all slow the firing rate of the pacemaker cell; whereas raising the membrane potential toward the threshold potential, increasing the slope of phase 4, or lowering the threshold potential so that it is closer to the membrane potential all increase the firing rate (Fig 10-1). Variables that affect the automaticity of pacemaker cells are listed in Table 10-1.

Conduction

The ability of cardiac tissue to conduct an impulse is dependent upon phase 0 (the rate of change of voltage) and the amplitude of the action potential. Slowing the rate of phase 0 or decreasing the amplitude of the action potential (or both) decreases the speed of conduction of an impulse through the tissue (conduction delay) and favors the development of failure of impulse transmis-

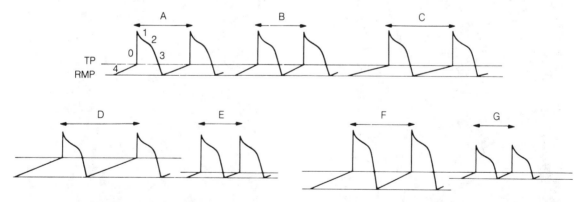

Figure 10-1. Schematic drawing of action potentials and the determinants of intrinsic firing rate. Phase 4 represents diastolic depolarization; RMP, resting membrane potential; and TP, threshold potential. *A:* Impulse formation is determined by the slope of phase 4 and by the levels of RMP and TP. *B:* An increase in the slope of phase 4 results in an increase in firing rate (enhanced automaticity). *C:* A decrease in the slope of phase 4 results in a decrease in firing rate (decreased automaticity). *D:* Raising the threshold potential toward 0 mV, resulting in a longer time required until the cell achieves threshold and is activated, with a consequent decrease in automaticity. *E:* Lowering the threshold potential toward resting membrane potential, resulting in less time required for the cell to reach threshold and depolarize (enhanced automaticity). *F:* Lowering of resting membrane potential away from threshold potential, resulting in a longer time required for threshold to be reached (decreased automaticity). *G:* Raising of resting membrane potential closer to threshold potential, requiring a shorter time necessary to attain threshold (enhanced automaticity).

sion (conduction block). A progressive decrease in the rate of rise of phase 0 and the action potential amplitude leads to **decremental conduction**, in which impulses fail to be conducted further.

If decremental conduction occurs in only one direction (**unidirectional block**), an impulse that has failed to be conducted in that direction may still be capable of being propagated in the opposite direction, thus initiating a **reciprocating** (or reentry) **arrhythmia** (Fig 10–2). In some experimental situations, local circuit current continues to flow intercellularly despite the block in impulse conduction. This current flow can reexcite these cells by a process known as **reflection**.

Table 10-1. Variables that affect automaticity of pacemaker cells.[1]

Increased Firing Rate	Decreased Firing Rate
Sympathetic nervous system activity	Parasympathetic nervous system activity
Hypoxia	Hypothermia
Hypercapnia	Hyperkalemia
Cardiac dilation	Antiarrhythmic agents
Ischemia/necrosis	(eg, quinidine,
Hypokalemia	procainamide)

[1]These variables affect both automaticity and conduction properties of different portions of the specialized conduction system to varying degrees; thus, the net effect on pacemaker rate will depend upon their interaction.

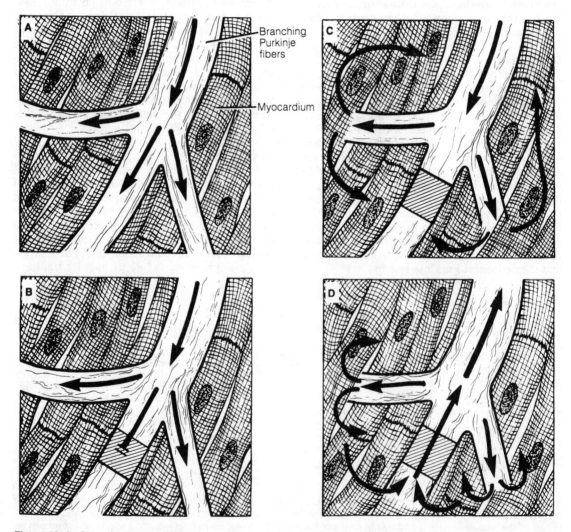

Figure 10-2. Schema of a reentrant (reciprocating) arrhythmia caused by decremental conduction, with unidirectional block and reentry. *A:* Normal propagation of an impulse through branching Purkinje fibers, with activation of the neighboring myocardium. *B:* A zone of decremental conduction (hatched area) causes unidirectional block of the impulse. *C:* Propagation of the impulse through normally conducting fibers activates the myocardium. *D:* The impulse that has spread through the myocardium penetrates the zone in which depressed antegrade conduction was present and is propagated in a retrograde direction, thus reactivating the Purkinje fibers and producing a second (reentry or reciprocating) response. Maintenance of this circuit leads to reciprocating tachyarrhythmias.

Concealed conduction occurs when an impulse penetrates a portion of the conduction system (most commonly the AV junction) but is not propagated further; its presence is inferred from its effects on subsequent electrocardiographic events, where it usually slows conduction in some portion of cardiac tissue.

Triggering

Triggered activity refers to cell depolarizations iniated by a stimulus (the drive stimulus) that produces an action potential which displays an **afterdepolarization** wave (Fig 10–3). An afterdepolarization wave is actually a voltage oscillation. It may occur early or late relative to the total duration of the action potential. If early, the afterdepolarization has occurred before complete repolarization of the cell; if late, or delayed, the afterdepolarization has occurred after complete repolarization of the cell. If the after depolarization waves reach the depolarization threshold, the cells can depolarize spontaneously for a brief period of time. The rhythms of digitalis toxicity, as well as some catecholamine-stimulated arrhythmias, are thought to be due to triggering mechanisms.

THE SINUS RHYTHMS

The P waves of the surface ECG represent atrial depolarization. Actual pacing activity occurring within the sinus node precedes atrial depolarization and is therefore not seen in the ECG. That P waves result from impulses generated in the sinus node is therefore inferred from their morphology and axis.

Sinus rhythm is the normal cardiac rhythm, and its rate is usually 60-100/min. **Sinus tachycardia** is present when the resting sinus rate exceeds 100/min; with exercise the sinus rate can approach 200/min. **Sinus bradycardia** is present when the resting sinus rate is less than 60/min. Neither sinus tachycardia nor sinus bradycardia per se indicates organic heart disease.

The sinus P wave has a mean frontal plane axis of between $+15$ and $+75°$, and is thus upright in leads I, II, and aVF, inverted in aVR, and variable in III and aVL. In the horizontal plane the sinus P wave may be inverted in lead V_1 but is upright in V_{3-6}. Some variability in sinus P wave contour in the inferior leads may be present with respiration.

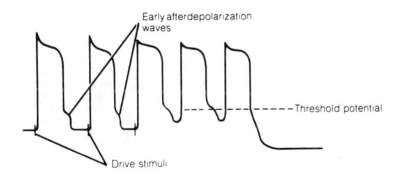

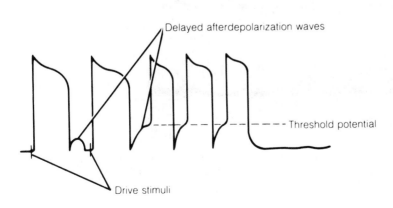

Figure 10-3. Schema of a triggered rhythm due to early and late afterdepolarization waves. The driven action potentials are followed by small afterdepolarization waves. If the drive stimulus is followed by an action potential with a sufficiently large afterdepolarization wave to reach threshold, (triggering) a self-terminating burst of tachyarrhythmia will be initiated.

Sinus arrhythmia is present when the PP interval varies by more than 0.16 s and the P wave morphology is normal and consistent. In **respiratory sinus arrhythmia** the sinus rate varies with respiration, with slower rates being present during expiration and more rapid rates during inspiration. Respiratory sinus arrhythmia is not an abnormal rhythm, and is most commonly seen in young subjects. In **nonrespiratory sinus arrhythmia** phasic changes in sinus rate do not accompany respiration. The mechanism is unknown, and the rhythm may be accentuated by the use of vagal agents such as digitalis and morphine. Patients with the nonrespiratory form of sinus arrhythmia are more likely to be older and to have

underlying cardiac disease, but the rhythm does not predict its presence. Fig 10–4 illustrates the sinus rhythms, and Fig 10–5 illustrates variability in P wave configurations with respiration.

Ventriculophasic sinus arrhythmia occurs when sinus rhythm and high grade or complete atrioventricular block coexist (see Chapter 11). The arrhythmia is characterized by the PP intervals enclosing QRS complexes being shorter than the PP intervals not enclosing QRS complexes. The precise mechanism for the shorter PP intervals is not known with certainty, but is probably related to the effects of the mechanical ventricular systole itself. Ventricular contraction may produce greater blood supply to the sinus node thereby in-

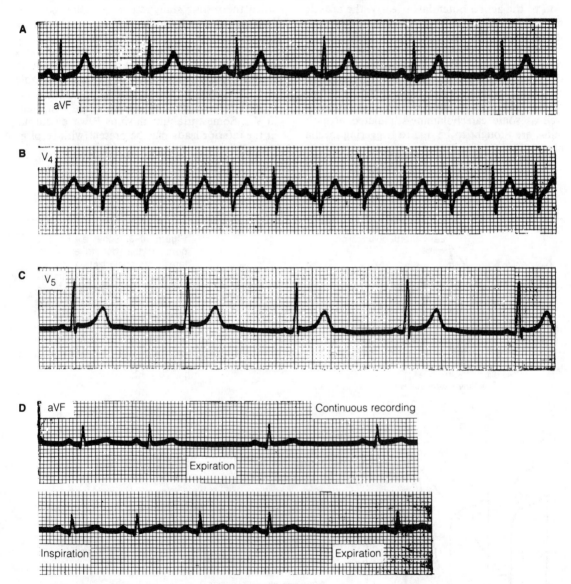

Figure 10–4. *A.* Normal sinus rhythm, rate, 63/min. *B:* Sinus tachycardia, rate, 125/min. *C:* Sinus bradycardia, rate, 50/min. *D:* Sinus arrhythmia with increase in rate during inspiration and decrease during expiration. The P wave contours are identical, and the PR intervals are constant.

creasing its firing rate, may produce traction on the sinoatrial area which imposes a mechanical stimulus to increase its rate, and may lead to vagal inhibition of sinus rate in response to the transient increase in intra-atrial pressure caused by the prior ventricular systole. Ventriculophasic sinus arrhythmia per se is not a pathologic arrhythmia (although the AV block is), and should not be confused with atrial premature depolarizations or sinoatrial block.

Sinoatrial block exists when not all impulses generated by the sinus pacemaking cells leave the SA node to reach the atrial conducting tissue and depolarize the atria. In the absence of atrial depolarization, a P wave will not be inscribed on the ECG. SA block may take the form of *progressive delay in transmission* of the impulse through the sinus node to the atrium, resulting in a nonconducted sinus impulse (SA **Wenckebach**, or **type I**, exit block [see Chapter 11]) or *abrupt failure of transmission* of the impulse to the atrium (type II SA exit block [see Chapter 11]). Abrupt failure of conduction can take the form of 2:1, 3:1, etc., SA block. High-degree SA block will manifest itself on the surface ECG as pauses in sinus rhythm. These pauses cannot always be differentiated from either sinus arrest due to failure of impulse generation or from atrial standstill due to inability of the atrial muscle to be depolarized. Only if the pauses between sinus P waves are *multiples of a*

A

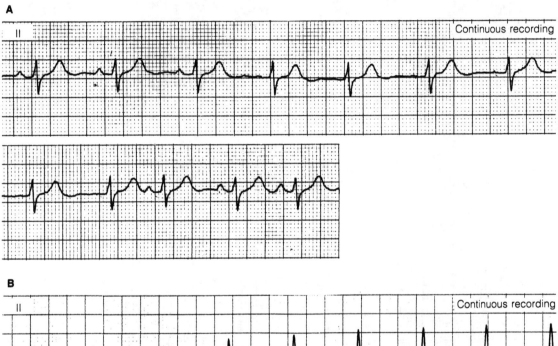

B

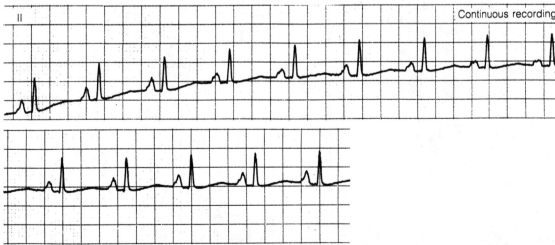

Figure 10-5. Lead II rhythm strips illustrating phasic variation in P wave contour during respiration. In (A) a phasic variation in sinus rate is present in association with the P wave changes (sinus arrhythmia). Changes in sinus rate are not present in (B) although P wave morphology changed consistently in relation to respiration. Since multiple wave configurations and varying PR intervals are not present in these rhythm strips, criteria for wandering atrial pacemaker are not met. Rate-dependent interatrial conduction delays may account for P wave contours that change with rate, but this is unlikely.

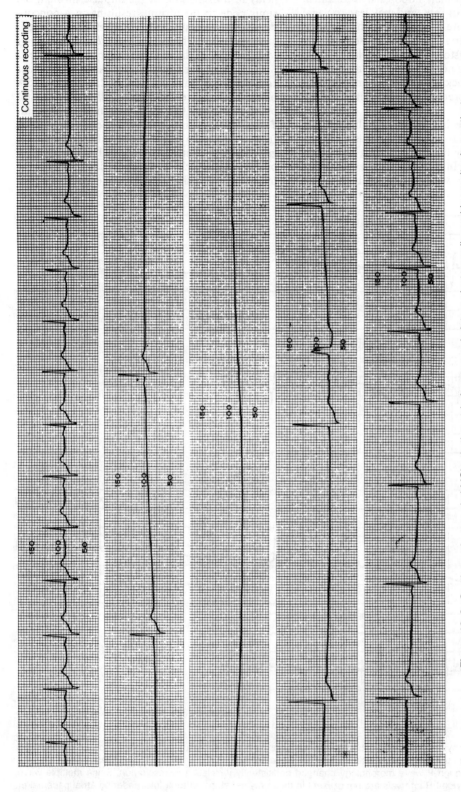

Figure 10–6. Continuously recorded MCL$_5$ rhythm strip from an ambulatory electrocardiographic monitor in a patient with syncopal and presyncopal spells. The rhythm in the top strip is sinus. Abrupt sinus bradycardia with a markedly prolonged pause in rhythm occurs during the second through fourth strips. The asystolic period is terminated by a junctional escape rhythm which demonstrates "warm-up" of its rate. Sinus rhythm is reestablished at the end of the bottom strip. The pause in sinus rhythm is not a multiple of the basic sinus rate and therefore likely represents failure of impulse generation within the sinus node. Atrial standstill, in which the atrial muscle is incapable of being depolarized despite its being stimulated, is also a possibility but only if underlying sinus arrhythmia is presumed to be present. (Rhythm strip reduced by 18%).

basic sinus rate is the diagnosis of type II SA block tenable. Figs 10–6 through 10–8 illustrate these points.

Sinoventricular conduction is the term used to describe sinus impulses that are conducted through the atrial conduction system and into the AV node but which fail to depolarize atrial tissue. This type of conduction is seen principally in hyperkalemia, which causes atrial muscle standstill even though intra-atrial conduction is preserved (Fig 10–9). Since the atria are not depolarized, the surface ECG shows QRS complexes without preceding P waves. Maneuvers that increase sinus rate might result in an increase in QRS rate, but the diagnosis can be made with certainty only if P waves that occur at the same rate as the prior QRS rhythm appear when the hyperkalemia is being treated (Fig 10–9).

ELECTROPHYSIOLOGIC EVALUATION OF SINUS NODE FUNCTION

Sinus node function can be evaluated in the electrophysiology laboratory by means of surface and intracardiac electrographic recordings obtained simultaneously during normal (basal) conditions, physiologic and pharmacologic interventions, and atrial pacing. This evaluation is usually undertaken in patients with symptomatic sinus bradycardia, bradycardia-tachycardia syndrome, and patients with recurrent syncope of unclear etiology. Measurements include the **intrinsic heart rate**, the **sinus node recovery time** (SNRT), the **sinoatrial conduction time** (SACT), and the response to parasympathetic (vagal) stimulation (assessed by carotid sinus massage).

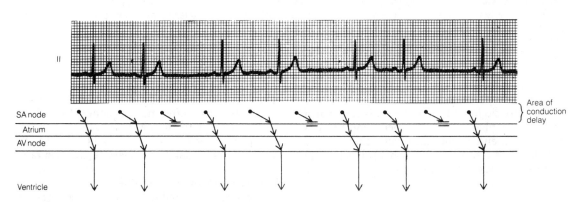

Figure 10–7. Sinus node exit block (3:2 type I [Wenckebach] block). Repetitively, 2 sinus-conducted impulses are followed by a pause. All P waves are of the same configuration, the PR intervals are constant, and no nonconducted atrial premature beats are evident. In type I SA exit block, the sinus node fires regularly (but cannot be seen in the ECG). The impulses encounter progressive delay in exiting the sinus node until one is not conducted to the atrium. In this instance, every third sinus impulse fails to be conducted to the atrium.

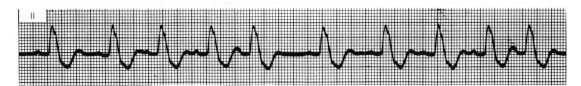

Figure 10–8. Type I (Wenckebach) SA exit block. Cycles of 5 sinus-conducted impulses are followed by a pause. The PR intervals are constant. No P wave fails to be conducted to the ventricles. The PP interval between the first 2 beats of the cycle is longest because the greatest increment of conduction delay occurs between the first 2 beats of the Wenckebach period (see Chapter 11). Left bundle branch block is also present.

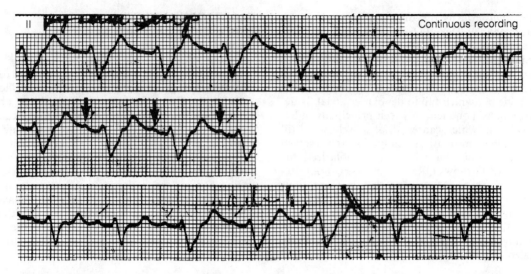

Figure 10-9. Probable sinoventricular conduction in a patient with hyperkalemia (serum K^+ = 6.7 meq/L). The rhythm strips were recorded within seconds of each other, during treatment of the hyperkalemia. In the top strip, the rhythm appears to be junctional (or ventricular) in origin, since no P waves precede the broad QRS complexes. Respiratory variation in the QRS duration is present. In the middle strip, P waves emerge (arrows) and precede the QRS complexes at regular PR intervals of about 0.19 s. The P wave rate is the same as the QRS rate in the top strip, suggesting that sinus impulses stimulated the QRS complexes by traversing the interatrial conduction pathways to enter the AV node–His-Purkinje system. Since atrial muscle is more sensitive to the effects of hyperkalemia than conduction system fibers, atrial muscle depolarization does not occur despite intact interatrial impulse conduction, and thus P waves are not inscribed in the ECG. In the bottom strip, sinus rhythm is established.

Intrinsic Heart Rate

The intrinsic heart rate is the sinus rate which results after pharmacologic denervation using a beta-blocker and atropine has been achieved. It is sometimes used to separate normal subjects from those with "sick sinus syndrome."

Sinus Node Recovery Time

The sinus node recovery time describes the interval between the end of a period of pacing-induced **overdrive suppression** of sinus activity and the return of sinus function, manifested by the appearance of a sinus P wave on the surface ECG. In normal subjects, atrial pacing at rates of 120-130/min for 15 or more seconds is followed by a return of sinus activity at a reproducible interval. The basic sinus rate is generally achieved within 3 post-pacing beats. In general, the sinus node recovery time is about 1.5 s although considerable variation may exist depending upon prevailing autonomic tone. The "corrected" sinus node recovery time is usually calculated by subtracting the basic sinus rate (in milliseconds) from the sinus node recovery time, and is generally between 350 and 550 msec. Several methods are available for calculating corrected sinus node recovery time, all intending to better separate abnormal from normal individuals.

Patients with sinus node dysfunction have sinus node recovery times that are not reproducible and tend to be longer after more prolonged periods of pacing. Return to the basic sinus rate within 3 post-pacing beats is inconstant and may be followed by additional ("secondary") pauses in rate.

Sinoatrial Conduction Time

The sinoatrial conduction time reflects (1) the time taken by a premature atrial pacing stimulus delivered near the sinus nodal area to traverse atrial tissue to reach the sinus node and prematurely depolarize it, (2) the time to the formation of the next sinus impulse following the premature depolarization, and (3) the return of the sinus-generated impulse to the recording atrial electrode. It may be prolonged in some patients with clinical evidence of sinus node dysfunction.

Tests of sinus node function may be abnormal in patients who do not have sinus bradycardias (the tests are nonspecific) and may be normal in patients who do have symptomatic sinus bradycardias (the tests are insensitive). The test results per se should therefore not be relied upon in clinical decision-making as to optimum treatment. Ambulatory electrocardiographic monitoring (see Chapter 20) is often needed to document the exact cardiac rhythm during symptoms. Often, the diagnosis of sinus node dysfunction is clear from the standard ECG.

ABNORMAL ATRIAL RHYTHMS

Atrial Premature Complexes

A premature atrial complex results from an impulse arising in an ectopic focus somewhere in the atria. Since the impulse is premature, atrial excitation is early relative to the sinus rate. A premature atrial impulse will usually initiate ventricular activation and produce a QRS complex. This QRS complex may be normal or aberrant, depending upon whether or not the bundle branches are refractory at the time of arrival of the impulse. A premature atrial impulse may be so early as to meet refractoriness in the AV node, in which case ventricular activation does not occur and no QRS complex results. The impulse is said to be **nonconducted** (Figs 10-10 and 10-11). *Nonconducted atrial premature impulses are the most common cause of pauses in cardiac rhythm.*

The P wave contour of the premature complex will depend upon the focus of origin of the impulse and on the intra-atrial spread of activation. Generally, atrial premature beats that arise near the sinus node have a normal mean frontal plane axis (upright in I, II, and aVF; negative in aVR) (Fig 10-12); those arising in the lower portion of the atrium have a superior axis (negative in II and aVF and upright in aVR), since the atria are depolarized in retrograde fashion (Fig 10-13), and those arising in the mid portion of the atria have an intermediate axis.

The PR interval depends upon the distance between the focus of origin of the ectopic impulse and the AV node, as well as on the RP interval that precedes it. Thus, the PR interval may be longer or shorter than the sinus PR interval (Figs 10-12 and 10-13).

Nonconducted P waves are followed by pauses

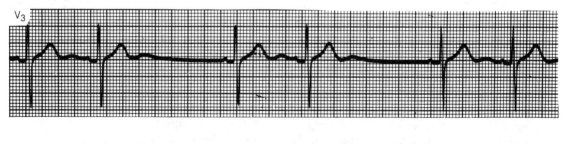

Figure 10-10. Conducted and nonconducted atrial premature impulses. In the lead II rhythm strip a mild sinus arrhythmia is present. The PR interval is 0.2 s. After the fourth P wave a premature atrial complex (first arrow) occurs at a coupling interval of 0.32 s. This P wave is conducted to the ventricles with a PR interval of 0.25 s due to partial refractoriness in the AV node–His-Purkinje system. The second premature P wave (second arrow) occurs at a coupling interval of 0.28 s. Since this P wave occurs so early, it encounters refractoriness in the AV node–His-Purkinje system due to normal conduction of the previous sinus impulse. This premature P wave is therefore not conducted (blocked).

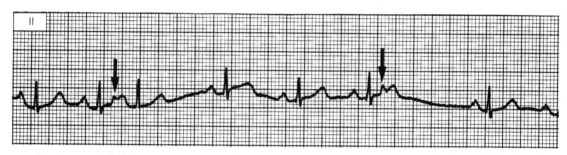

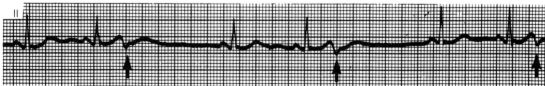

Figure 10-11. Nonconducted atrial premature complexes. The simultaneously recorded leads V₃ and II illustrate the point that not all electrocardiographic leads show events equally well. Groups of 2 sinus beats are followed by a pause. Whereas in lead V₃ the pause appears to result from sinus arrest, in lead II premature P waves are clearly seen in the T waves of the second of the pair of sinus beats (arrows). This grouping, in which 2 sinus beats are followed by an atrial premature beat, is called "atrial trigeminy."

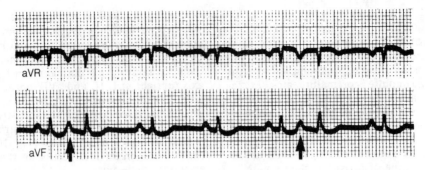

Figure 10-12. The rhythm is predominantly sinus at a rate of 75/min (the PP interval is 0.8 s). Premature waves occur 0.64 s after preceding sinus P waves (arrows). The PR intervals of these premature P waves are longer than the sinus PR intervals, reflecting delayed AV nodal conduction due to conduction of the preceding atrial impulse through it. Since the premature waves are inverted in aVR and upright in aVF, the focus of origin is high in the atrium.

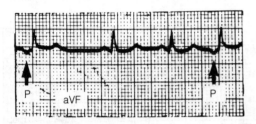

Figure 10-13. Sinus rhythm at a rate of 80/min is present. The premature P waves are inverted in aVF, suggesting a focus of origin low in the atrium with retrograde atrial depolarization. Since the premature P wave falls late in diastole, it does not encounter delay in the AV node, and its PR interval is therefore normal.

that are described as **fully compensatory** or **less than fully compensatory.** If the premature impulse fails to penetrate the sinus node, the sinus firing rate continues undisturbed, and the interval from the sinus beat preceding the atrial premature beat to the next sinus beat will equal 2 sinus PP intervals (fully compensatory). If the premature impulse penetrates the sinus node, it discharges the sinus pacemaker cells prematurely and resets their cycle. Since the sinus node is discharged early and reset, the interval between the sinus P wave preceding the atrial premature beat and the next sinus P wave will be less than 2 sinus PP intervals (less than fully compensatory). Pauses that are less than fully compensatory or fully compensatory depend only upon whether or not the sinus node has been penetrated by an ectopic impulse and *not* by the site of origin of the premature impulse.

Wandering Atrial Pacemaker

In this arrhythmia, some atrial impulses originate in the sinus node and others in various portions of the atria and AV junction. Recent data suggest that "wandering" of the atrial pacemaker can occur entirely within the sinus node and produce similar electrocardiographic findings. Multiple P wave contours and variability in atrial rate and PR intervals are seen (Fig 10-14).

Multifocal Atrial Tachycardia

Multifocal atrial tachycardia, as its name implies, is an atrial arrhythmia characterized by varying P wave contours reflecting different foci of origin, and by variable PP and PR intervals (Figs 10-15, page 164; and 10-16, page 165). It is similar to wandering atrial pacemaker, but the rate is faster, exceeding 100/min and often reaching 150-180/min. Occasionally, P waves are not conducted to the ventricles because of their prematurity. Intraventricular conduction is often aberrant. Multifocal atrial tachycardia is most commonly seen in patients with chronic obstructive pulmonary disease or severe congestive heart failure. It is important to recognize this rhythm, as it is easily confused with atrial fibrillation yet does not respond to digitalis therapy, which may mistakenly be given in toxic doses in an attempt to slow the ventricular rate.

Automatic (Ectopic) Atrial Rhythm

Automatic (ectopic) atrial rhythm is rhythm generated in an ectopic focus. The P wave rate can exceed the sinus rate (accelerated atrial rhythm). If the ectopic atrial rhythm follows an atrial escape beat resulting from a slowing of sinus rate, the rhythm is termed an **atrial escape rhythm.** The rate of an ectopic atrial rhythm is generally regular, and the P wave morphology and PR intervals are constant. The P wave morphology will depend upon the focus of origin of the rhythm and the pathway of atrial depolarization (Figs 10-17, page 166 and 10-18, page 167).

Automatic (Ectopic) Atrial Tachycardia

Automatic atrial tachycardia is a rhythm arising in an ectopic atrial focus. Its rate is usually 150-200/min and may be slightly irregular. The usual AV conduction ratio is 1:1, but type I (Wenckebach) AV block or type II AV block can occur, depending upon the tachycardia rate and integrity of AV conduction (Fig 10–19, page 167) (see Chapter 11). The PR interval is often prolonged because of the rapid atrial rate and also possibly because of abnormal atrial and AV nodal depolarization pathways.

The ectopic P waves are generally directed inferiorly and leftward, resulting in a normal mean frontal plane P wave axis. However, they are characteristically peaked and of brief duration, thus distinguishing them from sinus P waves. An ectopic atrial rhythm arising near the sinus node, however, may not be easily distinguishable from sinus tachycardia. Carotid sinus massage may be of value in differentiating between the two: Sinus tachycarida is expected to slow slightly, whereas the atrial rate of an atrial tachycardia will not change even though AV block with slowing of ventricular rate is produced. (In contrast, AV nodal reentry tachycarida may be abolished by carotid sinus massage, as the AV block produced by the maneuver disallows reentry of the tachycardia impulse within AV nodal tissue [see below].)

Atrial Flutter

Atrial flutter is a regular atrial rhythm resulting from intra-atrial reentry ("circus movement") of impulses. The rate is usually 220-350/min but may be as low as 175 or as high as 430/min. Slow atrial

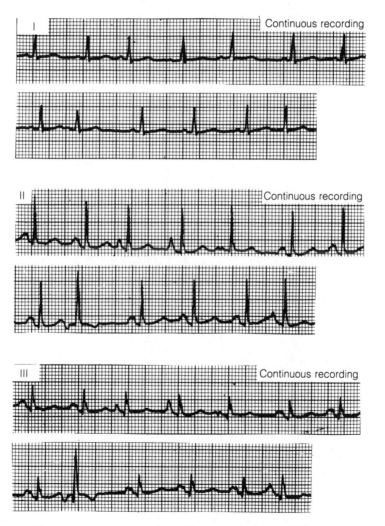

Figure 10–14. Wandering atrial pacemaker. Each QRS complex is preceded by a P wave, but the P wave contours vary, as do the PP and PR intervals. Changing P wave contours reflect the different foci of origin of the P waves. Identification of a given P wave as originating in the sinus node is not always possible.

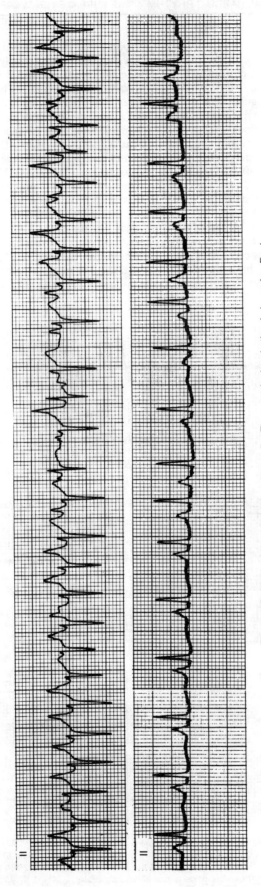

Figure 10–15. Multifocal atrial tachycardia. The ventricular rhythm is irregular. Each QRS is preceded by a P wave, but P wave contours and PR intervals vary.

164

flutter rates occur in patients with large or hypertrophied atria and in those receiving quinidine or procainamide (Table 10–2). The most commonly observed atrial rate is 300/min. The AV conduction ratio of the flutter impulses is usually 2:1 or 4:1 in patients receiving no treatment; thus, the ventricular rate is usually regular at 150/min or 75/min (Fig 10–20, page 168). However, because of varying AV conduction ratios as well as type I (Wenckebach) block at the AV node, the ventricu-

Table 10-2. Causes of slow (< 280/min) atrial rates in atrial flutter.

Atrial enlargement
Atrial hypertrophy
Interatrial conduction delay
Type I antiarrhythmic drugs

lar rate in atrial flutter may be irregular. Identification of the flutter waves will serve to distinguish

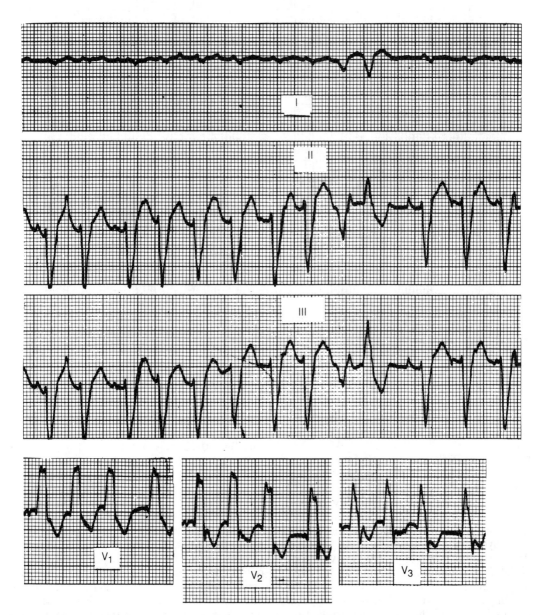

Figure 10-16. Multifocal atrial tachycardia. The ventricular rate is irregular at about 130/min. Each QRS is preceded by a P wave, but the P waves are of varying configurations, and the PR intervals vary. Right bundle branch block is present, and the superior axis deviation is compatible with left anterior fascicular block. Further intraventricular aberration is seen in the ninth and tenth QRS complexes in the simultaneously recorded leads I, II, and III.

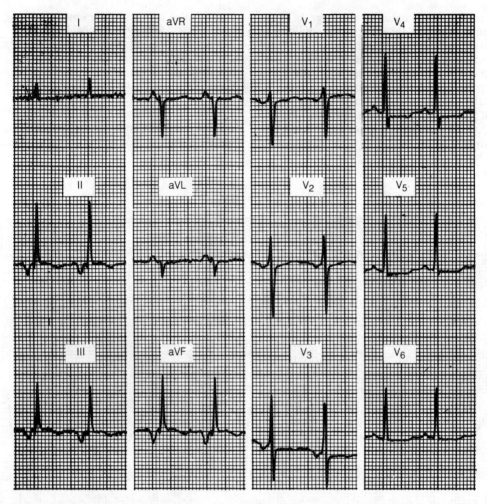

Figure 10-17. Automatic (ectopic) atrial rhythm with inverted P waves in leads II, III, aVF, and V_{2-3}, indicating an inferior to superior and anterior to posterior depolarization sequence in the atria. The focus of origin is presumably low in the atrium or in or near the AV junction but cannot be known with certainty since the P wave morphology depends not only on site of origin but also on pathway of atrial activation.

this rhythm from atrial fibrillation, the hallmark of which is an irregular ventricular rate (see below).

The atrial waves in atrial flutter (F waves) are classically "saw-toothed" in appearance, reflecting atrial depolarization and repolarization (T_a) waves. This characteristic morphology is most easily seen in leads II, III, and aVF and may not be apparent at all in V_1 or may mimic ectopic atrial tachycardia in this lead (Fig 10-20). In other leads, the F waves may resemble the wavy baseline of atrial fibrillation (Fig 10-20). Carotid sinus massage will result in AV block of some of the flutter impulses, allowing the atrial waves to be more clearly seen and the correct diagnosis of the atrial rhythm to be made (Fig 10-21, page 168). Atrial flutter can mimic not only atrial tachycardia and atrial fibrillation, but can also deform

QRS complexes, ST segments, and T waves to mimic intraventricular delays or myocardial ischemia (Fig 10-22, page 169).

Recent studies of atrial flutter have suggested that 2 types of flutter exist. **Type I** is the classically described flutter, having rates between 250 and 350/min (usually 300/min) and a saw-toothed appearance usually best seen in the inferior leads. It is thought to be due to a macro-reentry mechanism. **Type II** flutter occurs at faster atrial rates (350-430/min). The classic saw-toothed pattern is not inscribed; rather, the flutter waves appear as regular upright deflections in the inferior leads and in V_1. Although atrial fibrillation might be mimicked by this rhythm, type II flutter is more regular than fibrillation, and the baseline does not undulate. Differentiation of these types of flutter has potential therapeutic value.

Atrial Fibrillation

Atrial fibrillation is a very rapid, irregular atrial rhythm. Most of the fibrillatory impulses (f waves) fail to be propagated through the AV node to the bundle of His (**decremental conduction**) to stimulate the ventricles; thus, the ventricular response is irregular and occurs at rates as low as 50/min and as high as 200/min in the unmedi-

cated patient. The ventricular response to atrial fibrillation depends upon the integrity of AV nodal conduction and autonomic nervous system input, with sympathetic stimulation increasing the ventricular rate and parasympathetic stimulation decreasing it. Slow ventricular rates in atrial fibrillation in the unmedicated patient who does not have high vagal tone suggest underlying conduc-

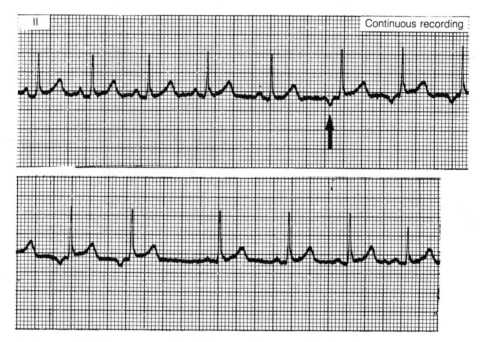

Figure 10–18. Lead II rhythm strip. Sinus rhythm is present at the beginning of the tracing. The P waves are upright. A slight slowing of sinus rate leads to the emergence of an ectopic atrial rhythm (arrow) characterized by an inverted P wave, indicating inferior to superior (retrograde) direction of atrial depolarization. (The distinction from a junctional rhythm cannot always be made.) The ectopic rhythm terminates spontaneously and is followed by the resumption of sinus rhythm. There is minor variation in the sinus P wave configuration which could result from respiratory variation or changes in interatrial conduction.

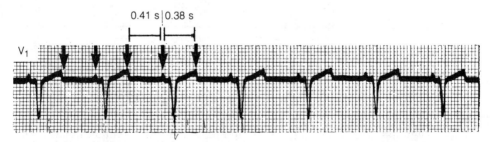

Figure 10–19. Atrial tachycardia with 2:1 AV conduction. The ventricular rhythm is regular at 75/min. The atrial rate varies: the PP intervals enclosing a QRS complex are 0.38 s and the PP intervals not enclosing a QRS complex are 0.41 s (arrows). This phenomenon, in which the PP intervals vary depending upon the presence or absence of QRS complexes, is termed **ventriculophasic arrhythmia** and is thought to result in part from reflex mechanisms induced by the ventricular contraction resulting from the QRS complex. Whereas in this V$_1$ lead the rhythm suggests atrial tachycardia with block, confirmation of the atrial mechanism requires analysis of the atrial waves in II, III, and aVF to exclude the saw-toothed pattern of atrial flutter, which can occasionally occur at this slow rate.

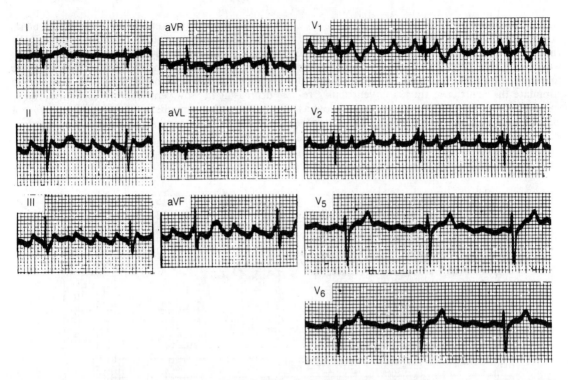

Figure 10-20. Atrial flutter with 4:1 AV conduction. The atrial rate is regular at 240/min, and there is a characteristic saw-toothed appearance to the flutter waves that is best seen in leads II, III, and aVF. In contrast, the atrial waves do not have this appearance in the precordial leads, where atrial tachycardia (V_1) or atrial fibrillation (V_6) might be mimicked.

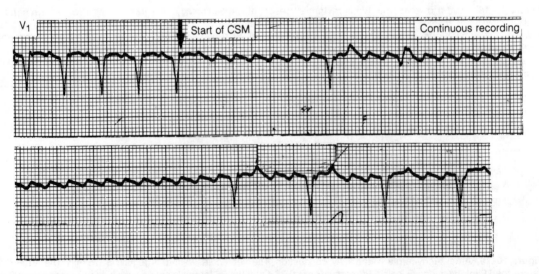

Figure 10-21. Response of atrial flutter to carotid sinus massage. At the beginning of the V_1 rhythm strip atrial flutter with 2:1 AV conduction is present; the ventricular rate is 150/min. Alternate flutter waves are buried within the QRS complexes and are not appreciated; sinus tachycardia is mimicked. At the arrow, carotid sinus massage is begun, resulting in AV block of flutter impulses. The long pauses in ventricular rhythm allow the atrial rhythm to be clearly appreciated as flutter occurring at a rate of 300/min. (CSM = carotid sinus massage.)

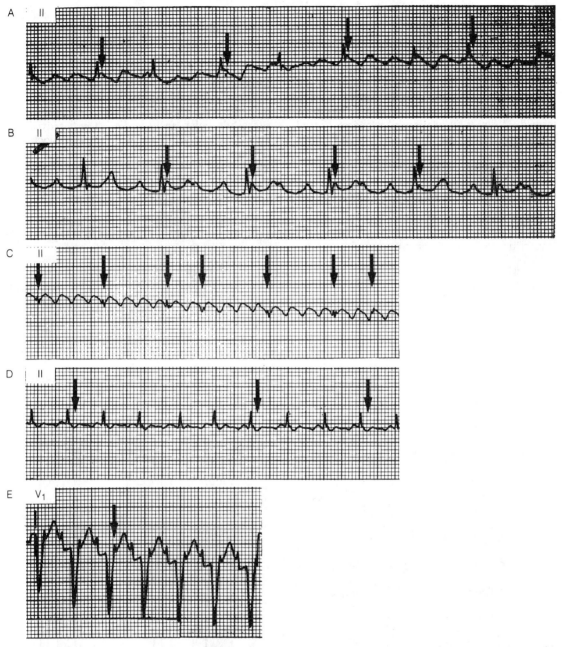

Figure 10–22. Various electrocardiographic patterns produced by atrial flutter. *A:* Atrial flutter showing the typical saw-toothed pattern is present. The atrial rate is unusually slow at about 220/min. The flutter waves deform the ST segments, mimicking ST elevation (arrows). Careful attention to the *variation* in QRST morphology should provide a clue to the correct diagnosis. The ventricular rate shows group beating characteristic of type I (Wenckebach) second-degree block of the flutter impulses (see Chapter 11). Type I AV block of flutter impulses which occurs within the AV node has no clinical significance since the AV nodal block often occurs in response to rapid atrial rates. *B:* Flutter waves superimposed upon QRS complexes deform them (arrows), mimicking an intermittent intraventricular conduction delay. Careful measurement of the atrial rate will provide evidence that the wave deforming the downstroke of the QRS complexes is a flutter wave. Note the unusually slow flutter rate of about 190/min. *C:* Flutter waves having the same amplitude as the QRS complexes (arrows) mimic a period of ventricular asystole. Simultaneous recording of other leads will more clearly define the QRS complexes. *D:* Flutter waves superimposed upon the downstrokes of the QRS complexes (arrows) mimic ST segment depression. *E:* Flutter waves occurring at the ends of the QRS complexes (arrows) mimic a Qr configuration and an intraventricular conduction delay. Since the ventricular rate is regular at 150/min, the diagnosis of atrial flutter with 2:1 AV conduction should always be strongly considered.

tion system disease in the AV node–His bundle area (Fig 10–23).

Atrial fibrillatory waves may be "fine," resulting in a wavy baseline in the surface ECG (Fig 10–24), or "coarse," resulting in defined atrial waves that, although they may resemble atrial flutter waves (especially type II flutter), are too rapid (Fig 10–25). The latter rhythm has been termed "flutter-fibrillation," "coarse atrial fibrillation," and "impure flutter," but it behaves like atrial fibrillation rather than flutter in its response to treatment. The f waves of atrial fibrilla-

tion are usually most prominent in V_1, and the saw-toothed configuration of atrial flutter waves is not seen in II, III, and aVF. '

Bradycardia-Tachycardia Syndrome

Bradycardia-tachycardia syndrome is characterized by periods of bradycardia and episodes of supraventricular tachycardia. The bradycardia may be due to sinus arrest or SA exit block, reflecting sinus node dysfunction ("sick sinus syndrome") with subsequent junctional or ven-

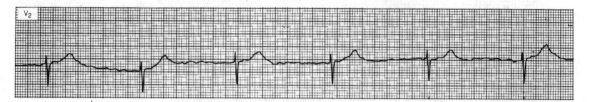

Figure 10–23. Lead V_2 rhythm strip illustrating atrial fibrillation with slow ventricular rate (37/min) in a patient receiving no medications. In addition to its slow rate, the ventricular rhythm is regular, indicating the presence of complete AV block with an ectopic subsidiary (escape) pacemaker stimulating the ventricles. Since the QRS duration is normal, the origin of the ventricular rhythm is likely to be within the AV node–His bundle area (see Chapter 11).

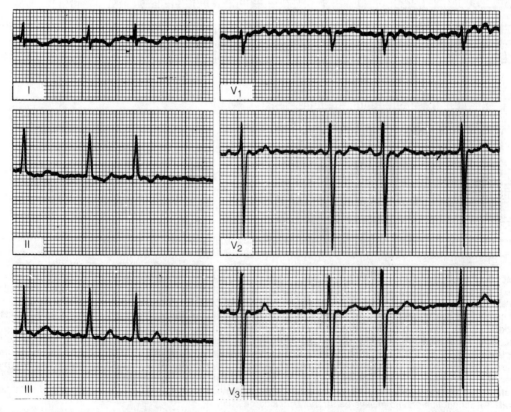

Figure 10–24. Atrial fibrillation. Atrial activity is manifested by rapid, small, irregular atrial (f) waves. The ventricular rhythm is irregular.

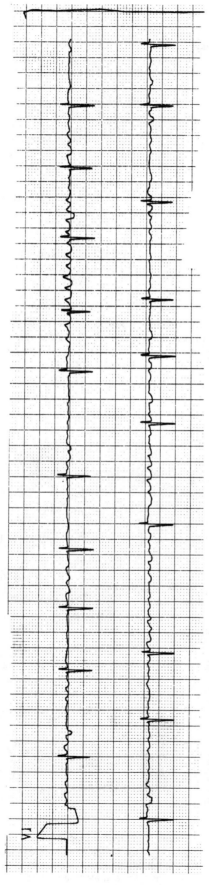

Figure 10–25. Atrial flutter-fibrillation. In the first portion of the strip, fine atrial fibrillatory waves are seen. In the latter portion of the strip, the atrial waves have a more organized configuration and appear to occur at regular intervals at a rate of 500/min. This rate is too rapid to be atrial flutter, although another term to describe it is "impure flutter." A hallmark of atrial fibrillation is the variation in contour as well as rate of the fibrillatory impulses.

tricular escape rhythms. The supraventricular tachycardias may be automatic, atrial flutter, atrial fibrillation, or reentry AV nodal tachycardia, singly or in combination (Fig 10–26). The pauses in rhythm are often associated with symptoms of cerebral insufficiency, and cardiac pacing is required. The tachycardias may be associated with palpitations and usually require suppression with antiarrhythmic agents.

Bradycardia-tachycardia syndrome represents diffuse disease of the conduction system of the heart but is not necessarily associated with structural heart disease.

PAROXYSMAL REENTRANT SUPRAVENTRICULAR TACHYCARDIA

Paroxysmal reentrant supraventricular tachycardia is characterized by a regular tachycardia, usually occurring at rates of 150- 250/min. Unlike automatic atrial tachycardia, which results from enhanced automaticity of an atrial focus, or triggerd atrial arrhythmias, the underlying mecha-

nism of paroxysmal supraventricular tachycardia is more complex (Fig 10–27). In paroxysmal reentrant supraventricular tachycardia, a premature impulse fails to propagate down a pathway (**unidirectional block**) because of a *long refractory period* in that pathway. The impulse therefore proceeds down a second pathway having *slow conduction velocity* and is *conducted with delay* in this pathway. Because the impulse conducts slowly in the antegrade direction, it has the opportunity to turn around and be conducted retrograde (reenter) in the first pathway, which has now recovered from its refractory state (Fig 10–27). Maintenance of this "reentry" phenomenon constitutes a *reentry*, or *reciprocating*, tachycardia. The tachycardia rate will depend upon the conduction velocity and refractory times of the involved pathways, as well as upon autonomic nervous system input.

Paroxysmal reentrant supraventricular tachycardias often involve pathways within the AV node itself (*intra–AV nodal* reentry tachycardia) but may also involve *extra–AV nodal* bypass tracts (see Chapter 15). In the latter instance, antegrade conduction to the ventricles may proceed down

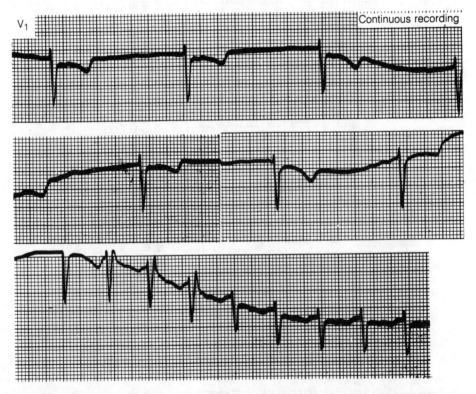

Figure 10–26. Bradycardia-tachycardia syndrome. In the top 2 strips, a regular narrow-QRS rhythm is present at a rate of 38/min. The narrow complexes suggest a junctional origin; each complex is followed by a P wave within its T wave, suggesting that retrograde atrial activation is occurring. (However, confirmation of retrograde depolarization must be sought in superior-inferior leads such as II or aVF.) In the bottom strip, a supraventricular tachycardia at a rate of 125/min occurs abruptly; this could be sinus tachycardia or automatic atrial tachycardia.

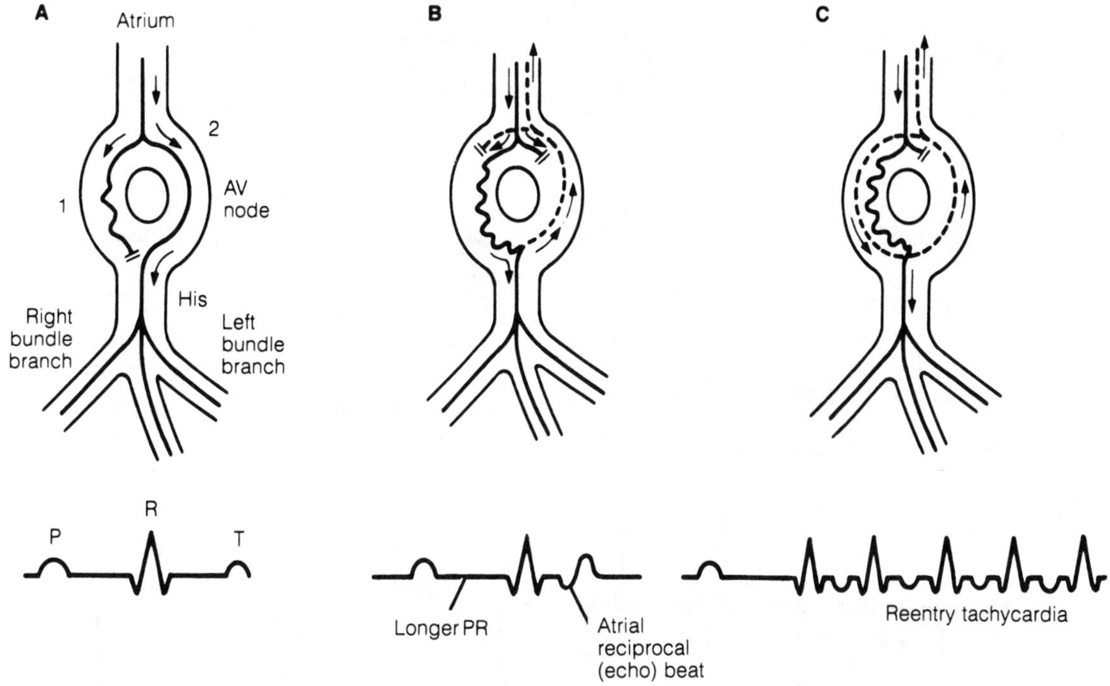

Figure 10-27. Schema of a reentry (reciprocating) tachycardia involving 2 pathways in the AV node but which could represent other areas of conduction tissue within the heart. Pathway 1 is capable of conducting an impulse but with delay. Pathway 2 can conduct the impulse without delay but has a long refractory period. *A:* Sinus rhythm, in which the impulse is transmitted down the fast pathway to the ventricles. *B:* A premature impulse fails to be conducted in pathway 2 because of its long refractory period; it is conducted slowly to the ventricles in the slow pathway. The delay in conduction in pathway 1 is manifested by the prolonged PR interval associated with the premature impulse. *C:* Initiation of reentry tachycardia. The premature impulse, which was originally blocked in the fast pathway (pathway 2) and is conducted with delay in the slow pathway (pathway 1), is able to turn around and conduct in retrograde fashion in the fast pathway, which is now no longer refractory. When the impulse reaches a certain level in the reentry pathway, it turns around again and is now conducted in antegrade fashion. Continuation of these events constitutes a reentry (reciprocating) tachycardia. (Schema adapted from Goldreyer BN, Bigger JT Jr: Site of reentry in paroxysmal supraventricular tachycardia in man. *Circulation* 1971;**43:**15.)

the normal AV node–His-Purkinje system and retrograde conduction via the bypass tract, or antegrade down the bypass tract and retrograde via the normal conduction system. The QRS complex morphology will be determined by the pathway of ventricular depolarization. Most reciprocating tachycardias occur within the AV node.

In AV nodal reentrant tachycardia, the surface ECG shows a regular, usually narrow QRS tachycardia (Fig 10–28) unless preexistent bundle branch block is present, in which case the QRS complexes will be wide (Fig 10–29). The P waves, if they are seen, are *inverted* in II, III, and aVF, since the atria are depolarized in retrograde manner. The relation of the P waves to the QRS complexes (preceding, superimposed on, or following) depends upon the retrograde pathways used, and on the relative conduction times from the reentry sites (levels) to the atria and ventricles, respectively.

Anything that blocks conduction of impulses within the AV node (such as carotid sinus massage, edrophonium, digoxin, beta-blocking drugs, and some calcium channel–blocking agents) either terminates the paroxysmal reentrant supraventricular tachycardia or has no effect, in distinct contrast to such effects in automatic atrial tachycardia, atrial flutter, and atrial fibrillation, in which the atrial rate and rhythm remain essentially unchanged, although AV block is produced and slowing of the ventricular rate occurs.

Reentrant tachycardias are not confined to the AV node or extra–AV nodal bypass tracts but may involve the sinus node (sinus node reentry tachycardia), bundle of His and bundle branches (bundle branch reentry tachycardia), and Purkinje-myocardial tissue (some forms of ventricular tachycardia). Atrial flutter is another form of reentry tachyarrhythmia in which the atria participate.

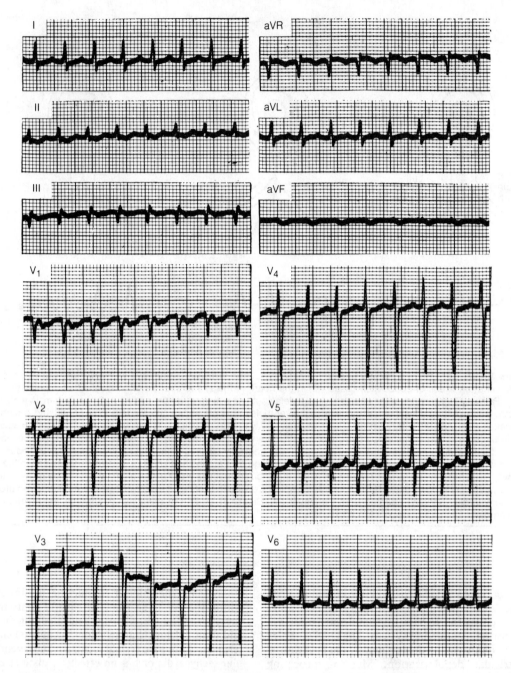

Figure 10–28. Paroxysmal supraventricular tachycardia. A regular, narrow complex tachycardia at a rate of 190/min is present. P waves immediately follow the QRS complexes (best seen in V_1 and V_2). Verification of this tachycardia as paroxysmal supraventricular tachycardia would depend on identifying inverted P waves in the inferior leads.

JUNCTIONAL RHYTHMS

Junctional Impulses

The AV node is divided into the **atrionodal (A-N)** region, the **"N" region**, and the **nodal-His (N-H)** region. As the "N" region of the AV node is thought not to contain pacemaker cells, rhythms originating in this area are currently termed **"AV junctional"** rather than "nodal" rhythms.

Impulses arising in the A-N and N-H regions are conducted to the atria in retrograde fashion, producing inverted P waves in leads II, III, and aVF. They are conducted to the ventricles over the

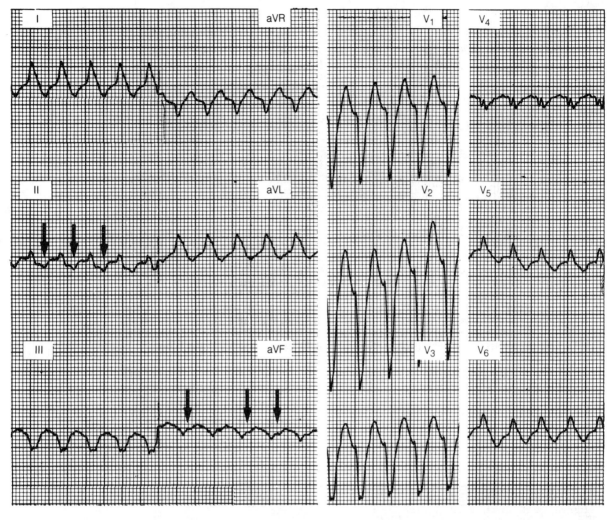

Figure 10-29. Regular wide QRS complex tachycardia which could represent ventricular tachycardia or supraventricular tachycardia with intraventricular aberration (see below and also Chapter 13). The QRS morphology indicates left bundle branch block (notched R wave in leads I, aVL, and V_{5-6} and broad S waves in the right precordial leads); the QRS duration is 0.16 s. Inverted P waves can be best discerned deforming the ST segments in leads II and aVF (arrows). Delta waves (see Chapter 15) are not present. The patient had a known prior pattern of left bundle branch block. The rhythm is reentry supraventricular tachycardia, confirmed at electrophysiologic study to be occurring within the AV node.

normal His-Purkinje pathways. The relation between the P waves and QRS complexes will depend upon the relative conduction times from the junctional focus to the atria and ventricles, respectively; thus, the P waves can precede, be superimposed upon, or follow the QRS complexes (Fig 10-30). If the P waves precede the QRS complexes, differentiation from an ectopic atrial rhythm originating in the inferior portions of the atria may not be possible.

Junctional impulses can be premature or can occur as a result of slowing of the sinus rate, in which case they are termed **escape** beats. A junc-

tional premature beat, which results from enhanced automaticity of the AV junction, can initiate an **accelerated junctional rhythm**, which usurps the sinus rhythm, resulting in *AV dissociation* (Fig 10-31) (see Chapter 12). A junctional escape beat can initiate a junctional **escape rhythm** with rates of 35/min to 60/min (Fig 10-31). A junctional impulse can also cause a **reciprocal (echo) beat**: If the junctional impulse is conducted slowly in the AV node in retrograde fashion to the atria, it can turn around within the AV node to initiate ventricular activation a second time (Fig 10-32).

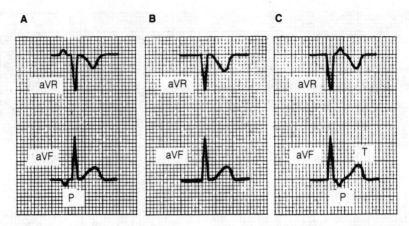

Figure 10-30. Electrocardiographic patterns of impulses arising in various sites within the AV junction. *A:* High AV junctional focus (A-N). Note the upright P in aVR and the inverted P in aVF preceding the QRS complex. The impulse is activating the atria before the ventricles. *B:* AV junctional focus. The P wave is buried in the QRS complex. The impulse is arising in either the A-N or N-H zones and activating the atria and ventricles simultaneously. *C:* Low AV junctional focus (N-H). Note the upright P in aVR and the inverted P in aVF following the QRS complex. The impulse is activating the ventricles before the atria. Because activation times of the atria and ventricles relative to each other determine where the P waves are located relative to the QRS complexes, precise site of origin (high or low junctional, for example) is not always known.

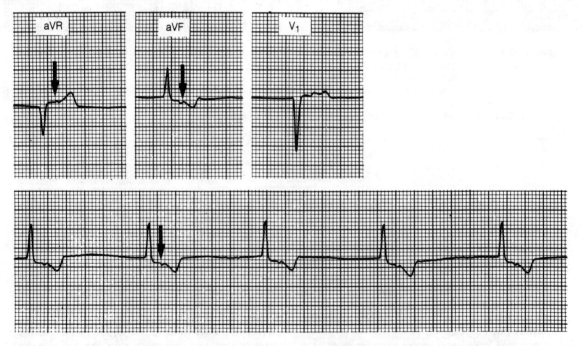

Figure 10-31. AV junctional rhythm. A regular QRS rhythm at a rate of 47/min is present. The QRS complexes are of normal duration. No atrial activity precedes the QRS complexes. P waves are seen in the T waves following each QRS complex (arrows). The P waves are upright in aVR and inverted in II and aVF, indicating retrograde atrial depolarization.

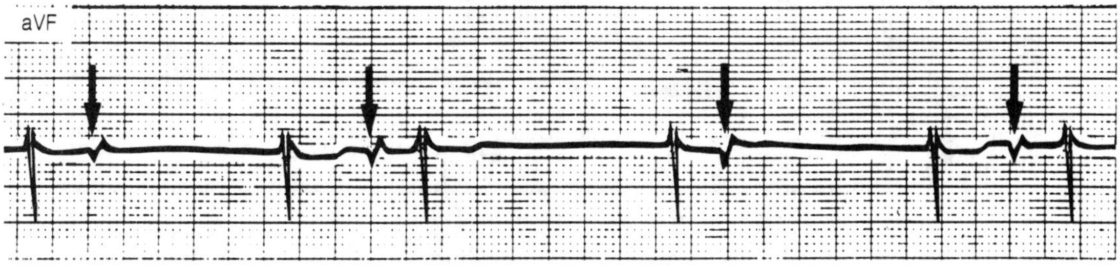

aVF

Figure 10-32. AV junctional rhythm with retrograde atrial activation and reciprocal ("echo") beats. Each QRS complex is followed by an inverted P wave in its T wave, indicating retrograde atrial activation (arrow). The RP interval is long, reflecting delayed retrograde conduction. The second and fourth retrograde P waves occur at even longer RP intervals, allowing time for the impulse to turn around within the AV node and be conducted in antegrade fashion to the ventricles ("echo" phenomenon). If these events are sustained, a reciprocating tachycardia could develop. (Tracing retouched for clarity.)

Junctional Tachycardia

Junctional tachycardia is usually due to enhanced automaticity of the AV junction and may be seen as a manifestation of digitalis toxicity or in patients with severe congestive heart failure or those who have had cardiac surgery. Whereas an accelerated junctional rhythm has a rate of 60-120/min, junctional tachycardia has a rate of 120-200/min. Junctional tachycardia may be virtually impossible to differentiate from paroxysmal reentry supraventricular tachycardia on the ECG; however, the clinical circumstances as well as the response to vagal maneuvers (termination of paroxysmal supraventricular tachycardia but no effect on junctional tachycardia) are important distinguishing points.

ABERRANCY OF INTRAVENTRICULAR CONDUCTION IN ASSOCIATION WITH SUPRAVENTRICULAR ARRHYTHMIAS

Wide, notched, bizarre QRS complexes may be seen in association with any atrial of AV junctional rhythm and may thus simulate a ventricular arrhythmia. The abnormal QRS configuration may be due to preexisting bundle branch block or ventricular preexcitation (see Chapters 8 and 15), in which case it will be present during sinus rhythm; or, it may be seen only during an arrhythmia, with normal intraventricular conduction being present at other times. When atrial activity is seen to precede the abnormal QRS complexes, the diagnosis of intraventricular aberration may easily be made (Fig 10-33). However, when atrial activity is not easily seen to be related to ventricular activity, the differential diagnosis of intraventricular aberration and ventricular arrhythmia may be difficult (Fig 10-34). Carotid sinus massage may be helpful if the expected AV block is

achieved (Fig 10-35) but is not helpful when this response does not occur. Comparison with prior ECGs to establish the presence or absence of preexisting intraventricular conduction delay will aid in ascertaining the origin of the QRS complexes. Special leads (intracardiac or esophageal) may clarify the presence and rate of atrial activity but will not aid in determining the relationship (antegrade or retrograde) between atrial and ventricular activity if there is one P wave associated with each QRS complex.

An important morphologic feature that favors intraventricular aberration over ventricular ectopy is a *typical* right bundle branch block configuration of the premature QRS complexes (Fig 10-36). A right bundle branch block configuration occurs because the right bundle branch normally has the longest refractory period of the intraventricular conduction system (followed in turn by the anterior division of the left bundle branch and the posterior divison of the left bundle branch). Thus, premature impulses are more likely to arrive at the right bundle branch when it is still refractory, and their conduction in this bundle branch is therefore more likely to be delayed or blocked.

Another feature of intraventricular abberation is termed the **long-short rule (Ashman's phenomenon)**. When a QRS complex follows another QRS complex at a given interval (cycle length) and a third QRS has a short coupling interval to the second, the third QRS may show aberrant intraventricular conduction. This occurs because the duration of the refractory period of the bundle branches is related to the heart rate: Slowing the heart rate (increasing the RR cycle length) lengthens the refractory period; thus, if the next impulse is early, it is more likely to be blocked in the refractory bundle branch and conducted to the ventricles aberrantly (Fig 10-37). However, since a long RR cycle length also favors the appearance of a premature ventricular complex, the long-short rule may not always be helpful in differentiating

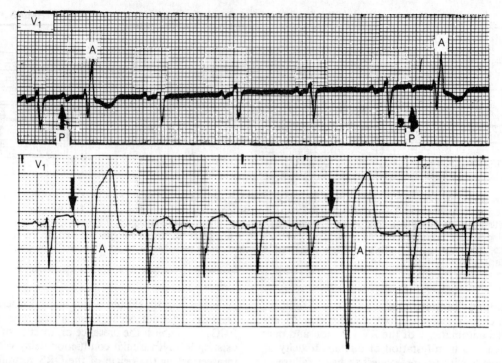

Figure 10-33. Premature atrial complexes with aberrant intraventricular conduction. *A:* The rhythm is sinus, and the PR interval is 0.16 s. Premature atrial complexes (P) (arrows) are conducted to the ventricles with a PR interval of 0.24 s, reflecting conduction delay in the AV node due to depolarization by the preceding sinus impulse. The QRS complexes stimulated by the P waves have a right bundle branch block pattern, reflecting refractoriness in this bundle branch at the time of arrival of the premature atrial impulses. *B:* The rhythm is sinus and the intraventricular conduction of the sinus impulses is normal. The atrial premature complexes (arrows) that occur at short coupling intervals to the preceding sinus P waves are conducted to the ventricles with a left bundle branch block pattern due to refractoriness in this bundle branch at the time of arrival of the atrial impulse. Whether aberrant intraventricular conduction shows right or left bundle branch block patterns is of little clinical significance, but merely reflects variations in refractory periods within these bundle branches. (A = aberrant intraventricular conduction.)

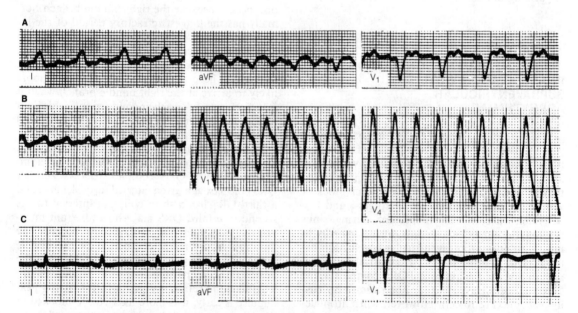

Figure 10-34. Automatic atrial tachycardia with changing AV conduction ratios and intraventricular aberration. *A:* A wide complex tachycardia (rate, 100/min) suggesting left bundle branch block is present; P waves are occurring at 200/min (best seen in V₁). Thus, the rhythm is atrial tachycardia with 2:1 AV conduction. *B:* Acceleration of the ventricular rate to 200/min as the AV conduction ratio becomes 1:1. The QRS complexes are broader and more bizarre; the rhythm now cannot be distinguished from ventricular tachycardia based on this recording alone. *C:* Restoration of sinus rhythm.

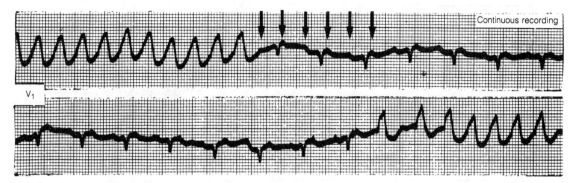

Figure 10-35. Effect of carotid sinus massage on a wide QRS complex tachycardia. Broad, bizarre QRS complexes having a pure R wave configuration in V₁ occur at a regular rate of 200/min. It is not possible to tell whether this represents ventricular tachycardia or supraventricular tachycardia with intraventricular aberration. Carotid sinus massage results in slowing of the ventricular rate to 100/min and the appearance (arrows) of a discernible atrial tachycardia (or slow atrial flutter) at a rate of 200/min; thus, 2:1 AV conduction of the atrial impulses has been produced, and the wide complex tachycardia represented intraventricular aberration. Upon cessation of carotid sinus massage, 1:1 AV conduction of the atrial impulses resumes, with reappearance of the wide QRS complexes. This tracing illustrates that intraventricular aberration is often a rate-dependent (tachycardia-dependent) phenomenon.

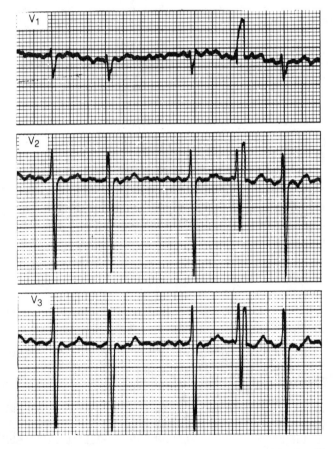

Figure 10-36. Atrial fibrillation with aberrant intraventricular conduction. The fourth QRS complex has an rsR' pattern in V₁₋₃, indicating right intraventricular conduction delay. This complex follows the preceding QRS complex by a short interval, which in turn follows the one preceding it by a longer interval, illustrating the "long-short" rule (Ashman's phenomenon). Right bundle branch block pattern in an early QRS complex is related to the longer refractory period in the right bundle branch compared to that in the other fascicles and indicates aberrancy of intraventricular conduction.

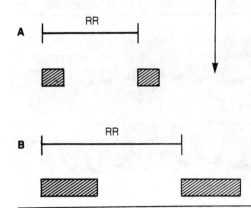

Figure 10-37. Schema of the refractory period (hatched areas) of a bundle branch in relation to heart rate (RR cycle length). *A:* At a faster heart rate (shorter RR cycle length) the refractory period is short. An early impulse (arrow) arrives at the bundle branch when it is no longer refractory, and intraventricular conduction is normal. *B:* Slower heart rate (longer RR cycle length) with proportionately longer refractory period of the bundle branches. The premature impulse now arrives during the refractory period of a bundle branch and is not conducted down that bundle branch. Ventricular depolarization will be aberrant.

Table 10-3. Features differentiating intraventricular aberration from ventricular ectopy.

ABERRATION	ECTOPY
Preceded by premature P wave (unless AV junctional in origin).	Not preceded by premature P wave.
Triphasic rSR' in V_1; Rs with wide s in V_6.	R, RR', QR in V_1; rS or QR in V_6.
Initial vector of depolarization in V_1 the same as during normal intraventricular conduction.	Initial vector of depolarization in V_1 opposite to that during normal intraventricular conduction (unless an initial q wave is present).
Absence of fixed coupling interval between normally conducted and wide QRS complexes.	Fixed coupling interval between wide QRS complexes and normally conducted complexes.
Ashman's phenomenon.	
QRS duration often less than 0.14 s.	QRS duration often greater than or equal to 0.14s.
Often resembles a defined bundle branch block pattern.	Superior frontal plane QRS axis.
Absence of long interval between wide QRS complex and subsequent QRS complex in atrial fibrillation (may not be present).	Long interval between wide QRS complex and subsequent normal QRS complex in atrial fibrillation (may not be present).

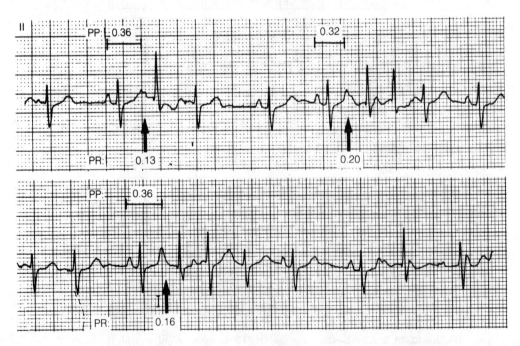

Figure 10-38. Multifocal atrial tachycardia with intraventricular conduction patterns that are aberrant to varying degrees. Early atrial premature impulses that are conducted to the ventricles with a normal PR interval are associated with more aberrancy than those conducted with a longer PR interval. This indicates that the premature impulses which do not encounter delay in conduction at the AV node arrive at the bundle branches while they are partially refractory (and thus depolarize the ventricles aberrantly), whereas those which do encounter conduction delay at the AV node (manifested by a longer PR interval) arrive at the bundle branches when they are recovered from their refractoriness.

supraventricular impulses with intraventricular aberration from ectopic ventricular complexes.

Table 10–3 lists those features that help to distinguish intraventricular aberration from ventricular ectopy. Different degrees of aberrant intraventricular conduction are often seen, and depend upon the coupling intervals of the premature P waves to the preceding P waves, and on the PR intervals. The earlier the premature P wave, the greater the likelihood of aberrant intraventricular conduction. However, if the premature impulse encounters sufficient conduction delay in the AV node (long PR interval), it may reach the bundle branches when they have recovered from their refractory state. The resulting QRS complex will be normal or near normal. If, on the other hand, the premature impulse does not encounter delay within the AV node (normal PR interval), it will reach the bundle branches when they are refractory and the QRS complexes will be aberrant (Fig 10–38).

A third, much less useful feature suggesting (but not proving) intraventricular aberration is the interval between the wide QRS complex and the following QRS complex. If this is short, intraventricular aberration may be more likely, whereas if it is long, ectopy may be more likely.

Aberration Versus Ectopy in Atrial Fibrillation

If the atrial rhythm is fibrillation and the presence of atrial premature complexes cannot be used to distinguish intraventricular aberration from ventricular ectopy, the configuration of the premature ventricular complexes becomes the prime criterion for the correct diagnosis. Another helpful feature in differentiating aberration from ectopy in atrial fibrillation is the absence of a **fixed coupling** interval of the wide QRS complex to the preceding normally conducted complex in the former; fixed coupling suggests ventricular premature impulses due to a ventricular reentry mechanism (Figs 10–39 and 10–40). Ashman's phenomenon, in which a wide QRS complex occurs at short coupling interval to a preceding one which has itself terminated a long RR interval, can also suggest intraventricular aberration.

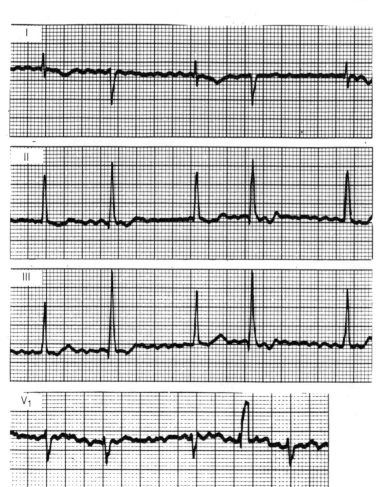

Figure 10-39. Atrial fibrillation with premature ventricular complexes versus supraventricular complexes with intraventricular aberration. The second and fourth QRS complexes are wide and have a pattern of left posterior fascicular block, suggesting possible origin in the anterior fascicle of the left bundle branch. There is a long interval between these wide complexes and the subsequent normally conducted complexes, suggesting retrograde conduction of premature ventricular beats into the AV node, delaying antegrade conduction of the fibrillatory impulses. However, the lack of a fixed coupling interval between the normal and aberrant QRS complexes favors intraventricular aberration of supraventricular impulses. Sometimes an intracardiac electrogram is required to arrive at the proper diagnosis.

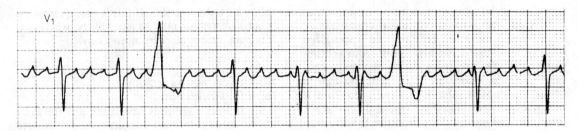

Figure 10-40. Atrial fibrillation with closely coupled wide QRS complexes. The broad QRS complexes have a fixed coupling interval to the preceding normal QRS complexes of 0.39 s and a pure R wave configuration in V₁. Each is followed by a relatively longer cycle length than preceding or following ones. These features suggest that they represent ventricular premature complexes.

REFERENCES

Bär FW et al: Differential diagnosis of tachycardia with narrow QRS complex (shorter than 0.12 second). *Am J Cardiol* 1984;**54**:555.

Chan AQ, Pick A: Reentrant arrhythmias and concealed conduction. *Am Heart J* 1979;**97**:644.

Cranefield PF: Action potentials, afterpotentials, and arrhythmias. *Circ Res* 1977;**41**:415.

Fisch C, Knoebel SB: Recognition and therapy of digitalis toxicity. *Prog Cardiovasc Dis* 1970;**13**:71.

Fisher, JD: Role of electrophysiologic testing in the diagnosis and treatment of patients with known and suspected bradycardias and tachycardias. *Prog Cardiovasc Dis* 1981;**24**:25.

Josephson ME, Kastor JA: Supraventricular tachycardia: Mechanisms and management. *Ann Intern Med* 1977;**87**:346.

Kastor JA, Yurchak PM: Recognition of digitalis intoxication in the presence of atrial fibrillation. *Ann Intern Med* 1967;**67**:1045.

Lown B, Wyatt NF, Levine HD: Paroxysmal atrial tachycardia with block. *Circulation* 1960;**21**:129.

Rosen KM: Junctional tachycardia: Mechanisms, diagnosis, differential diagnosis, and management. *Circulation* 1973;**47**:654

Shine KI, Kastor, JA, Yurchak PM: Multifocal atrial tachycardia: Clinical and electrocardiographic features. *N Engl J Med* 1968;**279**:344.

Singer DH, Ten Eick RE: Pharmacology of cardiac arrhythmias. *Prog Cardiovasc Dis* 1969;**11**:488.

Vassalle M: The relationship among cardiac pacemakers: Overdrive suppression. *Circ Res* 1977;**41**:269.

Wells JL Jr et al: Characterization of atrial flutter: Studies in man after open heart surgery using fixed atrial electrodes. *Circulation* 1979;**60**:665.

Wit Al, Rosen MR: Pathophysiologic mechanisms of cardiac arrhythmias. *Am Heart J* 1983;**106**:798.

Figure 10-T1.
TEST TRACINGS

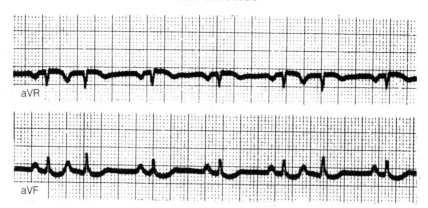

What is the rhythm?	Sinus with atrial premature beats.
Explain the variation in PR intervals.	The sinus beats have a constant PR interval of 0.16 s. The premature complexes have a longer PR interval reflecting the delay in transmission of the premature impulse through the AV node. This delay is caused by prior transmission of the sinus impulse through the node.
Is intraventricular aberraton present?	There is mild alteration in the premature QRS complex; it is slightly wider than the sinus-stimulated QRS complex, and is notched in its terminal portion.

Figure 10-T2.
TEST TRACINGS

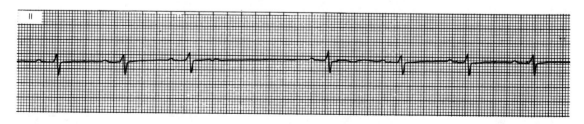

What is the cause of the pause?	A nonconducted atrial premature complex, which arrives at the AV node–His-Purkinje system while it is still refractory. The premature P wave deforms the T wave of the third QRS complex.
What is the underlying rhythm?	Sinus, with first-degree AV block (PR interval 0.26 s).

Figure 10-T3.
TEST TRACINGS

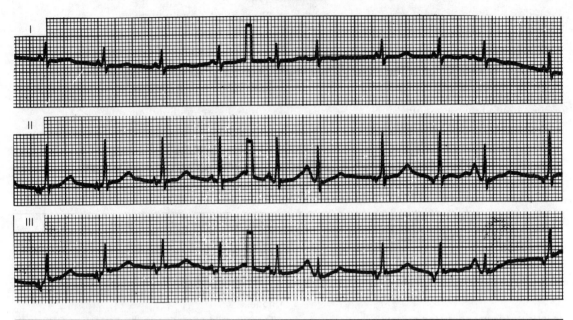

Is the atrial rhythm regular or irregular?	Irregular.
Are the P waves constant in morphology?	No.
Are the PR intervals constant?	No.
How many P wave configurations can you identify?	At least 4.
What is the diagnosis?	Wandering atrial pacemaker.

Figure 10-T4.
TEST TRACINGS

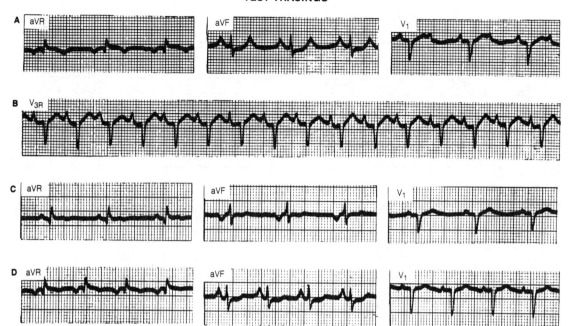

This series of tracings was recorded from a patient receiving digitalis.

Describe the atrial rhythm and rate in rhythm strips A–D.	A: 142/min. The P waves are upright in aVF and V_1. The atrial rhythm could be sinus tachycardia or automatic (ectopic) atrial tachycardia. B: No change in atrial rhythm or rate. C: The P wave rate is now 75/min and the P waves are inverted in aVF and upright in aVR and V_1. D: The P waves are now normally upright in aVF and the atrial rate is 100/min.
What is the AV conduction ratio in strips A–D?	A: 2:1, B–D:1:1.
What is the diagnosis in strips A–D?	A: Automatic atrial tachycardia with 2:1 AV block. B: Same atrial mechanism, with 1:1 AV conduction. C: Low atrial or high junctional ectopic atrial rhythm. D: Normal sinus rhythm.
What is the likely cause for this series of tracings.	Digitalis toxicity.

Figure 10-T5.
TEST TRACINGS

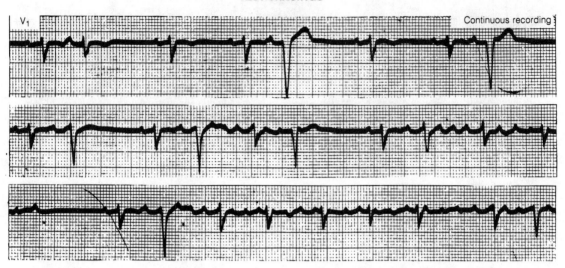

Describe the rhythm in the top strip.

Sinus with atrial premature complexes.

Explain the presence of the broad QRS complexes in the top strip.

The atrial premature impulses are conducted with a left bundle branch block pattern, due to their reaching it during its refractory state.

Do the wide QRS complexes in the top strip represent premature ventricular complexes or aberrant intraventricular conduction? Why?

They are aberrantly conducted since they are preceded by a premature P wave.

Describe the events in the bottom 2 strips.

Atrial premature depolarizations initiate bursts of flutter-fibrillation, the first 2 of which are nonsustained. This results from an atrial premature impulse falling in the atrial vulnerable period.

Figure 10–T6.
TEST TRACINGS

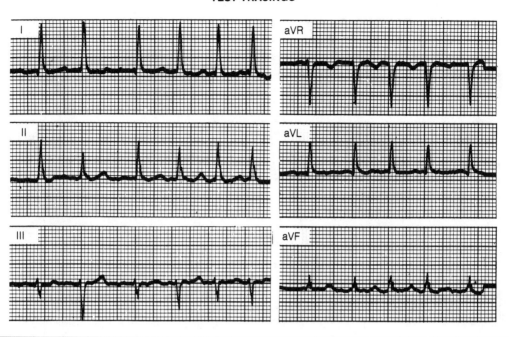

Is the ventricular rhythm irregular or regular?	Irregular.
Is atrial activity present?	Yes, the baseline displays fine undulations representing fibrillatory waves.
What is the rhythm diagnosis?	Atrial fibrillation.

Figure 10–T7.
TEST TRACINGS

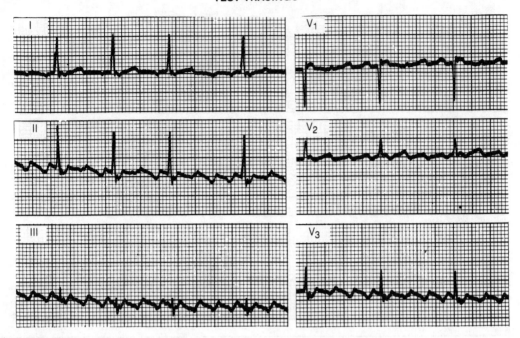

Is the ventricular rhythm regular or irregular?	Irregular.
Is atrial activity present?	Yes.
Describe the atrial rate and rhythm.	Saw-toothed waves in II, III, and V_3. The rate is 300/min.
What is the rhythm diagnosis?	Atrial flutter with 3:1 and 4:1 AV conduction.
Is inferior wall myocardial ischemia present?	Slight deformities of the ST segments by the flutter waves are present. There is no apparent deviation of the true ST segment.

Figure 10-T8.
TEST TRACINGS

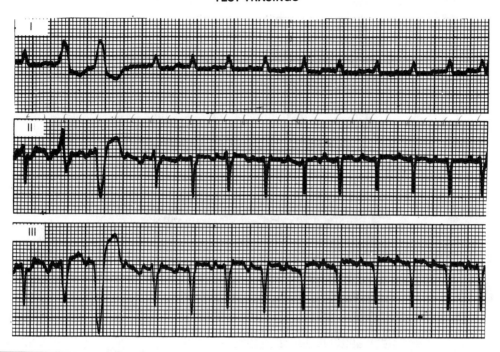

What is the ventricular rate?	150/min.
Is the ventricular rhythm regular or irregular?	Regular, except for the broad, bizarre complexes which are premature.
What might the atrial rhythm be, given this ventricular rate?	Atrial flutter with 2:1 AV conduction (this diagnosis should be considered in all cases when the ventricular rate is regular at 150/min).
How is the diagnosis of atrial flutter substantiated in these rhythm strips?	In leads II and III, flutter waves are clearly seen following the postextrasystolic pause. The flutter rate is 300/min.

Figure 10–T9.
TEST TRACINGS

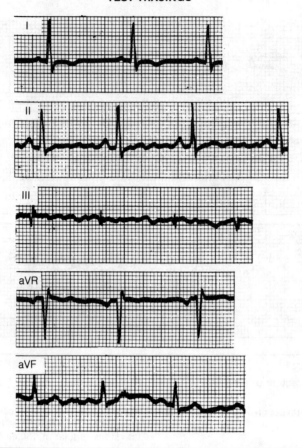

Is the ventricular rhythm regular or irregular?	Regular.
What is the rhythm diagnosis in leads II, III, and aVF?	Sinus. Undulations deform the baseline in these but P waves can be seen in lead II despite the baseline artifact, and are clearly visible in leads I and aVR.
What could account for the findings in the inferior leads?	Artifact involving the lower extremity electrodes. This patient had a cast on his left leg.

Figure 10–T10.
TEST TRACINGS

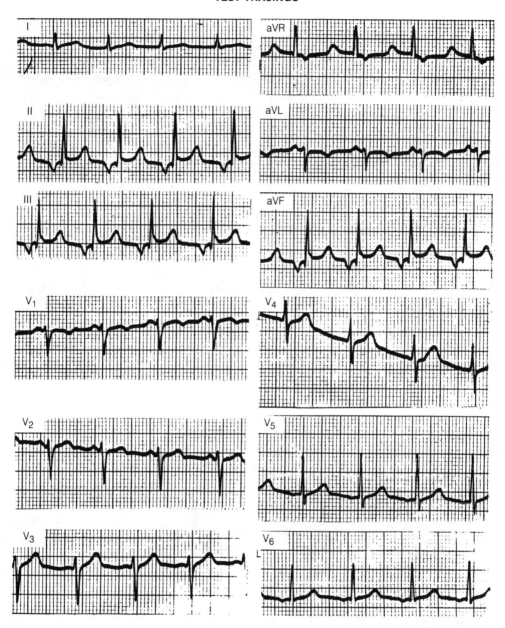

Is this sinus rhythm? Why or why not?

The P waves have a normal PR interval but they are inverted in leads II, III, and aVF. The rhythm is therefore originating low in the atrium, or in the AV junction.

What is the orientation of the atrial depolarization vector?

Rightward (negative P in lead V_6) and superior (negative P in II, III, and aVF).

How could this rhythm originate?
Can you tell from this tracing?

Either by enhanced automaticity of an ectopic focus, or as an escape rhythm following a slowing or pause in sinus rhythm. Since the mode of onset of the rhythm is not seen in this ECG, the exact diagnosis cannot be known.

Figure 10-T11.
TEST TRACINGS

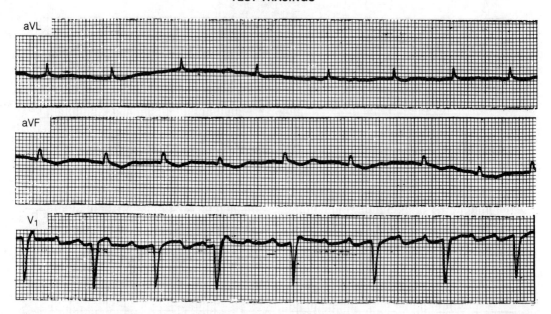

Is the ventricular rate regular or irregular?	Irregular.
Is atrial activity discerned?	Not in leads aVL or aVF, but it is in V₁.
What is the atrial rhythm?	Flutter, but this is obscured in aVL and aVF, where the mistaken diagnosis of atrial fibrillation could easily be made.

Figure 10-T12.
TEST TRACINGS

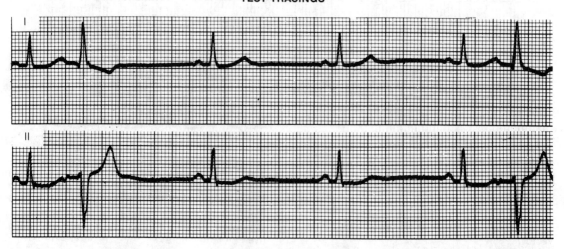

What is the atrial rhythm?	Sinus bradycardia, with atrial premature depolarizations.
What accounts for the broad bizarre QRS complexes?	The atrial premature impulse is arriving at the bundle branches when they are partially refractory.
What is the pattern of intraventricular conduction of the premature broad QRS complexes?	The axis in lead II is superiorly directed. This pattern is consistent with left anterior fascicular conduction delay.

Figure 10-T13.
TEST TRACINGS

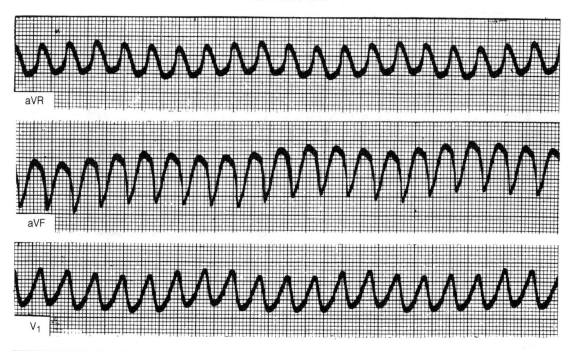

aVR

aVF

V₁

Describe the ventricular rhythm.	Wide complex tachycardia, regular, rate about 200/min.
What is the differential diagnosis?	Ventricular tachycardia or supraventricular tachycardia with aberrant intraventricular conduction.
What is the mean frontal plane QRS axis?	Superiorly directed, since QS complexes are present in lead aVF, and pure R wave complexes are present in lead aVR.
What is the morphology of the complexes in V₁?	Pure R wave.
What is the likely diagnosis?	Ventricular tachycardia.
Why is it unlikely that the atrial rhythm is flutter?	The atrial rate would have to be 400/min if 2:1 AV conduction were present; this is relatively fast for flutter. The atrial rate would have to be 200/min if 1:1 AV conduction were present; this is relatively slow. Atrial flutter remains a possibility, however.
How would you go about making the correct rhythm diagnosis?	Carotid sinus massage, AV nodal blocking agents, intravenous lidocaine.

The tracing shown in Fig 10–35 was recorded just after these rhythm strips were obtained, establishing the diagnosis of supraventricular tachycardia with intraventricular aberration.

Figure 10-T14.
TEST TRACINGS

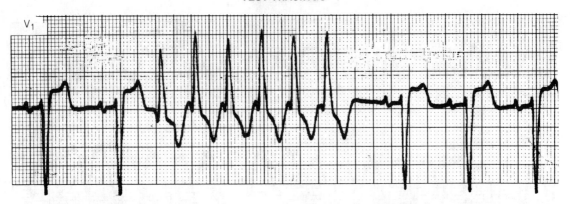

Why are the wide QRS complexes likely to be ventricular in origin?

They have a qR pattern in lead V_1, an initial vector opposite in direction to the sinus-stimulated QRS complexes, and there are no premature P waves.

Figure 10-T15.
TEST TRACINGS

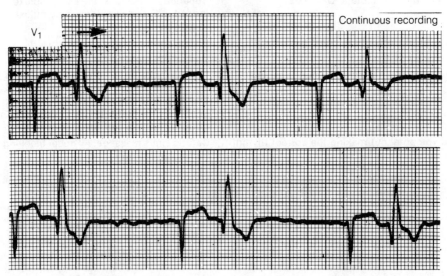

What is the atrial rhythm?

Fibrillation.

Describe the ventricular rhythm.

A normal-appearing QRS complex is followed at fixed coupling intervals by a broad bizarre QRS complex in bigeminal fashion.

What criteria for ventricular premature complexes are met in this tracing?

qR configuration in lead V_1, fixed coupling interval, different initial vector from the normal QRS complexes.

Abnormalities of Atrioventricular Conduction

11

Atrioventricular (AV) conduction delay ("block") is a disturbance in conduction of sinus (or atrial) impulses to the ventricles. The more common causes of AV block are listed in Table 11-1.

His Bundle Electrography

The technique of His bundle electrography was developed during the late 1960s and early 1970s, providing a great deal of information regarding normal and abnormal AV conduction in humans. The technique consists of placing a multipolar electrode cathether in proximity to the AV node–His bundle in order to record electrical activity as it passes through these structures (Fig 11-1). The electrical deflections recorded by this catheter are then related to events on the surface ECG. Several multipolar cathethers can be placed in both the right and left atria and ventricles, as well as in the coronary sinus in order to track the conduction

Table 11-1. Common causes of AV conduction disturbances.

Hypervagotonia (often associated with sinus bradycardia or sinus arrhythmia)
Digitalis
Beta-blocking drugs
Some calcium channel–blocking drugs (verapamil, diltiazem)
Coronary artery disease
  Inferior wall myocardial infarction (AV nodal ischemia)
  Right ventricular myocardial infarction (AV nodal ischemia)
  Anterior wall myocardial infarction (interventricular septal necrosis, often associated with bundle branch block)
Lenegre's disease (diffuse fibrosis of the conduction system)
Infiltrative heart disease
Aortic root disease (syphilis, spondylitis)
Calcification of the mitral aortic anulus (or both)
Acute infectious diseases
Myocarditis

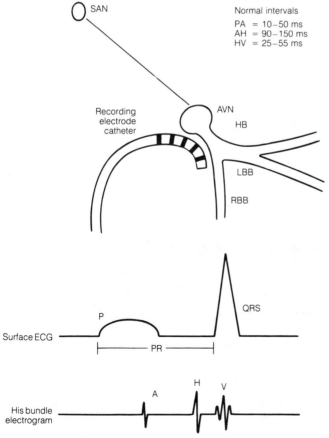

Normal intervals
PA = 10–50 ms
AH = 90–150 ms
HV = 25–55 ms

Figure 11-1. Schema of the technique of His bundle electrography. A multipolar electrode catheter is placed across the tricuspid valve in proximity to the His bundle. The catheter thus is capable of recording electrical activity at the level of the low right atrium, His bundle, and proximal right bundle branch, in addition to ventricular electrical activity. The sinus node pacemaker cells initiate an impulse which is not registered on either the surface ECG or the His bundle electrogram (recent data suggest that catheters placed at the level of the sinus node are capable of defining the sinus node potential). Atrial depolarization begins with the onset of the P wave on the surface ECG. Since the intracardiac catheter lies at the level of the low right atrium, the initial portions of atrial depolarization are not detected by it; it will register a deflection as the wave front passes through the area in which it is located, namely the low right atrium (A). As the impulse traverses the His bundle, a deflection is registered representing its depolarization (H). This is followed by a ventricular deflection which is registered at the time that the wavefront of depolarization of ventricular tissue reaches the electrodes (V), and therefore often follows the onset of inscription of the QRS complex on the surface ECG.

pattern of an impulse. In addition to defining the conduction pathway of impulse transmission during normal or baseline cardiac rhythm, electrical pacing through the intracardiac electrodes can be performed from different areas of the heart in order to study the pattern of conduction of stimuli applied with differing degrees of prematurity relative to a basic rate (or cycle length). Such "mapping" of cardiac conduction is useful in the diagnosis and management of certain arrhythmias and conduction system disorders, and has validated certain teachings based on the surface ECG alone, while invalidating others. His bundle electrography has also afforded insight into the refractory periods of cardiac tissue at various locations and has helped in evaluating the effects of cardiotonic and antiarrhythmic drugs.

First-Degree AV Block

First-degree AV block indicates a conduction delay between the atria and the ventricles; all atrial impulses are conducted. It is characterized by a *long PR interval,* which exceeds 0.2 s (Fig 11-2). The components of the PR interval are interatrial conduction (10-50 ms), AV nodal conduction (90-150 ms), and His-Purkinje conduction (25-55 ms). (Depolarization of the sinus node occurs prior to the inscription of the P wave and is not recorded on the surface ECG.) The prolonged PR interval of first-degree AV block can therefore reflect prolonged interatrial, intra–AV nodal, or His-Purkinje conduction; it usually represents delay in AV nodal conduction.

Second-Degree AV Block

Second-degree AV block describes a situation in which not all atrial impulses are conducted to the ventricles. **Type I (Wenckebach)** second-degree

AV block is present when atrial impulses encounter *progressive delay* in conduction to the ventricles because of AV nodal refractoriness, with eventual failure of conduction of an impulse (Fig 11-3). The ratio of P waves to QRS complexes describes the *AV conduction ratio* in type I second-degree AV block and may thus be 4:3, 8:7, etc. This ratio is also referred to as a **Wenckebach period.** Because type I second-degree AV block usually occurs within the AV node, the PR interval of the first conducted P wave of the Wenckebach period is often prolonged; and, because this form of conduction disturbance involves the AV node rather than the bundle branches, the QRS complexes are usually narrow and appear normal.

The Wenckebach period may be described as follows (Fig 11-4). The sinus rate is constant. As the sinus impulses are conducted through the AV node, they encounter increasing conduction delay (prolongation of PR intervals). However, the *increment* in conduction delay from one P–QRS complex to the next is slightly less each time, resulting in a shortening of the RR interval relative to the preceding RR interval. Finally, a P wave fails to be conducted. The RR interval encompassing the nonconducted P wave is twice the PP interval *minus* the total increment in the PR intervals of the Wenckebach period. In a typical or classic Wenckebach period, therefore, 3 "rules" obtain: (1) the PR intervals progressively lengthen; (2) the RR intervals progressively shorten; and (3) the RR interval encompassing the nonconducted P wave is less than twice the preceding RR interval. Whereas typical Wenckebach periods are usually seen with low AV conduction ratios (3:2, 4:3, or 5:4), as the AV conduction ratio increases (exceeding 6:5), many Wenckebach sequences are atypical and do not follow the classic "rules."

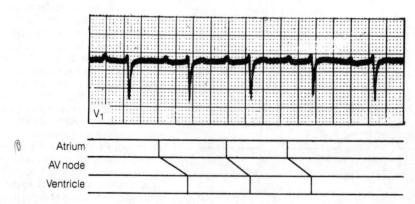

Figure 11-2. First-degree AV block. The PR interval is prolonged to 0.28 s. The laddergram beneath the ECG illustrates the 3 levels of AV conduction: the atrium, the AV node, and the ventricles, with the delay in AV conduction represented as occurring in the AV node.

Type II (Mobitz II) second-degree AV block is present when atrial impulses fail to be transmitted to the ventricles *without* prior progressive conduction delay. Thus, failure of antegrade conduction is often abrupt and unpredictable. In contrast to type I second-degree AV block, in which the conduction delay is in the AV node, the conduction block in type II second-degree AV block may be within the bundle of His or, more commonly, distal to the bundle of His in the bundle branches. Therefore, the QRS complexes often show a (preexistent) bundle branch block pattern, and the PR interval of the conducted P waves is constant and often normal (Fig 11–5).

2:1 AV Block

Second-degree AV block with a 2:1 AV conduction ratio may represent *either* type I (Wenckebach) or Type II (Mobitz II) second-degree AV block (Figs 11–6 and 11–7). Since 2 consecutive intervals are not recorded, the differential diagnosis may be difficult. However, certain general rules apply. If the PR interval of the conducted P waves is prolonged and the QRS complexes are narrow and appear normal, type I AV block (intra–AV nodal) is probably present. If the PR interval of the conducted P waves is normal and the QRS complexes show a bundle branch block pattern, type II AV block (distal to the bundle of His) is probably present. If the PR interval of the conducted P wave is prolonged and the QRS complexes show a bundle branch block pattern, or if the PR interval of the conducted P wave is normal and the QRS complexes appear normal, it may be impossible to distinguish between type I and type II second-degree AV block. Changing the AV conduction ratio from 2:1 to 3:2 or more by means of carotid sinus massage, intravenous atropine, or exercise will often unmask the nature and therefore the location of the AV block.

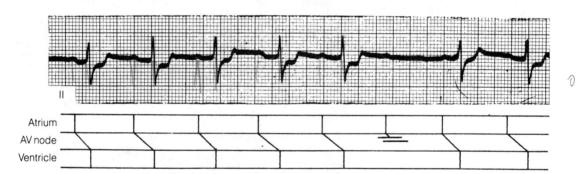

Figure 11–3. Type I (Wenckebach) second-degree AV block in which the sinus impulse is conducted to the ventricles with progressive delay (progressively increasing PR intervals) until an impulse fails to be conducted. Although type I AV block can occur in the His-Purkinje system, it most commonly represents AV nodal conduction delay, as illustrated in the laddergram.

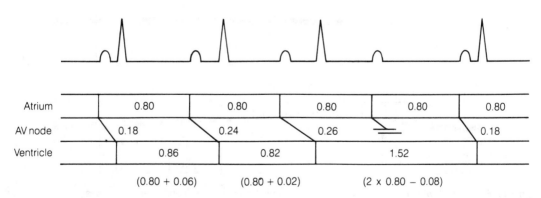

Atrium	0.80		0.80		0.80		0.80		0.80
AV node	0.18		0.24		0.26				0.18
Ventricle		0.86		0.82		1.52			
	(0.80 + 0.06)		(0.80 + 0.02)		(2 × 0.80 − 0.08)				

Figure 11–4. A *typical* Wenckebach period with a 4:3 AV conduction ratio (4 P waves and 3 QRS complexes). The sinus cycle length is constant at 0.8 s. The PR intervals progressively increase from 0.18 to 0.24 to 0.26 s; however, the *increment* in increase in PR intervals is 0.06 s between the first and second PR intervals and 0.02 s between the second and third PR intervals. Thus, the increment in PR interval increase is less each time. The RR cycle lengths equal the PP cycle lengths plus the *increment* in PR interval; thus, the RR cycle lengths get progressively shorter. The RR interval encompassing the nonconducted P wave is twice the sinus cycle length less the *total increment* in all PR intervals during the Wenckebach period.

High-Grade & Complete AV Block

In *high-grade* AV block, the AV conduction ratio is 3:1 or greater. Occasional conduction of atrial impulses to the ventricles does occur. In *complete* AV block, no atrial impulses are conducted to the ventricles, despite the temporal opportunity for this to occur, and the atria and ventricles are depolarized independently of each other (Figs 11–8 and 11–9). "Temporal opportunity" is a term used to describe a particular set of electrophysiologic conditions that must be present in order to allow transmission of the atrial impulse through the AV node–His-Purkinje system. The atrial rate in complete AV block is almost always faster than the ventricular rate. The ventricular pacemaker originates distal to the site of block and may be in the AV junction, bundle of His, bundle branches, or distal Purkinje system. In

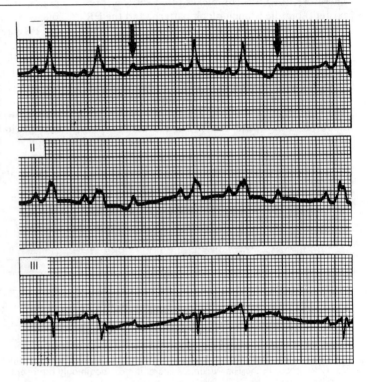

Figure 11-5. Type II (Mobitz II) second-degree AV block, with a 3:2 AV conduction ratio. The atrial rhythm is sinus. The PR intervals of the conducted beats are normal and constant. Every third P wave fails to be conducted to the ventricles (arrows). In addition to the AV block, left bundle branch block is present, with the second of each set of QRS complexes being more aberrant than the first. This suggests a progressive degree of conduction delay in the left bundle branch itself, ie, Wenckebach type block in the left bundle branch.

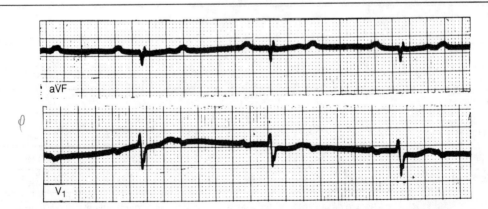

Figure 11-6. AV block with a 2:1 AV conduction ratio. The PR interval of the conducted P waves is prolonged, and the QRS complexes are narrow and appear normal. (The Q wave in aVF suggests inferior wall myocardial infarction.) When the conduction ratio is 2:1, it is often not possible to tell with certainty whether the block is in the AV node or in the His-Purkinje system. A change in the AV conduction ratio with a consequent demonstration of Wenckebach periodicity or type II block would be required for the precise diagnosis. However, 2:1 AV block in which the QRS complexes are of normal duration and the PR interval of the conducted beats is prolonged is usually occurring within the AV node; whereas 2:1 AV block in which the QRS complexes show a bundle branch block pattern and the PR interval of the conducted beats is normal often indicates a block below the level of the AV node.

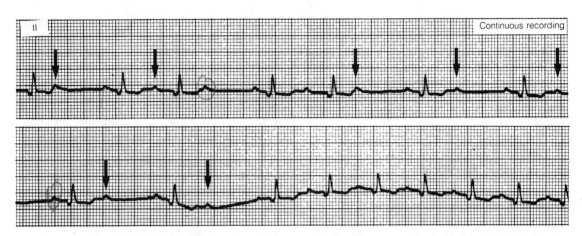

Figure 11-7. Type I (Wenckebach) second-degree AV block with varying AV conduction ratios. The atrial rhythm is sinus at a rate of 94/min. Nonconducted P waves are indicated by arrows. The rhythm strip begins with a nonconducted P wave following a narrow QRS complex (the Q wave indicates an inferior wall myocardial infarction, which was the cause of this rhythm disturbance in this patient). There follow 2 Wenckebach periods with a 3:2 AV conduction ratio, after which 3 Wenckebach periods with a conduction ratio of 2:1 occur. The PR intervals of these 2:1 conduction sequences is 0.2 s. If seen in isolation, the type of second-degree AV block might not be known with certainty. Subsequently, perhaps due to sympathetc stimulation caused by hemodynamic instability resulting from the pauses in QRS rhythm, a period of 1:1 AV conduction occurs (sympathetic stimulation enhances AV conduction). The second PR interval of this period shows the expected prolongation relative to the first. Variability in AV conduction ratios in an acute clinical setting is common in type I second-degree AV block.

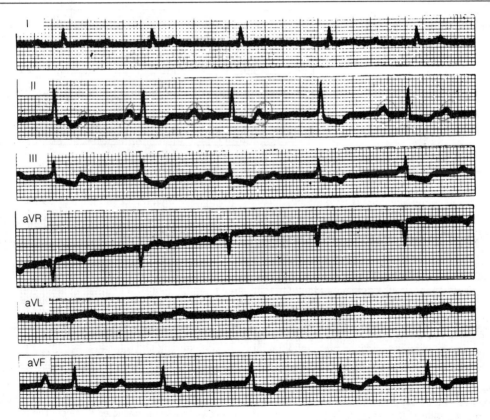

Figure 11-8. Complete AV block. The atrial rhythm is regular at a rate of 82/min. The ventricular rhythm is regular at a rate of 60/min. There is no relation between the 2 rhythms; the atria respond to the sinus node and the ventricles respond to an independent pacemaker. Since the QRS complexes are of normal duration and configuration, the ventricular pacemaker is likely to be originating in the AV junction or bundle of His. The apparent widening of some of the QRS complexes (fifth QRS in lead III and third QRS in lead aVF) is the result of fortuitous superimposition of the P wave upon the QRS complex.

complete AV block, the QRS rhythm is an **escape rhythm**; the morphology of the complexes and their rate will depend upon the site of origin of the rhythm (Fig 11—10). In high grade AV block escape rhythms will occur if the ventricular rate slows below the firing rate of the escape pacemaker due to changes in the AV conduction ratio (Fig 11-10).

Vagotonic Block

A high degree of vagal tone, such as occurs with sympathetic withdrawal during sleep, may be associated with (1) slowing of sinus rate; (2) pauses in sinus rhythm; (3) variable degrees of delay in AV conduction, manifested by (often irregular) prolongation of the PR interval; and (4) failure of conduction of P waves in a manner resembling type I (Wenckebach) or even type II AV block (Fig 11-11). It is important to recognize vagotonic block, since it often occurs in normal individuals as well as in patients with inferior or right ventricular myocardial infarction (or both) or any other clinical condition in which hypervagotonia is present. It not uncommonly accompanies the use of certain medications, notably beta-adrenergic blocking agents and some antihypertensive drugs. It can also be seen during swallowing ("deglutition" bradycardia), coughing ("tussive" bradycardia), and yawning. In the critical care setting, vagotonic block can occur during suctioning in patients with endotracheal tubes and in patients with elevated intracranial pressure.

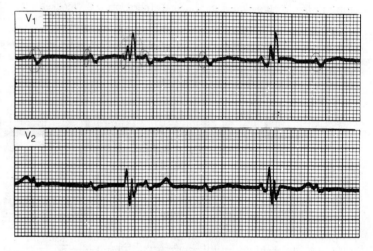

Figure 11-9. Complete AV block. The atrial rhythm is sinus at a rate of 88/min. The ventricular rhythm is regular at a rate of 37/min and is completely independent of the atrial rhythm. The QRS complexes are wide and show a right bundle branch block pattern. The long QRS duration and the slow rate of the QRS rhythm suggest a ventricular focus of origin.

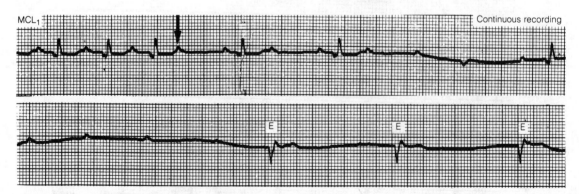

Figure 11-10. High-grade AV block progressing rapidly to complete AV block. Sinus rhythm with prolonged PR interval (first-degree AV block) is present in the beginning of the strip. A nonconducted P wave (arrow) is followed by a period of 2:1 AV conduction (second-degree AV block). This is in turn followed by 3 nonconducted P waves. The fourth P wave is conducted to the ventricles at a PR interval of 0.33 s, producing a QRS complex identical to those in the beginning of the strip (high-grade AV block). Following this, several nonconducting P waves result in the emergence of an escape rhythm (E). The broad QRS morphology of the escape rhythm and its slow rate suggest that the escape focus is in the distal Purkinje tissue. His bundle electrography could help to localize the site of origin of the escape pacemaker. Note that the P wave rate slows considerably concomitantly with the complete AV block. This suggests a vagal component of the block.

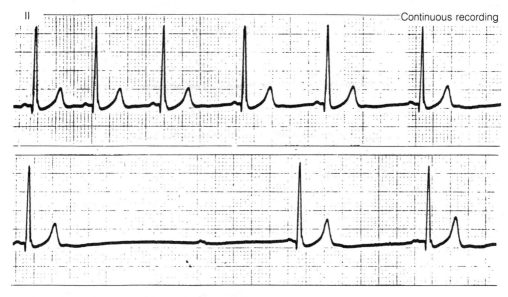

Figure 11-11. Vagotonic block in a young postoperative herniorrhaphy patient, recorded during sleep. The atrial rhythm is sinus. Slowing of the sinus rhythm occurs gradually, eventuating in a pause of almost 2 s. This pause is accompanied by failure of conduction of the P wave to the ventricles. Following the pause, sinus rhythm with normal AV conduction is again present. Vagotonic AV block should not be confused with type I or type II AV block. The diagnosis depends upon the demonstration of slowing of the sinus rate in association with failure of AV conduction, if present.

REFERENCES

Dhingra RC et al: Incidence and site of atrioventricular block in patients with chronic bifascicular block. *Circulation* 1979;**59**:238.

Dreifus LS et al: Atrioventricular block. *Am J Cardiol* 1971;**28**:371.

El-Sherif N et al: Atypcial Wenckebach periodicity simulating Mobitz II AV block. *Br Heart J* 1978;**40**:376.

James TN: Morphology of the human atrioventricular node, with remarks pertinent to its electrophysiology. *Am Heart J* 1961;**62**:756.

Kastor JA: Atrioventricular block (2 parts.) *N Engl J Med* 1975;**292**:462, 572.

Mangiardi LM et al: Bedside evaluation of atrioventricular block with narrow QRS complexes: Usefulness of carotid sinus massage and atropine administration. *Am J Cardiol* 1982;**49**:1136.

McAnulty JH, Murphy E, Rahimtoola SH: Prospective evaluation of intrahisian conduction delay. *Circulation* 1979;**59**:1035.

Martin P: The influence of the parasympathetic nervous system on atrioventricular conduction. *Cir Res* 1977;**41**:593.

Narula OS et al: Atrioventricular block: Localization and classification by His bundle recordings. *Am J Med* 1971;**50**:146.

Figure 11–T1.
TEST TRACINGS

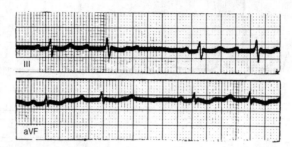

What is the atrial rhythm? What features substantiate this diagnosis?	Sinus, in view of the normal rate and P wave axis.
What are the PR intervals?	0.18 and 0.36 s.
What is the AV conduction ratio?	3:2.
What type of AV block is present?	Type I (Wenckebach).
What are the criteria for this diagnosis?	Progressive prolongation of PR intervals, progressive shortening of the increment in the PR intervals, and the RR interval encompassing the nonconducted P wave is less than twice the preceding RR interval.
Are most Wenckebach sequences typical or atypical?	Atypical.
Where is the conduction delay in the typical AV Wenckebach sequence?	The AV node.

Figure 11-T2.
TEST TRACINGS

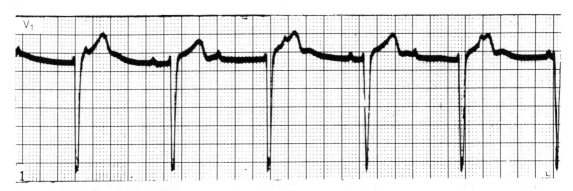

What is the atrial rate and rhythm?	Sinus, rate 72/min.
What type of AV block is present? Why?	Complete AV block. The P waves are independent from the QRS complexes.
Where is the QRS rhythm likely to be originating? Why?	In the AV junction or bundle of His, since the QRS duration is normal and the morphology is normal, and the rate is 54/min.

Figure 11-T3.
TEST TRACINGS

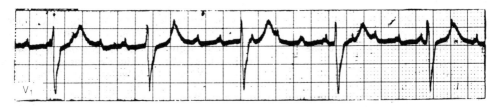

What is the atrial rate and rhythm?	Atrial tachycardia or flutter, rate 225/min.
Describe the ventricular rhythm.	Regular, rate about 55/min. The QRS complexes have a relatively normal appearance and duration.
Is AV block present?	Yes, since there is no relationship between the atrial impulses and the regularly occurring QRS complexes.
What is the likely origin of the ventricular rhythm? Why?	His bundle. The rate is 55/min and the QRS complexes are narrow and normal-appearing.

Figure 11–T4.
TEST TRACINGS

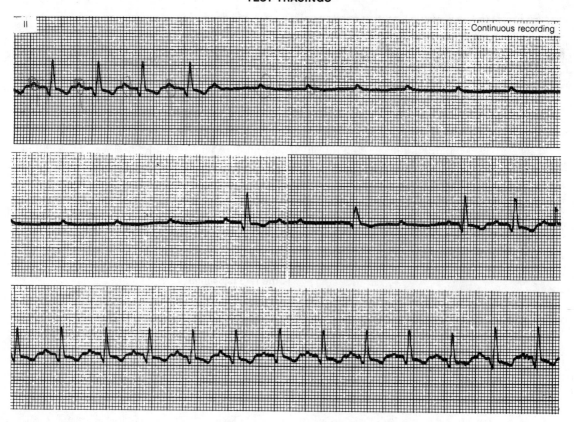

What characterizes the PR intervals prior to the group of nonconducted P waves?	The last PR interval prior to the pause in QRS rhythm is longer than the preceding ones.
Describe 2 types of AV block present in this strip.	The prolongation of the past PR interval prior to the pause in QRS rhythm suggests that type I second-degree AV block is present in the beginning of the rhythm strip. This is followed by a period of high grade AV block, which is terminated by two escape complexes and finally by resumption of 1:1 AV conduction.
What is the name of the QRS complexes that terminate the pauses in QRS rhythm?	Escape complexes.
Is an escape rhythm present?	No.
Is vagal tone playing a role in the AV block?	No. There is no decrease in sinus rate accompanying the AV block, so this diagnosis cannot be made.
Where is (are) this (these) conduction delay(s) likely to be?	The type I sequence may be occurring in the AV node or the bundle of His. The development of the high-grade AV block is probably occurring in the bundle of His.

Figure 11–T5.
TEST TRACINGS

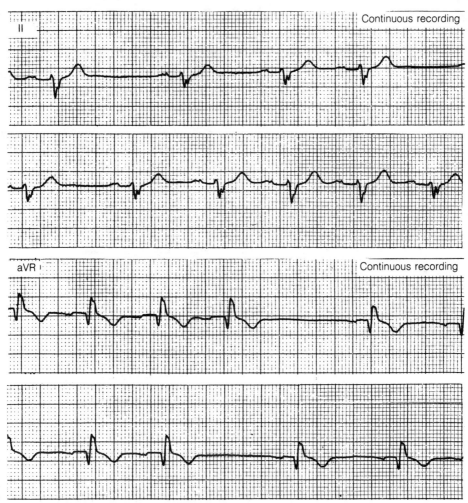

What is the atrial rhythm.	Sinus.
Is it regular?	No.
What is the AV conduction ratio?	1:1. No P waves fail to stimulate QRS complexes.
What is the pattern of intraventricular conduction?	The superior axis indicates left anterior fascicular block, and the delayed R wave in lead aVR indicates right bundle branch block.
Describe the sinus rhythm.	Progressive shortening of PP intervals occurs, followed by a pause in P wave rate.
What type of conduction block is suggested by progressive shortening of P waves or QRS complexes?	Type I (Wenckebach) second-degree block, in this case occurring in the sinoatrial area.
What is the diagnosis?	Type I (Wenckebach) sinoatrial block.

12

Atrioventricular Dissociation

AV dissociation is present when one pacemaker activates the atria and a second, *independent*, pacemaker activates the ventricles. The atrial pacemaker is usually the sinus node, but any atrial rhythm can be present. The ventricular pacemaker can originate in the AV junction, bundle of His, bundle branches, or peripheral Purkinje tissue (Figs 12–1 and 12–2). Its rate is usually faster than that of the atria. When the 2 rates are about the same, resulting in *apparent association* of the rhythms, the AV dissociation is termed **isorhythmic**. If the atrial rhythm is an ectopic tachycardia and the ventricular rhythm represents acceleration of a subsidiary pacemaker, **double tachycardia** is said to be present.

Emergence of the ventricular pacemaker can come about as a result of acceleration of the rate of the subsidiary pacemaker because of enhanced automaticity (**accelerated rhythm**) (Figs 12–1 and 12–2) or as a result of slowing of the atrial below the intrinsic rate of the lower pacemaker, which will take over as an **escape rhythm** (Figs 12–3 and 12–4) (Table 12–1).

AV dissociation is *not* a form of complete AV block. In AV block, atrial impulses *cannot* be conducted to the ventricles despite temporal opportu-

nity for this to occur. In contrast, in AV dissociation atrial impulses will *capture* (be conducted to and stimulate) the ventricles if temporal opportunity is provided.

Capture beats occur *prematurely* relative to the rate of the subsidiary pacemaker (Figs 12–1 and 12–3). They are a hallmark of AV dissociation. They often have morphologic features which are

Table 12-1. Some common causes of AV dissociation.

I. Due to slowing of atrial impulses with emergence
   of a subsidiary pacemaker
      Sinus bradycardia with sinus arrhythmia
      Sinoatrial exit block
      Sinus arrest
      High vagal tone
      Postcardioversion
      Beta-blocking drugs
      Some calcium channel–blocking agents
         (verapamil, diltiazem)
II. Due to acceleration of the rate of a subsidiary
   pacemaker
      Myocardial ischemia
      Digitalis toxicity
      Postoperative state
      Catecholamine stimulation
      Atropine

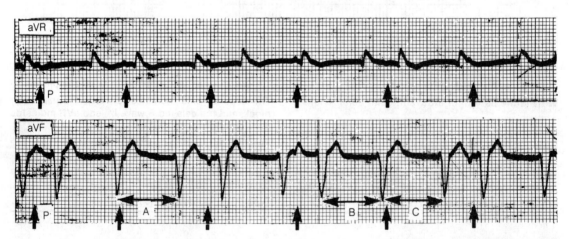

Figure 12-1. AV dissociation with capture. Two rhythms are present. A regular atrial rhythm (arrows) is present at a rate of 60/min. The P waves are upright in aVR and inverted in lead aVF, indicating retrograde atrial activation, presumably from a focus low in the atrium. The QRS rhythm occurs at a rate of 85/min (determined from the regular RR intervals shown at [A], [B], and [C]). The rate of the QRS rhythm and the normal duration of the QRS complexes indicate a focus of origin in the AV junction or bundle of His. In aVF, the second, fifth, seventh, and tenth QRS complexes occur early relative to the prevailing QRS rate and are preceded by P waves at intervals of 0.12 s. These early QRS complexes represent *capture* beats, that is, they are stimulated by the P waves that precede them. Ventricular capture is the hallmark of AV dissociation.

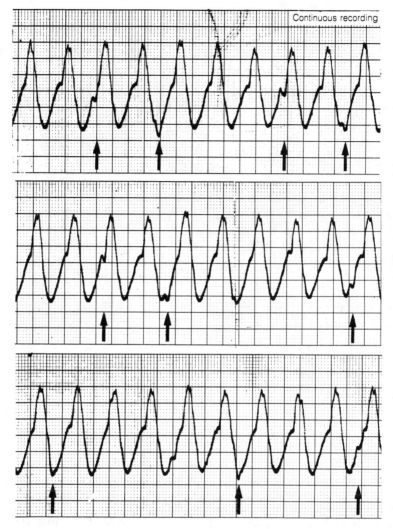

Figure 12-2. Wide QRS complex tachycardia at a rate of about 125/min. No clear P waves are seen preceding or following the QRS complexes. P waves do deform some of the ST–T waves of the tachycardia complexes (arrows); the P wave rate is about 75-85/min; their onsets are not clearly seen. The tracing illustrates dissociation between the wide QRS complexes and P waves. The rhythm is ventricular tachycardia with AV dissociation. In general, wide QRS complex tachycardias with AV dissociation are ventricular in origin.

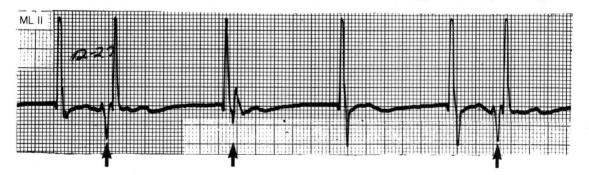

Figure 12-3. Narrow, normal-appearing QRS rhythm at a rate of 48/min (cycle length, 1240 ms). P waves are present at varying cycle length but each exceeding 1400 ms (arrows); they are exaggerated in this monitor lead. Earlier-than-expected QRS complexes are preceded by P waves at PR intervals of 0.12 s. These represent capture complexes (C). The rhythm is thus junctional rhythm with AV dissociation and capture.

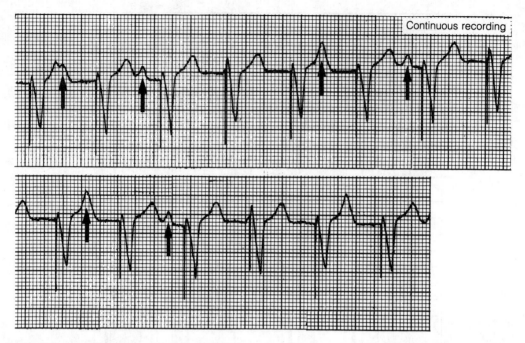

Figure 12-4. AV dissociation due to stimulation of the ventricles by a ventricular pacemaker. The atrial rhythm is sinus at a rate of 66/min (arrows). P waves do not stimulate QRS complexes. The ventricles are paced at a rate of 72/min. The longest P-to-pacing stimulus interval is 0.66 s (last complexes in the rhythm strip); since this interval is terminated by a paced QRS complex, the degree of intrinsic AV conduction block is unknown, although first-degree AV block is by definition present. Since the degree of AV block is not known from paced rhythms such as these, complete AV block cannot be said to be present. Since the sinus rhythm is independent from the paced ventricular rhythm, AV dissociation is present.

intermediate in configuration between complexes which have been stimulated by atrial impulses and those which have been stimulated by ectopic foci [whether the focus is an accelerated, an escape one, or one originating from a ventricular pacemaker (see Chapter 17) (Fig 12–4)]. Such complexes are called **fusion** complexes (Fig 12–5). Since the occurrence of fusion *implies* capture of the ventricles, fusion complexes are also hallmarks of AV dissociation. Long rhythm strips must often be recorded in order to demonstrate their presence.

When the AV dissociation is due to acceleration of the rate of a subsidiary pacemaker, the PR interval of the captured complex is often longer than expected. This reflects depolarization of the AV conducting tissue by the immediately preceding QRS impulse, and *not* first-degree AV block.

REFERENCES

Schott A: Atrioventricular dissociation with and without interference. *Prog Cardiovasc Dis* 1959;2:444.

Schubart AF et al: Isorhythmic dissociation: Atrioventricular dissociation with synchronization. *Am J Med* 1958;24:209.

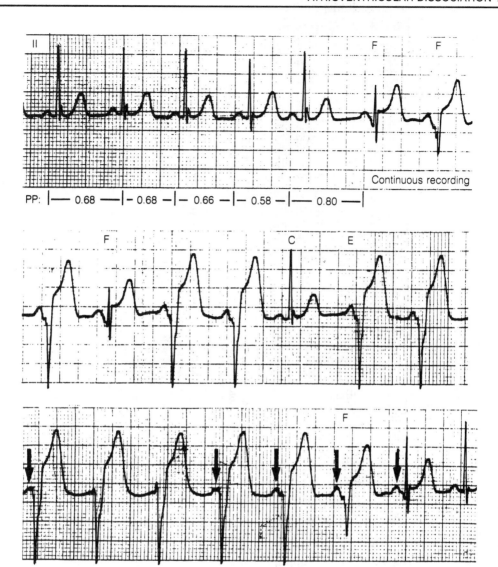

Figure 12-5. AV dissociation due to slowing of sinus rate and emergence of an escape rhythm. Sinus rhythm with a somewhat variable rate is present in the beginning of the rhythm strip. The PR intervals are 0.16 s. Between the fifth and sixth P waves there is a lengthening of the PP interval to 0.8 s. Following this P wave at short PR interval of 0.11 s is a QRS complex which is intermediate in configuration between the pure sinus-generated complexes and the broader QS complexes. This is a *fusion* complex (F), in which the ventricles have been depolarized both from the complex (F), in which the ventricles have been depolarized both from the sinus impulse and from the escape focus. An escape rhythm follows, which is interrupted by a capture beat (C). Sinus P waves can be seen at various times during the escape rhythm (arrows indicate some of them); their PR intervals vary, indicating that they are dissociated from the escape rhythm. At the end of the rhythm strip the sinus rate accelerates and reestablishes normal AV conduction. (F = fusion complexes; E = escape complex; C = capture complex.)

Figure 12-T1.
TEST TRACINGS

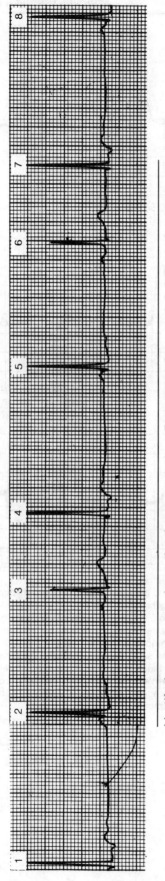

Identify the escape complexes, the sinus-generated complexes and the fusion complexes.

Escape complexes: 1, 2, 5, 8. The only *pure* escape complex is the 1st. Fusion complexes: 2, 5, 8. Sinus-generated complexes: 3, 6.

Identify the premature complexes. What is their probable origin? Why?

Premature complexes: 4, 7. They are probably originating near the AV junction since they have a normal duration but are slightly aberrant.

Explain the inverted P waves.

They represent retrograde atrial activation from the junctional premature focus.

Are the QRS complexes followed by inverted P waves dissociated from them?

No. Since the P waves are inverted the atria must have been depolarized retrogradely from the junctional focus. There is thus junctional-atrial association.

Is AV block present?

No.

Figure 12-T2.
TEST TRACINGS

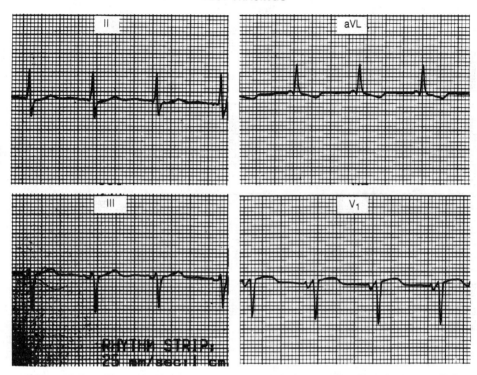

What is the rhythm?	Junctional is likely; low atrial rhythm is also possible.
Is AV dissociation present?	No. Each QRS complex has a P wave associated with it.
How are the atria depolarized?	Retrograde, since the P waves are inverted in lead III.
Is this an escape rhythm or an accelerated one?	Probably accelerated junctional rhythm, in view of its rate. However, since the onset is not seen, this is not known with certainty.

Figure 12-T3.
TEST TRACINGS

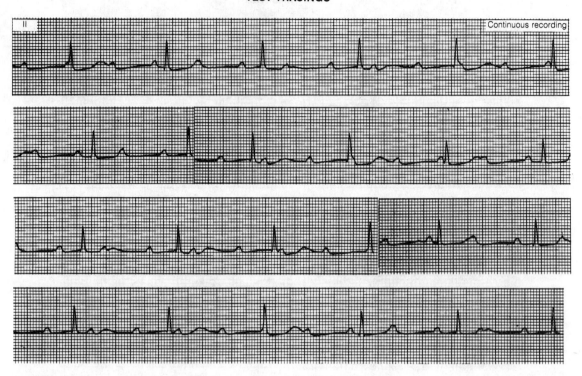

What is the atrial rhythm and rate?	Sinus, rate 100/min.
What criteria for AV dissociation are present?	An independent atrial and ventricular rhythm, and varying PR intervals.
What criteria for AV dissociation are not present?	Capture.
What criteria for AV block are present?	Independent atrial and ventricular rhythm without evidence of capture, and varying PR intervals.
What is the probable diagnosis?	AV block.
Where is the ventricular rhythm originating? Why?	Probably in the AV node–His bundle area, since the QRS duration and morphology are normal. The ventricular rate of 46/min is consistent with this focus of origin.

Figure 12–T4.
TEST TRACINGS

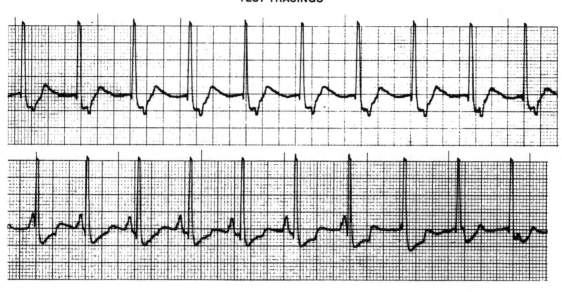

These 2 lead II rhythm strips were recorded from the same patient recorded seconds apart.

What is the rhythm in the top strip?	Junctional.
How are the atria depolarized? Why?	Retrogradely, indicated by the inverted P wave in lead II.
Is there AV dissociation or association?	Association, since each QRS is followed by an inverted P wave at relatively constant RP interval. The junctional focus has activated both ventricles and atria, including association between the two.
What is the atrial rhythm in the bottom strip?	Sinus.
Characterize the PR intervals.	Varying (shortening).
What occasions the emergence of the QRS rhythm not preceded by P waves?	Slowing of sinus rate.
Is the QRS rhythm at the end of the strip an accelerated one or an escape rhythm. Why?	It emerges with slowing of sinus rate. It is therefore an escape rhythm.
Where is it originating?	In the AV node or proximal His bundle, since the QRS morphology is identical to the sinus-generated QRS complexes.

Ventricular Premature Complexes

Ventricular premature complexes can arise from an **ectopic focus** in any portion of the ventricular myocardium or from **reentry** of an impulse (ventricular or supraventricular) into and through an area of ventricular tissue (Fig 13–1). Ectopic foci can be discharged by enhancement of automaticity or by triggering mechanisms (see Chapter 10). When ventricular premature complexes are due to reentry, the impulse conducted into the site of reentry is blocked in one area of ventricular tissue because of refractoriness, but is conducted through another area with some delay.

The impulse can then turn around and, because of its previously delayed transmission, reexcite the area that was previously refractory, resulting in a reentry beat. Premature ventricular complexes that have a **fixed coupling interval** to the QRS complexes preceding them are thought to arise by this mechanism (Fig 13–2).

Ventricular premature complexes may be conducted in retrograde manner into the His bundle and AV node, delaying or blocking antegrade conduction of the next sinus beat (Figs 13–2 through 13–4). They may be conducted to the atria and depolarize the atria in retrograde manner, result-

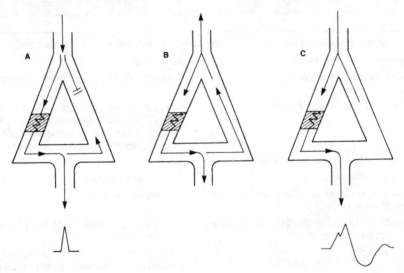

Figure 13-1. Reentry as a cause of ventricular extrasystoles. *A:* An impulse (supraventricular or ventricular) conducted from above into an area of ventricular tissue is blocked in one pathway and conducted with delay through another pathway (hatched area). The conducted impulse depolarizes myocardial tissue and also turns around and is conducted in a retrograde direction. *B:* The impulse has conducted in retrograde fashion through the area previously refractory and turns in antegrade fashion. *C:* The same impulse has again propagated through the area of conduction delay to the surrounding myocardium, in a particular temporal relationship to the original impulse (**coupled extrasystole**).

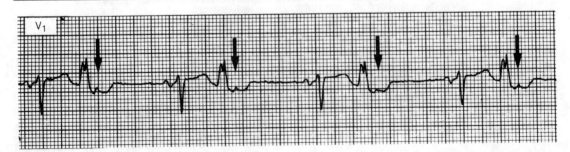

Figure 13-2. Premature ventricular complexes with fixed coupling intervals of 0.44 s to the QRS complexes preceding them. The atrial rhythm is sinus; the sinus impulses following the premature ventricular complexes are not conducted to the ventricles (arrows) due to refractoriness of the AV conduction system caused by the premature depolarizations.

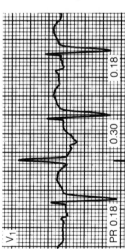

Figure 13–3. Premature ventricular complex causing delay in transmission of the next sinus impulse (concealed retrograde conduction into the AV node). This results in prolongation of the PR interval (in this example, from 0.18 s to 0.3 s). Concealed conduction causing delay in, or failure of, transmission of an antegradely conducting impulse should not be confused with AV block.

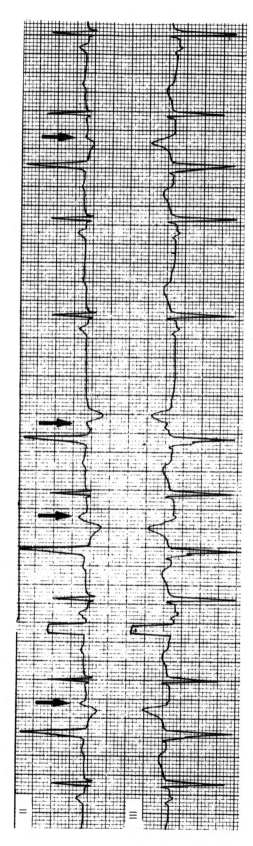

Figure 13–4. Pseudo–AV block due to concealed retrograde conduction. Sinus rhythm is present. Frequent uniform premature ventricular complexes are present. The P waves that follow them (arrows) are conducted to the ventricles with first-degree AV block (first, second, and fourth arrows) and are sometimes not conducted at all (third arrow). The AV block is due to concealed retrograde conduction into the AV node of the ventricular premature impulse, delaying or blocking subsequent antegrade impulse conduction.

ing in an inverted P wave in II, III, and aVF (Fig 13-5). They may invade the sinus node, depolarize it, and reset its timing, or they may depolarize the atria but not penetrate the sinus node and therefore not reset its timing (Fig 13-6). If the sinus node has been penetrated and reset by the ventricular premature impulse, the interval between the sinus beats enclosing the premature ventricular complex will be less than twice the sinus rate (**less than fully compensatory pause**). If the sinus node is not reset and the sinus firing rate is not disturbed, the next sinus impulse will occur on time. Thus, the interval between the sinus beats enclosing the ventricular premature complex will be twice the sinus rate (**fully compensatory pause**) (Fig 13-6).

Retrograde invasion of the AV node by a ventricular premature impulse can result in delay in antegrade transmission of the next sinus impulse or total failure of conduction of the impulse. Because the retrograde invasion of the AV node is not itself visible on the ECG but is recognized by its effect on subsequent electrocardiographic events, the phenomenon is known as **concealed conduction**. Delay in (or failure of) antegrade AV conduction due to concealed retrograde conduction of a ventricular premature impulse is termed **pseudo-AV block** (Figs 13-3 and 13-4).

Premature ventricular complexes may have similar configurations in a given electrocardiographic lead or more than one configuration. Uniform (**uni-morphic, monomorphic**) premature ventricular complexes may arise from a single focus or result from a reentry pathway (Fig 13-7). Premature ventricular complexes of varying configurations may arise from multiple foci (**multifocal**) or, more commonly, from a single focus but may be conducted through different pathways to depolarize the ventricular myocardium, resulting in different QRS configurations (Fig 13-8). The term **multiform** (or **polymorphic** or **multimorphic**), rather than multifocal, is therefore more precise in describing premature ventricular complexes of varying configurations in a given electrocardiographic lead.

Ventricular complexes are broad and bizarre in appearance and usually exceed 0.12 s in duration. They are often notched and slurred. The ST segment and T wave are usually displaced in a direction opposite to the main QRS deflection. If a P wave is associated with a premature ventricular complex, it may be a sinus P wave occurring in a fortuitous relation to the ventricular complex and therefore *dissociated* from it; or it may be a P wave caused by retrograde activation of the atria by the ventricular impulse (Fig 13-5). The retrograde atrial depolarization will result in an inverted P wave in II, III, and aVF; and its earlier occurrence in relation to the underlying sinus rate will distinguish it from a sinus impulse.

Occasionally, a premature ventricular complex will occur between 2 sinus impulses without disturbing the sinus rate. This is called an **interpolated premature ventricular complex** (Fig 13-9).

R-on-T Premature Ventricular Complexes

Since the QT interval approximates the refractory period of ventricular tissue, a premature ventricular complex is usually inscribed after the T wave of the preceding beat. However, a premature ventricualr complex will occasionally begin at the peak of the T wave or on its downstroke (Fig 13-10). R-on-T premature ventricular complexes may fall in the **vulnerable period** of ventricular tissue, initiating repetitive ventricular beating (tachycardia or fibrillation); they are thus considered to be of potentially serious clinical significance (Figs 13-11 and 13-12); however, many episodes of ventricular tachycardia or fibrillation are not preceded by R-on-T extrasystoles.

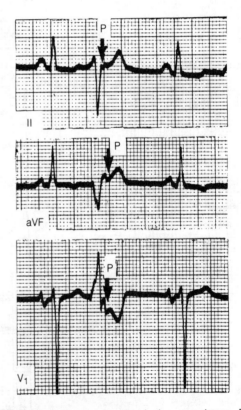

Figure 13-5. Premature ventricular complexes. The complexes are broad, bizarre, and prolonged. They are followed by P waves that are inverted in II and aVF, indicating retrograde atrial activation.

A

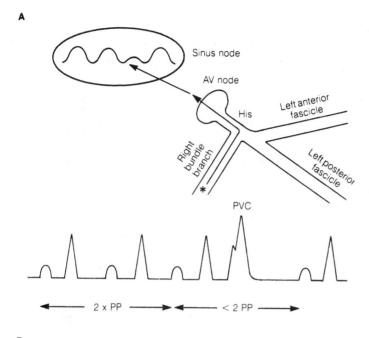

Figure 13-6. *A:* The premature ventricular impulse (*) is conducted in retrograde fashion to the atrium and through the SA area, depolarizing the sinus node and resetting its timing. (The partial premature depolarization of the sinus node does not result in atrial activation because of the suboptimal quality of the action potential.) The pause following the ventricular extrasystole is less than fully compensatory, as the PP interval encompassing the premature ventricular complex is less than twice the usual PP interval. *B:* The premature impulse has depolarized the atria in retrograde fashion but has not penetrated the SA area (entrance block); thus, the firing rate of the sinus node is not disturbed and the next sinus impulse occurs on time. The PP interval encompassing the premature ventricular complex is twice the normal PP interval, and the pause is fully compensatory.

B

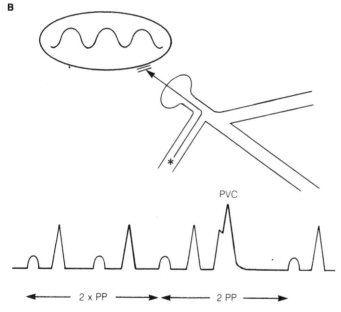

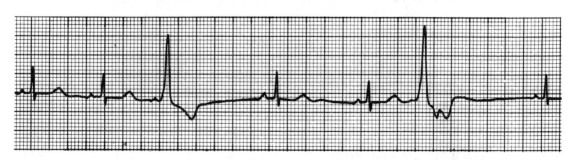

Figure 13-7. Uniform (''monomorphic'') premature ventricular complexes. These may arise from a single focus of origin or result from a reentry phenomenon. There is a fixed coupling interval between the sinus beats and the premature ventricular complexes, favoring the latter mechanism. (VPB = ventricular premature beats.)

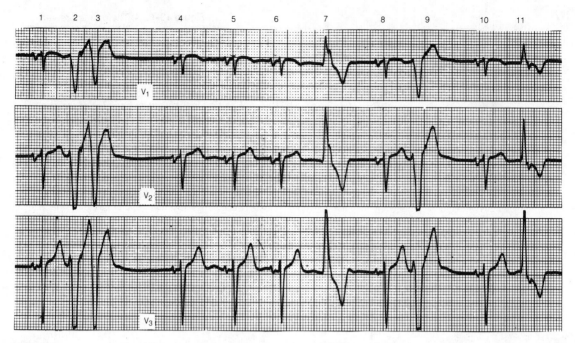

Figure13-8. Multiform premature ventricular complexes. QRS complexes 2, 3, and 9 are oriented posteriorly (deep S waves in V_{1-3}), suggesting a right ventricular focus of origin. QRS complexes 7 and 11 are oriented anteriorly (tall R waves in V_{1-3}) and suggest a left ventricular focus of origin. However, the site of origin of the ventricular complexes is difficult to tell with certainty, since the QRS configuration reflects intramyocardial impulse conduction and epicardial activation pattern rather than focus locations.

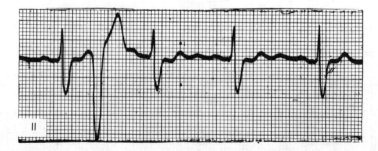

Figure 13-9. Interpolated premature ventricular complex. A broad, bizarre premature ventricular complex follows the first sinus-stimulated QRS complex but does not disturb the sinus rate. Thus, the premature ventricular beat is interpolated. The PR intervals of the first, third, and fourth sinus beats are 0.19 s, but that of the second sinus beat is 0.23 s. The prolongation in PR interval following the premature ventricular complex results from concealed retrograde conduction into the AV node by the premature complex, causing subsequent antegrade conduction delay. Note the prominent U waves following the T waves.

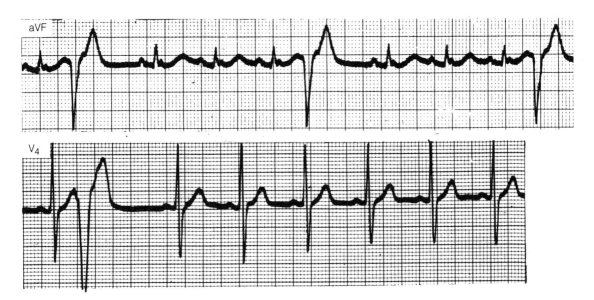

Figure 13–10. R-on-T premature ventricular complexes. The premature complexes are occurring near the peak of the T wave, during the time when the ventricles might be vulnerable to tachycardia or fibrillation. Since not all R-on-T premature ventricular impulses cause ventricular fibrillation, the vulnerable period must occupy an extremely critical time period during repolarization.

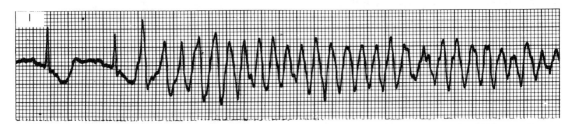

Figure 13–11. R-on-T premature ventricular complex occurring at the peak of the T wave of the preceding sinus beat. This premature complex falls during the vulnerable period of the ventricular tissue, resulting in polymorphic ventricular tachycardia.

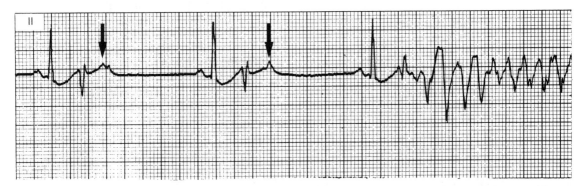

Figure 13–12. Ventricular bigeminy leading to ventricular fibrillation. The first 2 closely coupled premature ventricular depolarizations occur at intervals of 0.32 s to the preceding sinus complexes; the third premature complex occurs at a slightly shorter interval of about 0.3 s. Despite the fact that the first 2 premature ventricular depolarizations constitute the R-on-T phenomenon, only the third leads to a lethal arrhythmia. Thus, the vulnerable period to ventricular fibrillation is quite precise in a given clinical setting. P waves deform the T waves of the premature ventricular complexes (arrows), but it is not possible to tell from this tracing whether they are sinus in origin (with ventriculophasic sinus arrhythmia) or retrogradely conducted.

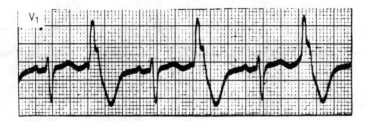

Figure 13-13. Ventricular bigeminy. After each sinus-conducted beat, a premature ventricular complex occurs at a fixed coupling interval. The sinus rhythm is undisturbed; however, in this arrhythmia the sinus *rate* cannot be ascertained, since consecutive sinus beats are not present.

Ventricular Bigeminy

In ventricular bigeminy, the rhythm alternates between a sinus beat (or any basic rhythm) and a ventricular premature complex (Fig 13–13). There is usually a constant interval between the sinus and ventricular complexes (**fixed coupling**), suggesting that reentry is the underlying mechanism for the ventricular impulse (Fig 13–1). Ventricular bigeminy is not itself a more dangerous rhythm than isolated premature ventricular beats; the significance of the arrhythmia will depend upon the present, type, and severity of underlying heart disease. Ventricular trigeminy (or quadrigeminy) describes an arrhythmia in which 2 (or 3) sinus beats are followed by a premature ventricular complex in repetitive fashion or in which one sinus beat is followed by 2 (or 3) consecutive premature ventricular complexes in repetitive fashion (Fig 13–14). Again, the prognosis depends on the underlying disease.

Premature Ventricular Complexes in Myocardial Infarction

In the presence of myocardial infarction, ventricular premature complexes may show some of the typical features of the infarction pattern, specifically a QR pattern. When myocardial infarction cannot be diagnosed from the ECG, as in left bundle branch block, the presence of premature ventricular complexes of QR or QRs (but not QS) configuration may confirm the diagnosis (Fig 13–15).

Postextrasystolic ST-T Wave Alterations

Occasionally, the ST-T wave of the sinus-stimulated QRS complex that follows a premature ventricular impulse will be different from that of other sinus-conducted beats (Fig 13–16). The difference may consist of more abnormal ST-T

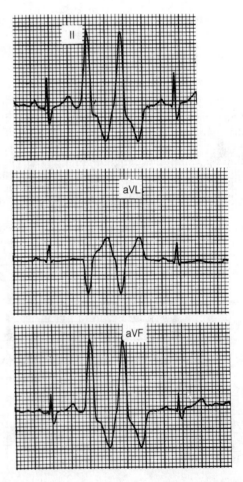

Figure 13-14. Ventricular doublet causing a pattern of trigeminy, in which 1 sinus-generated beat is followed by 2 consecutive premature ventricular complexes. The inferior and rightward direction of the ventricular complexes suggests a focus of origin in the right ventricular outflow tract, although this cannot be known with certainty.

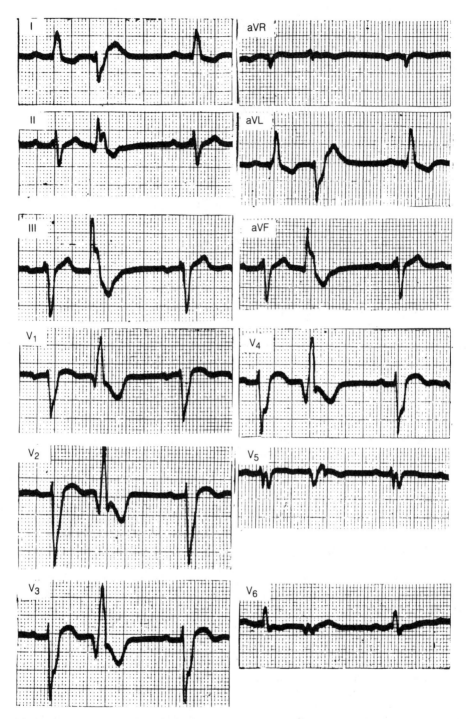

Figure 13-15. Premature ventricular complexes occurring in a patient with left bundle branch block pattern. The first and third complexes in each strip are sinus-stimulated, and the second QRS complex is a premature ventricular complex. The left bundle branch block pattern precludes the electrocardiographic diagnosis of myocardial infarction. However, the premature ventricular complexes have a QR pattern in the precordial leads, revealing underlying myocardial infarction (confirmed at autopsy).

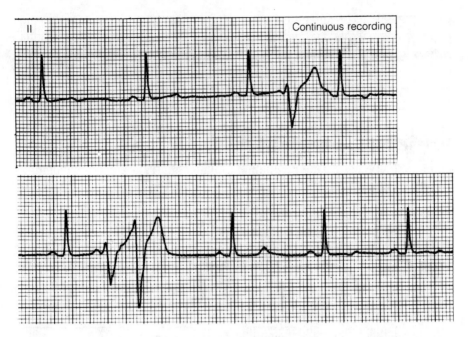

Figure 13–16. Postextrasystolic T wave alterations in a healthy 32-year-old man. The postextrasystolic T wave changes are themselves variable. Although this phenomenon was once thought to indicate coronary artery disease, it is now recognized to occur in normal individuals.

waves or "normalized" ST–T waves relative to the baseline. Although postextrasystolic ST–T wave changes are commonly seen in patients with coronary artery disease, they are nonspecific findings and therefore of no clinical significance.

VENTRICULAR TACHYCARDIA

Ventricular tachycardia is an arrhythmia originating in ventricular tissue, and may be sustained or non-sustained. It may originate in an automatic focus, from a reentry pathway, or by triggered automaticity (see Chapter 10). It may occur only within the ventricular myocardium, or it may involve the bundle branches and even the His bundle. Its rate exceeds the intrinsic ventricular rate of 20–50/min and usually ranges from 120 to 220/min. The rhythm may be irregular, especially if the tachycardia is short-lived. Although ventricular tachycardia is always a serious rhythm disturbance that requires early attention, it may or may not be associated with symptoms, depending upon the rate of the tachycardia, the relation of ventricular rate to atrial rhythm and rate, and the state of the myocardium. If there is AV dissociation, any atrial rhythm may be present; if a stable atrial rhythm such as sinus rhythm exists, adequate filling of the ventricles may occur and cardiac output will be maintained. However, if there is AV associ-

ation (as in ventriculoatrial conduction), ventricular and atrial systole may occur together, with insufficient time for ventricular filling via atrial systole to occur. Stroke output will fall rapidly, and cerebral hypoperfusion will result. Ventriculoatrial conduction may occur in a 1:1 relationship, a **ventriculoatrial Wenckebach** type of second-degree block, or a **fixed ventriculoatrial block** with 2:1 and 3:1 conduction ratios. Complete ventriculoatrial block may also occur.

Ventricular tachycardia complexes are broad and bizarre and resemble ventricular premature beats (Fig 13–17). The rate is often so rapid that the ST segment and T waves cannot be distinguished from the QRS complexes, and the ECG has the appearance of a series of wide, large undulations. If the atrial rhythm can be identified and AV dissociation demonstrated, the diagnosis of the wide complex tachycardia is ventricular tachycardia until proved otherwise (Fig 13–18).

Ventricular tachycardia may be **bradycardia-dependent**, that is, it may follow a pause in QRS rhythm. The pause may be due to SA block, sinus arrest, or AV block. Bradycardia-dependent ventricular tachycardia is thought to result from a premature ventricular impulse occurring during heterogeneous depolarization-repolarization sequences in ventricular myocardium. The heterogeneity in turn results from absence of a stimulus that would normally depolarize the tissue uniformly.

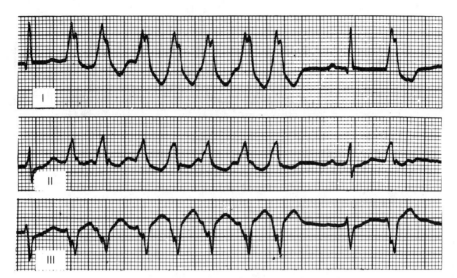

Figure 13-17. Sinus rhythm with a burst of ventricular tachycardia. Following the first sinus beat, there are 7 consecutive wide complexes occurring at a slightly irregular rate of 150/min. Following the burst of wide complex tachycardia, a premature ventricular complex is coupled to a sinus complex. Since the configuration of the premature ventricular complex is identical to the tachycardia complexes, the tachycardia is ventricular in origin.

Bidirectional ventricular tachycardia is the term applied to a rare form of ventricular tachycardia in which the QRS complexes in any one lead alternate in opposite directions (Fig 13-19). Its usual cause is digitalis toxicity.

Electrocardiographic Patterns in Ventricular Tachycardia

The QRS complex morphology in ventricular tachycardia is variable. Classic patterns have a superior mean frontal plane QRS axis, a qR, QR, or pure R wave configuraton in V_1, and an rS or QS

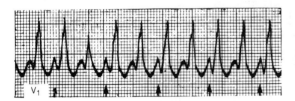

Figure 13-18. Ventricular tachycardia with AV dissociation. A wide complex rhythm is occurring at a rate of 173/min. The complexes have a pure R wave configuration in V_1. In alternate ST-T segments sharp deflections occur regularly at a rate of 95/min (arrows) and may be independent of the ventricular rhythm. If so, the atrial rhythm is sinus, the ventricular rhythm is ventricular tachycardia, and AV dissociation is present. An alternate explanation is that the wide complex tachycardia shows 2:1 ventriculoatrial conduction, with retrograde P waves occurring after every second tachycardia complex. Leads II or aVF would be required to ascertain the direction of atrial depolarization.

configuration in V_6 (Figs 13-20 and 13-21). Although tachycardias originating in the right ventricle are expected to have the configuration of left bundle branch block (since the right ventricular myocardium is activated in advance of the left ventricular myocardium) and those originating in the left ventricle are expected to have the configuration of right bundle branch block, electrode mapping studies of the endocardium and epicardium indicate that the tachycardia configuration does *not* necessarily indicate its origin. Whereas tachycardias with a right bundle branch block pattern often do originate in the left ventricular myocardium, most of those with a left bundle branch block pattern *also* originate in the left ventricular myocardium, particularly in the paraseptal area.

On occasion, the QRS configuration of ventricular tachycardia vary; the arrhythmia is then termed **polymorphic ventricular tachycardia**. Changes in QRS configuration do not indicate different foci of origin of impulses but rather reflect different pathways of myocardial activation taken by the tachycardia impulses.

A particular type of polymorphic ventricular tachycardia, in which the QRS complex configurations appear to undulate around an isoelectric baseline, is known as **torsades de pointes** (Fig 13-22). This form of ventricular tachycardia is seen in the presence of a long QTU interval due to any cause and may result from disparate depolarization-repolarization times in His-Purkinje tissue, reflected in the surface ECG as a long QTU interval. The tachycardia often occurs in self-terminating bursts but can degenerate into ventricular fibrillation.

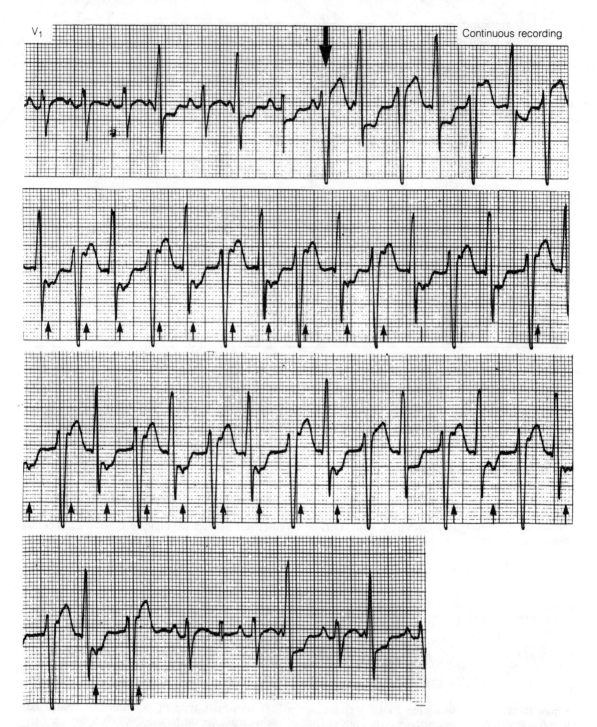

Figure 13-19. Bidirectional ventricular tachycardia in a patient with digitalis toxicity. The first 3 P–QRS complexes are sinus-stimulated, and the PR interval is 0.16 s. The fourth and sixth complexes are ventricular in origin and are dissociated from the P waves that precede them at short intervals. The third premature ventricular complex (large arrow) initiates a run of wide complex tachycardia with alternation of 2 QRS configurations. At the beginning of the second strip, 1:1 ventriculoatrial conduction occurs (small arrows). The tachycardia terminates spontaneously, and sinus rhythm resumes.

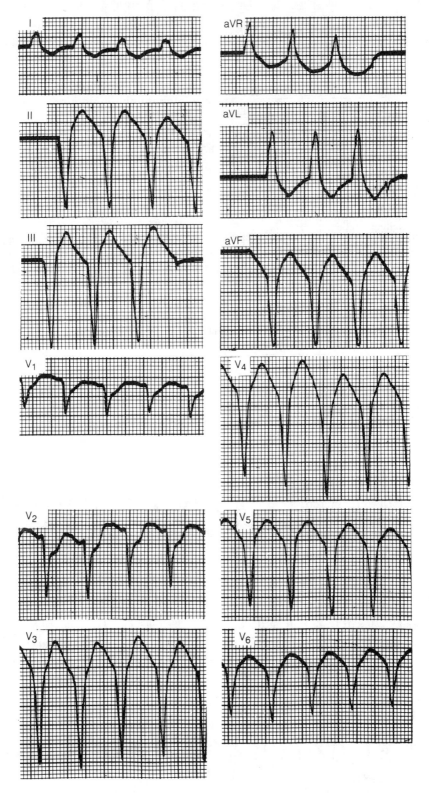

Figure 13-20. Ventricular tachycardia. The mean frontal plane QRS axis is directed superiorly and leftward. QS complexes are present in V$_{1-6}$ (*concordance* of QRS complex configuration). Atrial activity is discerned at times (eg, in the T wave of the second QRS complex in V$_2$) and is unrelated to the QRS rhythm.

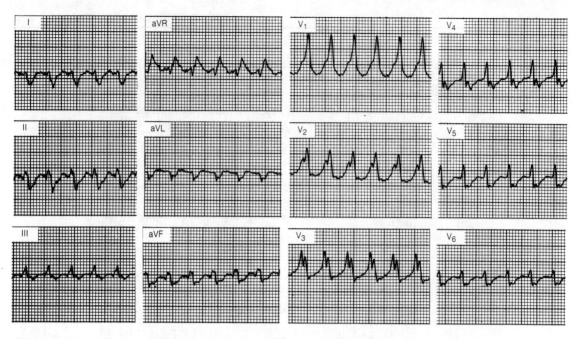

Figure 13-21. Rapid ventricular tachycardia (rate 215/min). The mean frontal plane QRS axis is directed rightward and superiorly. A pure R wave configuration is present in lead V_1, and an RS configuration in V_6. P waves occurring in 1:1 relationship to the tachycardia complexes are best seen in leads II and V_{1-2}; they appear to be inverted in lead II and thus represent retrograde atrial activation. The origin of this tachycardia was confirmed at electrophysiologic study.

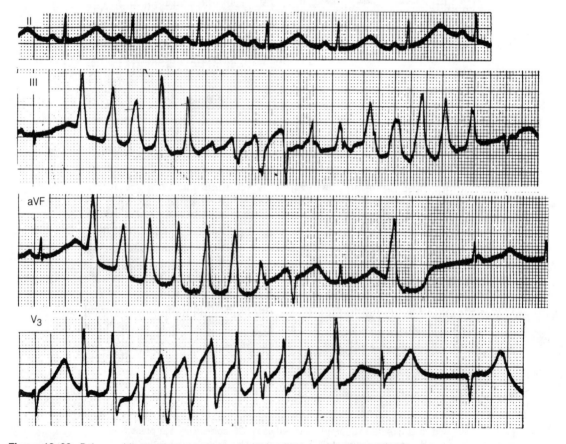

Figure 13-22. Polymorphic ventricular tachycardia. Sinus rhythm with a long QT interval is present. Self-terminating bursts of ventricular tachycardia are occurring, in which the QRS configuration is extremely variable and at times appears to rotate about an isoelectric point (**torsades de pointes**).

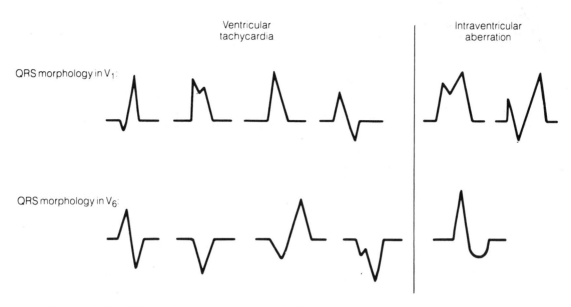

Figure 13-23. QRS complex morphology in ventricular tachycardia and in intraventricular aberration.

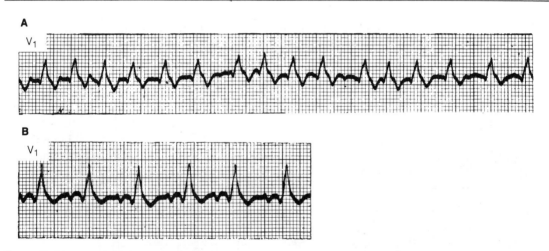

Figure 13-24. Atrial fibrillation with intraventricular conduction delay. *A:* Atrial fibrillation with wide complex ventricular rhythm at an irregular rate. The irregularity of the ventricular rhythm is evidence that it is not ventricular tachycardia. *B:* After sinus rhythm is restored, the pattern of intraventricular conduction is seen to be identical to that in *A.*

DIFFERENTIATION OF VENTRICULAR TACHYCARDIA FROM SUPRAVENTRICULAR TACHYCARDIA WITH INTRAVENTRICULAR ABERRATION

The differential diagnosis of ventricular tachycardia from supraventricular tachycardia with intraventricular aberration can be difficult (see Chapter 10), but certain clues can be helpful (Fig 13–23 and Table 13–1). If the atrial rhythm is fibrillation, the gross irregularity of the ventricular rhythm indicates that the QRS complexes are stimulated by the atrial fibrillation (Fig 13–24).

If the atrial rhythm is sinus, it will occur at a rate independent from that of the ventricular tachycardia and will therefore be dissociated from it. A wide complex tachycardia with AV dissociation is likely to be ventricular in origin. The same principle applies to an automatic atrial tachycardia. The simultaneous occurrence of an automatic atrial tachycardia and a ventricular tachycardia is known as **double tachycardia.**

If the atrial rhythm is flutter, differential diag-

Table 13-1. Wide QRS complex tachycardia: feature distinguishing ventricular tachycardia from supraventricular tachycardia with intraventricular aberration.

	VT	IV Aberration
QRS morphology	V_1: qR, R, RS, RR'	rSR'
	V_6: rS, QS, QR	Rs with wide S
QRS duration	> 0.14 s	< 0.14 s
Mean frontal plane QRS axis	Often superior	Depends upon prior bundle branch block and presence or absence of rate-dependent bundle branch block.
AV dissociation	Yes	No
Capture or fusion complexes	Yes	No

nosis of a wide complex tachycardia will depend primarily on the morphology of the QRS complexes (Fig 13–23) and the behavior of the rhythm during maneuvers that delay conduction at the AV node, such as carotid sinus massage. Carotid sinus massage is expected to slow the ventricular rate if the ventricular rhythm is stimulated by the flutter waves; it usually has no effect on ventricular tachycardia.

It may be impossible to distinguish between supraventricular reciprocating tachycardia with aberrant intraventricular conduction and ventricular tachycardia if ventriculoatrial association with 1:1 ventriculoatrial conduction of the tachycardia complexes to the atria is present (Figs 13–21 and 13–25). Again, QRS morphology and axis and response to vagal maneuvers may be helpful; increasing AV block by vagal maneuvers is expected to terminate a reciprocating supraventricu-

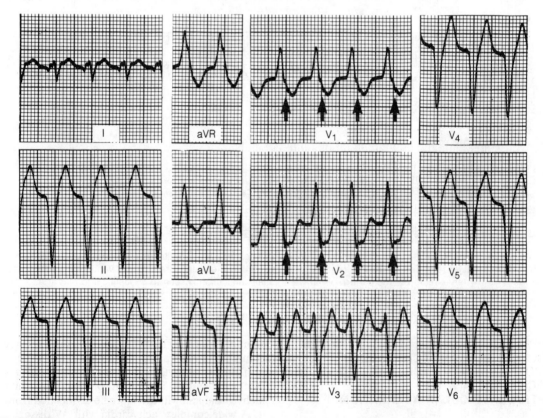

Figure 13-25. Wide complex tachycardia, which could be reciprocating supraventricular tachycardia with intraventricular aberration or ventricular tachycardia. The mean frontal plane axis of the tachycardia complexes is superior and rightward, and the precordial lead configuration suggests ventricular tachycardia (pure R wave in V_1 and a QS wave in V_6). P waves are seen following the QRS complexes in V_{1-2} (arrows), which, since they could represent either retrograde atrial activation from ventricular tachycardia or reciprocating supraventricular tachycardia, do not help to differentiate between the two. In this case, the configuration of the QRS complexes is the best evidence as to the ventricular origin of the tachycardia.

lar tachycardia, whereas no effect on ventricular tachycardia will be observed. Occasionally, vagal maneuvers will produce ventriculoatrial block and alter 1:1 ventriculoatrial conduction to 2:1, Wenckebach, or complete retrograde ventriculoatrial block; this will aid in establishing the diagnosis of ventricular tachycardia.

ACCELEREATED VENTRICULAR RHYTHM

Accelerated ventricular rhythm is a ventricular rhythm that is faster than an "idioventricular" rhythm (usual rate, 30-40/min) but slower than rapid ventricular tachycardia. It is characterized by 3 features: (1) emergence as a result of slight slowing of the sinus rate; (2) disappearance as a result of an increase in the sinus rate; and (3) onset and offset via fusion complexes, in which the ventricles are depolarized by both the sinus impulse and the ventricular focus (Fig 13-26). Since this rhythm is considered to be benign, its recognition is most important so as to avoid unnecessary treatment. Since it is actually an escape rhythm, treatment is not generally indicated. Accelerated ventricular rhythm must be distinguished from "slow" ventricular tachycardia (Fig 13-27), in which the onset is via a premature ventricular complex without prior fusion and the offset is spontaneous and unrelated to an increase in the sinus rate.

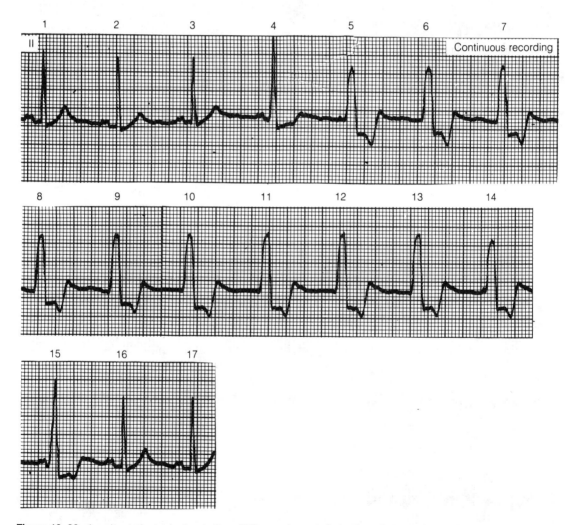

Figure 13-26. Accelerated ventricular rhythm. QRS complexes 1, 2, 3, 16, and 17 are sinus-conducted beats. Beats 5 through 14 have wide QRS complexes, are not preceded by P waves, and are regular at a rate of 75/min. Complexes 4 and 15 are preceded by sinus P waves but with shorter PR intervals and longer QRS intervals than the sinus-conducted beats. These are **fusion beats**, in which ventricular depolarization results in part from the sinus impulse and in part from the ventricular focus. Onset and offset of accelerated ventricular rhythm depends upon the slowing and subsequent increase in the sinus rate, respectively.

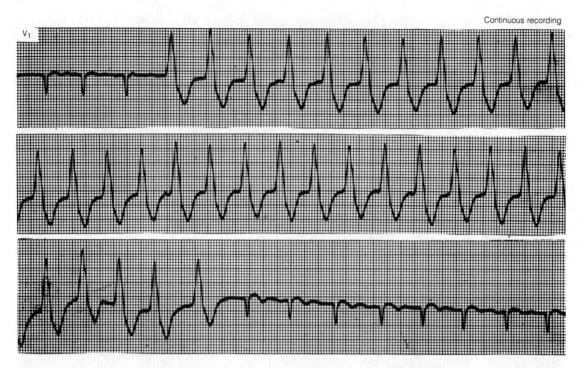

Continuous recording

V₁

Figure 13-27. ''Slow ventricular tachycardia.'' The rhythm is atrial fibrillation. A self-terminating wide complex rhythm of pure R wave configuration occurs, initially at a rate of about 100/min, and increases to 120/min. The QRS configuration of the wide complex rhythm suggests a ventricular origin; its somewhat irregular rate is not inconsistent with this diagnosis. ''Slow ventricular tachycardia'' must be distinguished from accelerated ventricular rhythm, as the former is not necessarily benign, whereas the latter more often is.

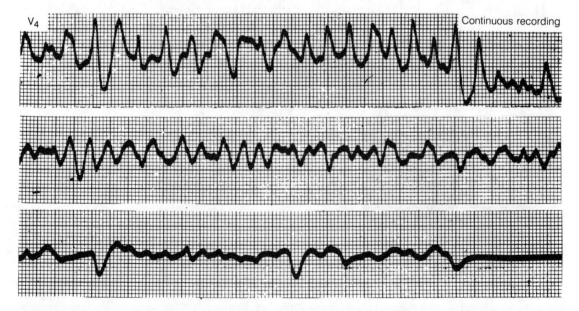

V₄   Continuous recording

Figure 13-28. Polymorphic ventricular tachycardia degenerating to ventricular fibrillation. The ventricular complexes in the second and third strips are rapid, irregular, and bizarre—typical of ventricular fibrillation. The rhythm terminates with asystole.

VENTRICULAR FIBRILLATION

Ventricular fibrillation is a rapid, irregular, disorganized ventricular rhythm resulting in lack of cardiac output and absent pulse and blood pressure. It usually results from a premature ventricular complex occurring in the vulnerable period of ventricular tissue. The ECG shows bizarre complexes of varying sizes and configurations (Fig 13–28). Electrical defibrillation is the only means of management; otherwise, death will result. Rarely, an episode of ventricular fibrillation is self-terminating. Ventricular fibrillation can follow a single closely coupled (R-on-T) ventricular depolarization (Fig 13–12), but more commonly results from the degeneration of monomorphic or polymorphic ventricular tachycardia. (Fig 13–29).

REFERENCES

Eysmann SB et al: Electrocardiographic changes after cardioversion of ventricular arrhythmias. *Circulation* 1986;**73**:73.

Fontaine G, Frank R, Grosgogeat Y: Torsades de pointes: Definition and management. *Mod Concepts Cardiovasc Dis* 1982;**51**:103.

Josephson ME et al: Sustained ventricular tachycardia: Role of the 12-lead electrocardiogram in localizing site of origin. *Circulation* 1981;**64**:257.

Langendorf R, Pick A, Winternitz M: Mechanisms of intermittent ventricular bigeminy: Appearance of ectopic beats dependent upon length of the ventricular cycle, the "role of bigeminy." *Circulation* 1955; **11**:422.

Schamroth L: Ventricular extrasystoles, ventricular tachycardia, and ventricular fibrillation: Clinical-electrocardiographic considerations. *Prog Cardiovasc Dis* 1980;**23**:13.

Wellens HJ, Bär FW, Lie KI: The value of the electrocardiogram in the differential diagnosis of a tachycardia with a widened QRS complex. *Am J Med* 1978;**64**:27.

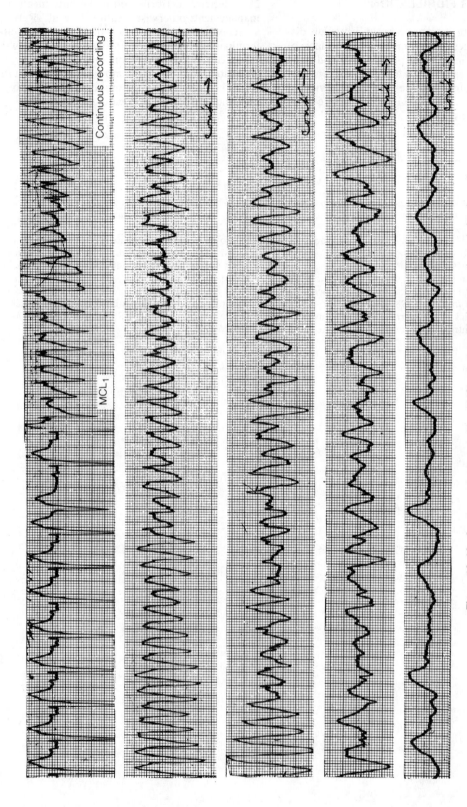

Figure 13-29. Continuously recorded lead MCL₁ rhythm strip from a patient admitted with acute myocardial infarction. Sinus rhythm is present at the beginning of the strip. A closely coupled ventricular depolarization (arrow) initiates a run of sustained polymorphic ventricular tachycardia which degenerates into ventricular fibrillation.

Figure 13–T1.
TEST TRACINGS

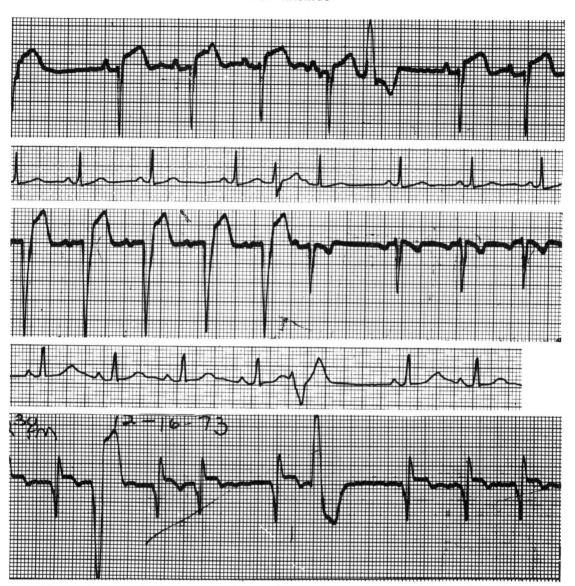

Identify the rhythm strip(s) which show the following:

Interpolated PVCs without concealed conduction	B
Multiform PVCs	A, E
Uniform (unimorphic) PVCs	C
Isorhythmic AV dissociation	C
Retrograde conduction to the atrium	None
Fully compensatory pause	D
R-on-T phenomenon	A (first PVC), D

Figure 13–T2.
TEST TRACINGS

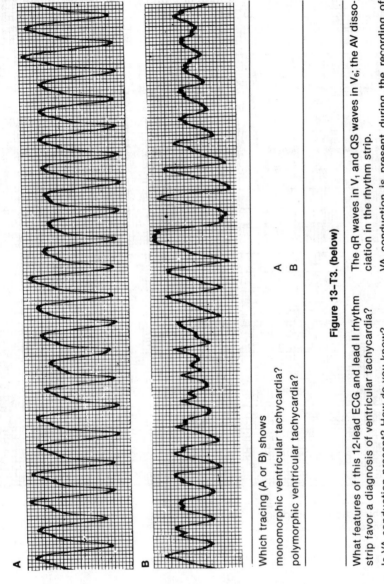

A

B

Which tracing (A or B) shows

monomorphic ventricular tachycardia?   A

polymorphic ventricular tachycardia?   B

Figure 13–T3. (below)

What features of this 12-lead ECG and lead II rhythm strip favor a diagnosis of ventricular tachycardia?	The qR waves in V_1 and QS waves in V_6; the AV dissociation in the rhythm strip.
Is VA conduction present? How do you know?	VA conduction is present during the recording of most of the 12-lead ECG. The P waves are inverted in II, III, and aVF.
Does VA conduction favor a ventricular rhythm or a supraventricular (junctional) one with intraventricular aberration?	Ventricular.
Is AV dissociation present?	Yes, in the rhythm strip.
Does AV dissociation favor a diagnosis of ventricular or supraventricular rhythm with intraventricular aberration?	Ventricular rhythm.

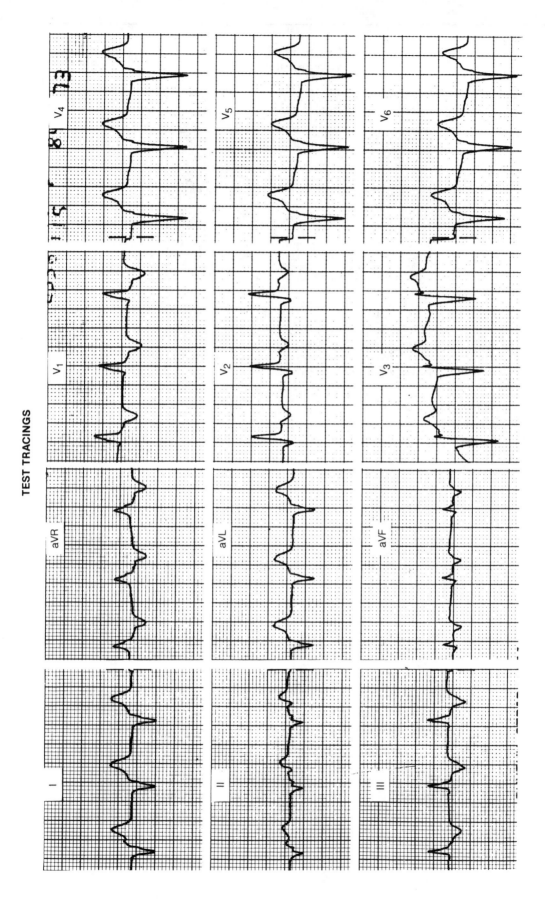

Figure 13–T4.
TEST TRACINGS

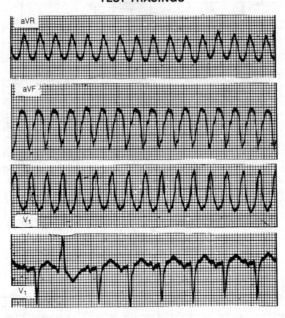

What is the mean frontal plane QRS axis?	Superior and rightward.
What is the QRS duration?	About 0.2 s.
What is the tachycardia rate?	250/min.
Does the rate favor ventricular or supraventricular tachycardia?	Neither one.
Is AV dissociation present?	Cannot tell.
What criteria favor a diagnosis of ventricular tachycardia?	The wide QRS duration, the superior axis, and the qR premature ventricular complex in V_1, which resembles the tachycardia complexes in V_1.

Figure 13–T5.
TEST TRACINGS

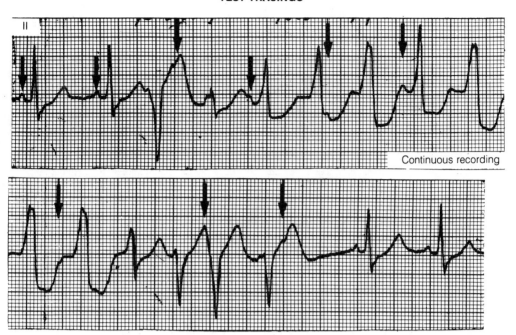

Continuous recording

Describe the run of ventricular tachycardia.	Polymorphic.
Is AV dissociation present?	Yes; the sinus P waves are denoted by the arrows.
Are fusion complexes present?	Yes; the fifth QRS complex is a fusion complex. The eighth may also be.

Figure 13–T6.
TEST TRACINGS

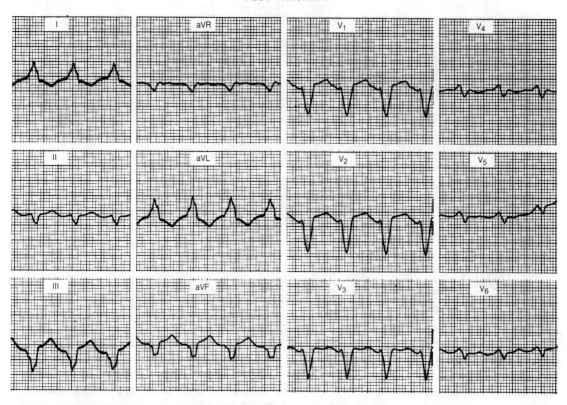

This ECG was recorded from a patient with congestive heart failure and renal failure, who was taking amiodarone for past ventricular tachycardia.

What is the mean frontal plane QRS axis?

Superior and leftward.

What is the QRS duration?

0.18 s.

What features favor ventricular tachycardia?

The QRS duration and the RS morphology in V_6.

What features favor supraventricular tachycardia with intraventricular aberration?

The pattern of intraventricular conduction resembles left bundle branch block; sinus P waves precede the QRS complexes (best seen in V_1).

Parasystole

14

Parasystole is an abnormal rhythm in which 2 pacemakers discharge independently of each other. One pacemaker is the dominant pacemaker of the heart and is therefore usually the sinus node. The parasystolic pacemaker may be located in the atrium (Fig 14-1), the AV junction, or the ventricles (Fig 14-2). Ventricular parasystole is the most common parasystolic rhythm observed.. Iatrogenic parasystolic foci are exemplified by cardiac pacemakers, functioning in a nonsensing (asynchronous) mode (see Chapter 17), which compete with spontaneous cardiac rhythm; and by heart transplantations, in which the atrial impulses from both the donor and recipient hearts

are visible on the surface ECG. (However, since one of these foci—the recipient's—is incapable of depolarizing the donor's ventricular myocardium, this does not represent true parasystole.)

A parasystolic focus generates impulses at about the same rate over long periods of time (up to years); the usual rates are 20/min to 100/min. Parasystolic tachycardia is rare. Parasystolic foci are usually not depolarized by the normal cardiac impulses because of a phenomenon known as **entrance block**, which prevents the normal cardiac depolarization wave front from penetrating the parasystolic foci to reset their rates. And, despite the continuous discharge of impulses by a para-

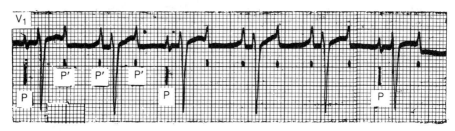

Figure 14-1. Atrial parasystole. Sinus P waves occur at a rate of 77/min. Not all sinus P waves (P) are seen, however, because of the presence of a parasystolic tachycardia (P') at 150/min. The AV conduction ratio of the parasystolic rhythm is 2:1.

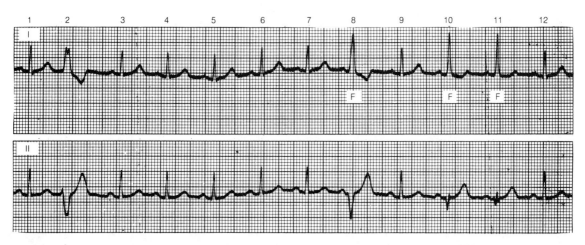

Figure 14-2. Ventricular parasystole. Most QRS complexes are sinus-stimulated. The second QRS complex is ventricular in origin and is not preceded by a P wave. The eighth, tenth, and eleventh QRS complexes are preceded by P waves and have configurations intermediate between the sinus-stimulated complexes and the ventricular complex; these are fusion complexes (F). The intervals between the ventricular and fusion complexes and the preceding normally conducted QRS complexes are not fixed coupled. The interectopic intervals between the second and eighth complexes is 3.9 s, between the eighth and tenth complexes is 1.3 s, and between the tenth and eleventh complex is 0.65 s. These intervals are all multiples of 0.65 s, indicating a parasystolic rate of 92/min.

systolic focus, most do not progagate very far out-side the focus (**exit block**) and thus do not depo-larize the surrounding myocardium to produce a complex on the surface ECG. Entrance and exit blocks surrounding a parasystolic focus are usu-ally of high degree, but occasionally first- and second-degree entrance and exit blocks can be demonstrated, and explain the occasional vari-ation in the parasystolic rate.

The activation of myocardium from a parasys-tolic focus will depend upon the state of refractor-iness of that myocardium. For example, a ventric-ular parasystolic complex will be seen on the surface ECG only when the ventricles are nonre-fractory and therefore capable of being depolar-ized. Since the discharge rate of a parasystolic fo-cus is constant, and since impulses do not exit the focus while others which do cannot depolarize the myocardium because of refractoriness, the com-plexes that are inscribed have *no constant relation* to preceding complexes, but are *multiples* of a ba-sic *interectopic rate*. Not uncommonly, *fusion* complexes, in which the ventricles (or atria) are stimulated by both the sinus-conducted impulse and the parasystolic impulse, occur. The 2 criteria for the electrocardiographic diagnosis of parasys-tole are, therefore, (1) *absence of a fixed coupling interval* between the normally conducted P wave or QRS complex and the parasystolic complex, and (2) demonstration of a *basic interectopic in-terval* of which the visible parasystolic complexes are multiples. The occurrence of atrial or ventric-ular fusion complexes is common, but not a crite-rion for diagnosis.

REFERENCES

Chung EK: Parasystole. *Prog Cardiovasc Dis* 1968;**11**:64.

Kinoshita S: Mechanisms of ventricular parasystole. *Circulation* 1978;**58**:715.

Langendorf R, Pick A: Parasystole with fixed coupling. *Circulation* 1967;**35**:304.

Singer DH et al: Ventricular parasystole and reentry: Clinical-electrophysiological correlations. *Am Heart J* 1974;**88**:79.

Watanabe Y: Reassessment of parasystole. *Am Heart J* 1971;**81**:451.

Figure 14–T1.
TEST TRACINGS

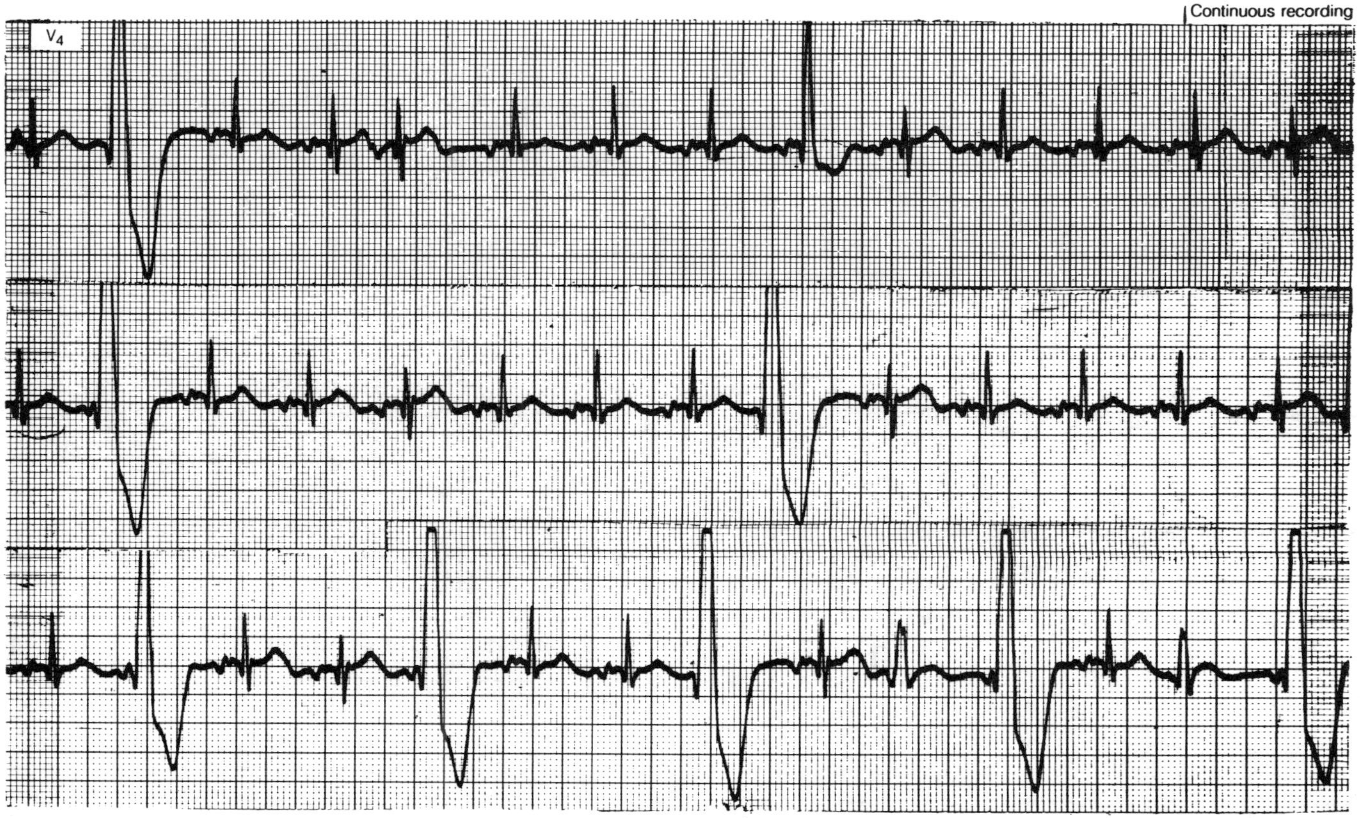

| Continuous recording

V₄

What criteria in this rhythm strip satisfy the diagnosis of a parasystolic rhythm?

What criteria for parasystolic rhythm are not satisfied?

Lack of fixed coupled interval between the premature ventricular complexes and the preceding QRS complexes; presence of fusion complexes.

There is no constant interectopic interval.

Figure 14-T2.
TEST TRACINGS

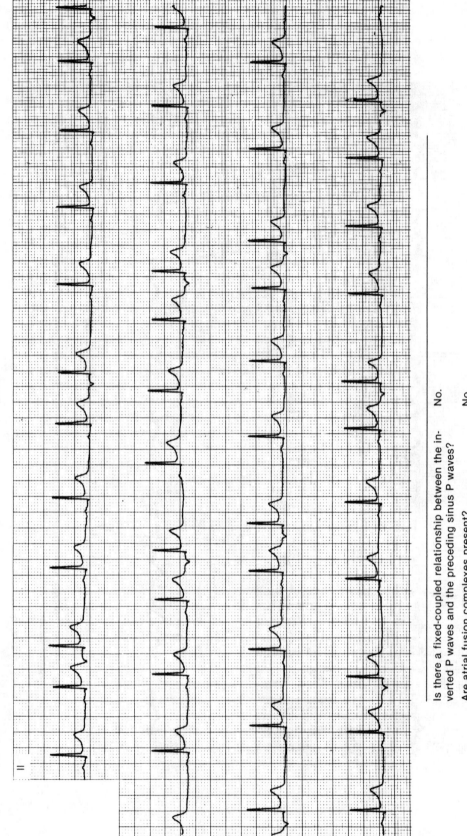

Is there a fixed-coupled relationship between the inverted P waves and the preceding sinus P waves?   No.

Are atrial fusion complexes present?   No.

Is there constant interectopic interval?   No.

Is this atrial parasystole?   Probably not.

Preexcitation Syndromes

15

Ventricular preexcitation is a term used to describe conditions in which ventricular activation occurs earlier than would be expected from activation via the normal AV node–His-Purkinje system. The preexcitation conduction patterns are characterized by specific electrocardiographic features which depend upon the particular pathway of ventricular depolarization. The syndromes are associated with a high incidence of tachyarrhythmias, which are usually reentrant in nature (see Chapter 10). Fig 15–1 illustrates some of the recognized accessory AV conduction pathways. Classification of ventricular preexcitation is as follows (Figs 15–1 and 15–2): (1) **Atrioventricular (AV) bypass tracts**, which connect atrial tissue directly with the ventricular tissue (Wolff-Parkinson-White [WPW] conduction); (2) **nodoventricular fibers**, which connect the AV node with the ventricular myocardium; (3) **fasciculoventricular fibers**, which connect a fascicle with the ventricular myocardium (Mahaim conduction); (4) **Atrionodal** or **atrio-His tracts**, which bypass much of the AV node and connect atrial fibers with the distal

portion of the AV node (James fibers) or His bundle; and (5) **intra–AV nodal fibers** in which rapid conduction occurs. Mapping of AV conduction pathways in the electrophysiology laboratory using multiple electrode catheters placed in various locations in the heart can define these pathways relatively precisely.

WOLFF-PARKINSON-WHITE CONDUCTION

In WPW conduction, the sinus impulse arises normally in the sinus node. It is then conducted through the atria to the accessory pathway in addition to the normal AV node. The accessory pathway may involve the left or right atrial and ventricular free walls or the interventricular septum. The impulse may then be conducted to the ventricles in 3 different ways. First, it can be conducted entirely in the accessory pathway, bypassing the AV node and thus the normally encountered AV nodal conduction delay. This results in a short PR

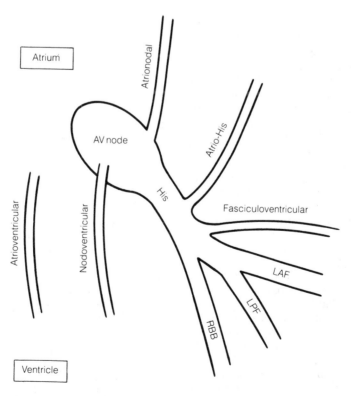

Figure 15–1. Diagram of accessory pathways. LBB, left bundle branch; LAF, left anterior fascicle; LPF, left posterior fascicle; RBB, right bundle branch.

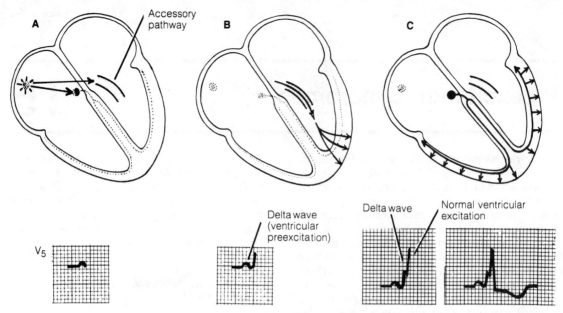

Figure 15-2. Diagram of one form of ventricular preexcitation. *A:* The sinus impulse traverses the normal pathways to the AV node and it also conducted to the accessory pathway. *B:* The impulse is conducted rapidly in the accessory AV pathway, directly from atrial to ventricular myocardium, without encountering the normal conduction delay within the AV node (ventricular preexcitation). A *delta wave* is inscribed in the QRS complex, reflecting early activation of the ventricular myocardium. *C:* The impulse is also conducted through the normal AV node–His-Purkinje system to the ventricular myocardium. Because this portion of the impulse does encounter the normal conduction delay in the AV node, it depolarizes a portion of the ventricular myocardium later than that conducted through the accessory pathway. The QRS complex inscribed is therefore a fusion complex, representing ventricular activation occurring via the normal AV node–His-Purkinje system and the accessory AV pathway. Pure normally conducted and pure preexcited complexes may occur; most WPW complexes are fusion complexes. Because ventricular depolarization is abnormal, repolarization is also abnormal, precluding interpretation of ST–T deviations.

interval (less than 0.1 s). Because AV nodal conduction of the impulse does not occur, the ventricular myocardium is depolarized earlier than normal; this results in the inscription of a slur at the beginning of the QRS complex—the **delta wave** (Fig 15-2). Second, the sinus impulse can be conducted entirely in the normal AV node–His-Purkinje system, resulting in a normal PR interval and QRS complex. Third, it can be conducted to the ventricles over both pathways, utilizing each to different degrees depending upon the location of the accessory pathway and the conduction velocities within the pathways; this results in a **fusion complex**, reflecting ventricular depolarization occurring via both the normal AV conduction pathway and the accessory pathway. The PR interval of the fusion complex will be shorter than normal, and the QRS complex may be less or more wide and slurred; the delta wave must be present, however, for the diagnosis of WPW conduction to be made (Fig 15-3).

The electrocardiographic patterns in WPW conduction may mimic myocardial infarction. The delta wave may be oriented superiorly, producing Q waves in II, III, and aVF (Fig 15-4) and simulating inferior' wall myocardial infarction; anteriorly, producing R waves in V_1 and simulating posterior wall myocardial infarction; or inferiorly and rightward, producing Q waves in I and

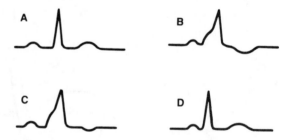

Figure 15-3. Patterns of ventricular preexcitation. *A:* Normal AV conduction. The P-QRS complex is normal, since the ventricles are depolarized via the normal AV node–His-Purkinje system. *B:* Accessory AV conduction (WPW). The PR interval is short (since the AV node has been bypassed), and the QRS complex has a slur on its upstroke (the delta wave), reflecting early ventricular activation. *C:* Nodoventricular conduction. The PR interval is normal, since the sinus impulse is conducted normally through the AV node. The QRS complex is slurred and exhibits a delta wave, since the ventricular myocardium has been preexcited via the nodoventricular pathway. *D:* Short PR interval with normal QRS complex. The PR interval may be short because of an anatomically short AV node, an intra-AV nodal bypass tract that bypasses the area of normal conduction delay, or a direct atrionodal or atrio-His connection. The QRS complex is normal, since the ventricles are depolarized via the normal His-Purkinje system.

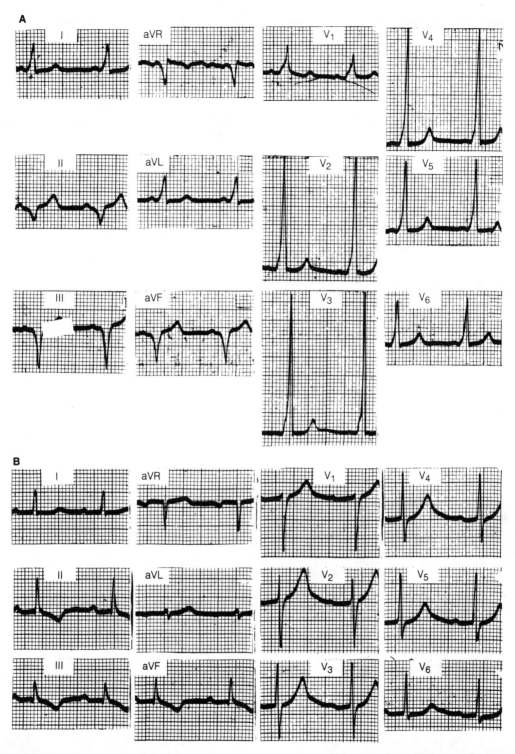

Figure 15-4. Ventricular preexcitation (WPW conduction) (A) reverting to normal (B). *A:* WPW conduction. The PR interval = 0.1 s. A positive delta wave is present in I, aVL, and V4-5, and a negative delta wave is seen in II, III, and aVF. The negative delta wave should not be confused with the Q wave of myocardial infarction. *B:* After treatment with quinidine, which has caused conduction delay in the accessory AV pathway to exceed that in the AV node, conduction of the sinus impulses is occurring normally via the AV node–His-Purkinje system. The PR interval is normal, and the QRS complexes do not show delta waves.

aVL, mimicking anterior wall infarction. When WPW conduction is present and ventricular depolarization is therefore abnormal, myocardial infarction *cannot be read* from the ECG. Conversely, an infarction pattern present during normal AV conduction can be masked by the development of WPW complexes.

The electrocardiographic patterns in WPW conduction can also mimic ventricular hypertrophy. An anteriorly oriented delta wave can produce a tall R wave in V_1, mimicking right ventricular hypertrophy. Similarly, a left and posteriorly oriented delta wave can inscribe deep QS waves in leads V_{1-3} and tall R waves in leads I, aVL, and V_{5-6} (as well as secondary ST–T wave abnormalities), mimicking left ventricular hypertrophy.

The electrocardiographic pattern of WPW conduction has no special clinical significance per se;

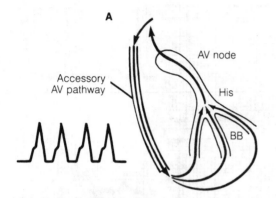
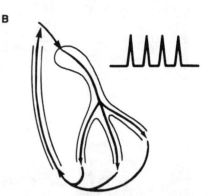

Figure 15–5. Diagrams of mechanisms of reciprocating supraventricular tachycardias in accessory AV conduction (WPW). *A:* Antegrade conduction over the accessory AV pathway and retrograde conduction through the bundle branches (BB), bundle of His, and AV node. The QRS complexes will show the preexcitation pattern. If the ventricles are depolarized via the accessory AV pathway and the patient develops rapid atrial arrhythmias such as flutter or fibrillation, the ventricular rate can be extremely rapid, leading to ventricular fibrillation. *B:* Antegrade conduction down the normal AV node–His-Purkinje system and retrograde conduction in the accessory pathway. The QRS complexes will appear normal. Retrograde conduction in an accessory pathway is *concealed*, since it is not visible on the surface ECG

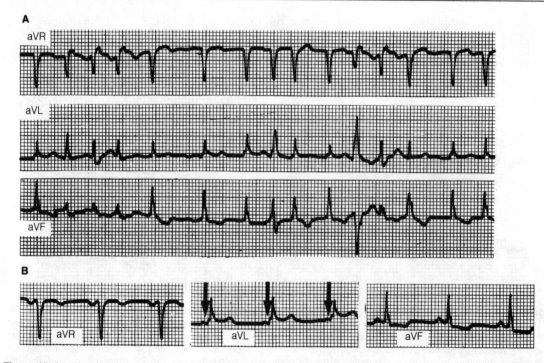

Figure 15–6. Atrial fibrillation in a patient with WPW syndrome. The QRS complexes reflect varying degrees of fusion. The ventricular rate is at times extremely rapid, approaching 240/min. Rapid ventricular rates reflect the direct transmission of atrial fibrillatory impulses into ventricular tissue via the AV bypass tract. *B:* After DC cardioversion, sinus rhythm is restored. The PR interval = 0.08 s, and a delta wave is seen in aVL (arrows).

however, patients with this type of ventricular pre-excitation are prone to develop paroxysmal reciprocating tachycardias (Fig 15–5) (see Chapter 10), as well as paroxysmal attacks of atrial fibrillation (Fig 15–6). One pathway of reciprocating tachycardia involves normal AV node–His-Purkinje conduction in an antegrade direction and bypass tract conduction in a retrograde direction. The resulting QRS complexes are narrow and normal-appearing, and the tachycardia responds to the usual maneuvers that terminate reentry supraventricular tachycardias. Since the bypass tract functions only to conduct impulses in a retrograde direction, it is referred to as a **concealed bypass tract**; delta waves are *not* seen during tachycardia. The second pathway of reciprocating tachycardia involves bypass tract conduction in an antegrade direction, and AV node–His-Purkinje conduction in a retrograde direction. The resulting QRS complexes will be broad and will have a delta wave, although the rate of the tachycardia may make the delta wave difficult to discern. This wide complex tachycardia, with its broad and bizarre QRS complexes, may be confused with ventricular tachycardia. Patients with either form of reciprocating tachycardia may conduct their normal sinus impulses to the ventricles over the normal AV pathways or over an accessory pathway: AV conduction during normal sinus rhythm does not predict the pathway of AV conduction during tachycardia (Fig 15–7).

If the patient develops atrial fibrillation and the impulses are conducted in antegrade fashion over the bypass tract, directly from atrial to ventricular myocardium, they do not encounter the normal conduction delay present in the AV node. Because of the direct insertion of the bypass fibers into ventricular tissue, extremely rapid ventricular rates (in excess of 250/min) can occur, resulting in ventricular fibrillation. In contrast, if the patient with atrial fibrillation conducts the fibrillatory impulses down the normal AV node–His-Purkinje system, conduction delay within the AV node will protect the ventricles from such rapid rates.

NODOVENTRICULAR & FASCICULOVENTRICULAR CONDUCTION

Nodoventricular and fasciculoventricular connections are relatively uncommon. They are recognized by a normal PR interval (since the atrial impulses pass through the AV node and encounter the normal delay in AV conduction) and a wide QRS complex with a delta wave (since the ventricles are preexcited via the nodoventricular fibers) (Figs 15–1 and 15–8). Like WPW conduction, the QRS complex configurations will reflect the degrees to which the ventricles are depolarized via the normal and accessory pathways.

SHORT PR INTERVAL & NORMAL QRS COMPLEX

The electrocardiographic pattern of a short PR interval and a normal QRS configuration could be due to an anatomically short AV node, an intra-AV nodal bypass tract having rapid conduction, or a direct connection between atrial fibers and the distal portion of the AV node (atrionodal connection) or His bundle (atrio-His connection) (Fig 15–1). Since ventricular depolarization occurs over the normal His-Purkinje pathways, the QRS complexes are normal (Fig 15–9).

Most patients with a short PR interval and a normal QRS complex have an intra–AV nodal bypass tract. Impulse conduction in this tract is very rapid and, because of preferential conduction of supraventricular impulses in this pathway, the normal conduction delay encountered in other portions of the AV node does not occur. Reentry tachycardias can occur in these patients, in which instance the **Lown-Ganong-Levine syndrome** is said to be present.

Table 15–1 summarizes the features of ventricular preexcitation.

Table 15–1. Electrocardiographic findings in ventricular preexcitation syndromes.

	Accessory AV bundle (WPW conduction)	Intra–AV nodal bypass tract, atrionodal or atrio-His conduction	Nodoventricular, nodofascicular connection
PR interval	Short (< 0.12 s)	Short	Normal
QRS duration	Broad (> 0.11 s)	Normal[1]	Broad
Secondary ST-T wave abnormalities	Yes	No	Yes
Delta wave	Yes	No	Yes
Can mimic myocardial infarction	Yes	No*	Yes
Can mimic ventricular hypertrophy	Yes	No*	Yes

[1]Unless prior abnormalities in intraventricular conduction are present.

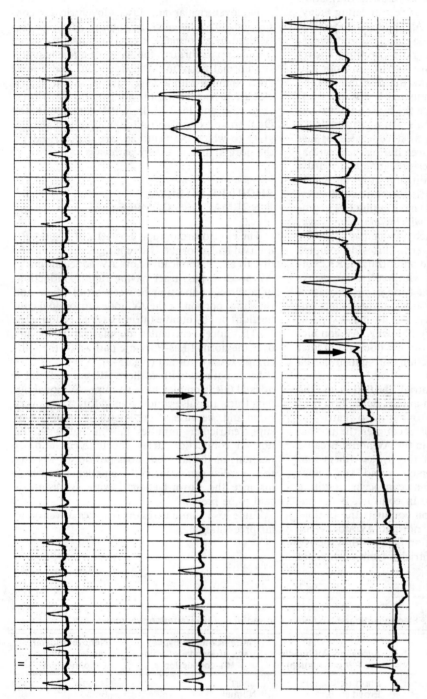

Figure 15–7. Reciprocating supraventricular tachycardia in a patient with Wolff-Parkinson-White conduction. The tachycardia complexes are narrow and normal-appearing. The P waves are inverted, indicating retrograde atrial depolarization. After intravenous administration of verapamil, tachycardia termination occurs (ARROW). The complex at tachycardia termination is a P wave, indicating that termination has been accomplished by failure of conduction of the reentrant supraventricular impulse to the ventricles. In the bottom strip, recorded seconds after recording the top two strips, a supraventricular escape rhythm with retrograde conduction is present. Sinus rhythm resumes (arrow); the sinus impulses are conducted to the ventricles over the accessory AV pathway, as illustrated by the short PR interval and the delta wave at the onset of the QRS complexes. These rhythm strips illustrate that AV conduction during normal sinus rhythm and during reciprocating supraventricular tachycardia may not occur over the same pathways. Tracing courtesy of Larry Epstein, MD.

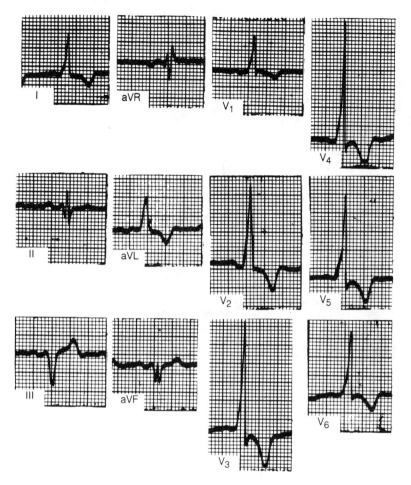

Figure 15-8. Nodoventricular conduction. A delta wave is seen in I, aVL, and all precordial leads; it is negative in II and aVF and should not be confused with the Q wave of myocardial infarction. Since the PR interval is normal at 0.14 s, the sinus impulse has been conducted through the AV node, after which it preexcites the ventricles.

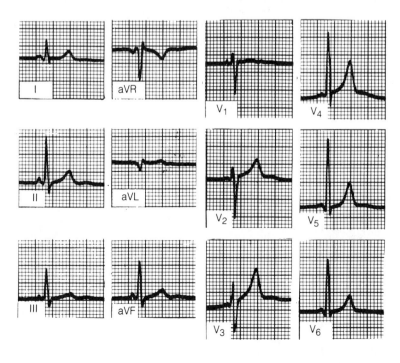

Figure 15-9. Short PR interval due to intra–AV nodal, atrionodal or atrio-His bypass tracts or to an anatomically short AV node. Since the ventricles are depolarized via the normal His-Purkinje system, the QRS complexes are normal.

Figure 15-T1.
TEST TRACINGS

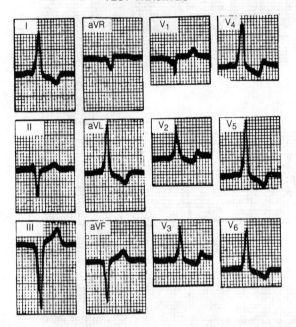

What is the atrial rhythm?	Sinus.
What is the PR interval?	0.1 s. (Best seen in V_{3-5}.)
What is the QRS duration?	0.12 s.
What is the direction of the mean frontal plane QRS axis?	Superior.
What is the QRS morphology in the inferior leads?	rS in II, QS in III and aVF.
Is a delta wave present? If so, what is its orientation?	Yes, Posterior (negative in V_1), left (positive in I and aVL), and superior (negative in III and aVF).
Is inferior wall or posterior wall myocardial infarction present?	This cannot be diagnosed since ventricular depolarization is abnormal, as is repolarization.
What is the pattern of AV conduction?	An accessory AV bundle is being utilized (short PR interval and delta wave) (Wolff-Parkinson-White conduction).

Figure 15-T2.
TEST TRACINGS

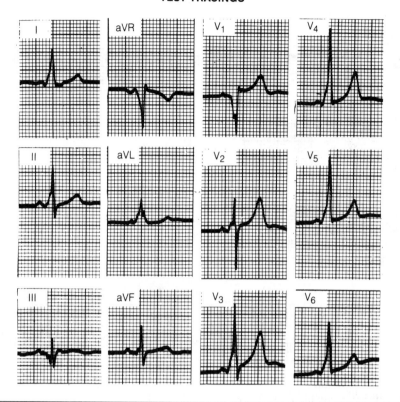

Are the ventricles depolarized via an accessory AV pathway or via a nodoventricular bundle? Why?

Since the PR interval is short, the AV node is bypassed, at least in part. Since nodofascicular conduction involves a pathway that arises below the AV node, the PR interval would be normal, and a delta wave would be present.

Is left ventricular hypertrophy present?

This cannot be diagnosed since ventricular depolarization is abnormal due to abnormal conduction pathways.

Are there QRS complexes, fusion complexes, or pure accessory pathway complexes?

Cannot tell from a single tracing, although most WPW complexes do represent fusion complexes.

Figure 15-T3.
TEST TRACINGS

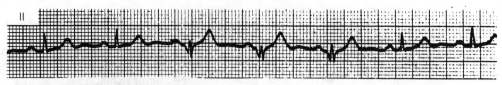

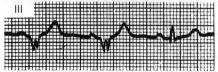

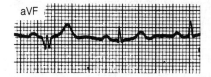

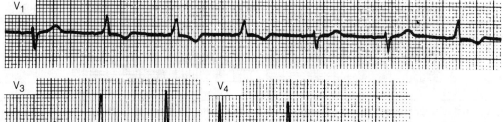

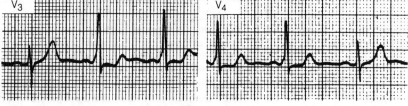

What is the atrial rhythm?	Sinus.
What are the PR intervals?	The PR intervals of the narrow QRS complexes are 0.16 s, and those of the broader QRS complexes are 0.11 s.
What characterizes the broad QRS complexes that is not found in the narrow complexes?	A delta wave, best seen in V$_{3-4}$.
Explain the rhythm. Is a rate-dependent phenomenon present?	The rhythm is sinus. Normal intraventricular conduction is interspersed with WPW conduction. The change in conduction pattern does not appear to be rate-dependent. This is termed "intermittent" WPW conduction.
What do the QS complexes in II, III, and aVF represent?	A negatively directed delta wave. Inferior wall myocardial infarction cannot be diagnosed.

Figure 15–T4.
TEST TRACINGS

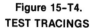

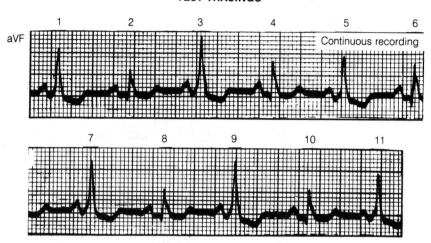

How do complexes 2,4,6,8 and 10 differ from the others?	They have a longer PR interval and a qR configuration; no delta wave is present.
Is inferior wall myocardial infarction present?	Since the normally conducted complexes have a qR morphology, inferior wall myocardial infarction might be present; however, the q waves are neither sufficiently deep nor wide to confirm this diagnosis from this lead alone.
Describe the type of conduction in the accessory pathway.	2:1.

Figure 15–T5.
TEST TRACINGS

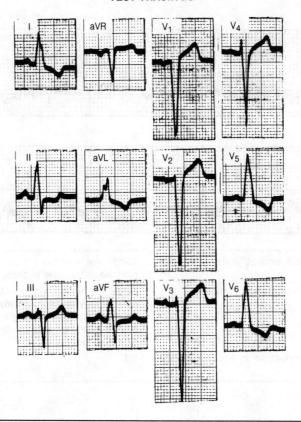

What is the atrial rhythm?	Sinus.
What is the PR interval?	0.12 s.
What is the QRS duration?	0.12 s.
What is the mean frontal plane QRS axis?	0°.
Is a delta wave present?	No.
What is the pattern of AV conduction?	AV conduction is normal; left bundle branch block pattern is present.

Figure 15-T6.
TEST TRACINGS

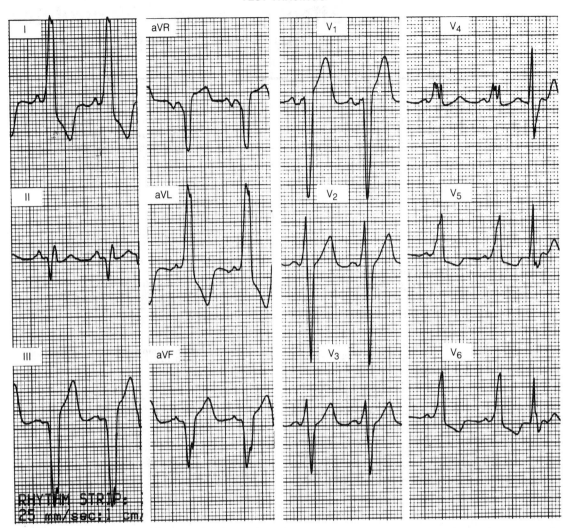

Which of the following are true of the tracing?

Left bundle branch block is present.	No.
Inferior wall infarction is present.	No.
Left ventricular hypertrophy is present.	No.
Sinus rhythm is present.	Yes.
Nodoventricular conduction is present.	No.
An intra-AV nodal bypass tract is present.	No.
A Kent bundle is present.	Yes.

16

Effect of Drugs & Electrolytes on the Electrocardiogram

Drug and electrolyte abnormalities affect the clinical ECG through their effects on intra- and extra-cellular ion movements and action potentials. Their effects can be manifested in alterations of P–QRST morphology, in PR, QRS, and QT intervals, and in alterations of cardiac rhythm and rate.

DIGITALIS

Digitalis Effect

Digitalis administration commonly produces ST segment depression in ventricular epicardial leads, which is unrelated to serum levels of the drug. The characteristic ST segment changes are a "scooped" ST configuration or an oblique line descending from the J point (Figs 16–1 and 16–2). Because of the ST segment depression, the T wave may be dragged downward, resembling T wave inversion. As a result of a shortening of electrical systole in digitalized patients, the QT interval shortens, but this is not often measurable from the routine ECG. Occasionally, the ST–T wave abnormalities related to digitalis use are not this characteristic, but may more closely resemble those of nontransmural ischemia or infarction.

PR interval prolongation (first-degree AV block) is an occasional finding in digitalized patients; some consider it a sign of digitalis toxicity. Measurement of the serum digitalis levels may be helpful in assessing whether or not the PR interval prolongation is due to digitalis effect or to toxic drug levels.

Digitalis Toxicity (Figs 16–3 through 16–7).

While many arrhythmias can result from digitalis intoxication, the most commonly encountered ones are listed in Table 16–1. Bundle branch

Table 16–1. Electrocardiographic manifestations of digitalis toxicity (Figs 16–3 through 16–7).

Automatic or triggered arrhythmias
Ventricular premature complexes
Bigeminy, trigeminy
R-on-T premature complexes
Multiform complexes
Ventricular tachycardia
Ventricular fibrillation
Atrial tachycardia (often with AV block)
Accelerated junctional rhythm (with AV dissociation)
Junctional tachycardia (with AV dissociation)
Bidirectional tachycardia
AV block
Second-degree, type I (Wenckebach)
High-degree or complete

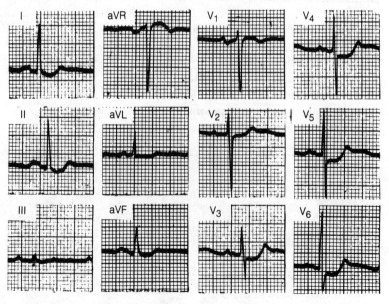

Figure 16–1. Digitalis effect. Scooped ST segment depression is present in I, II, aVF, and V$_{2-6}$.

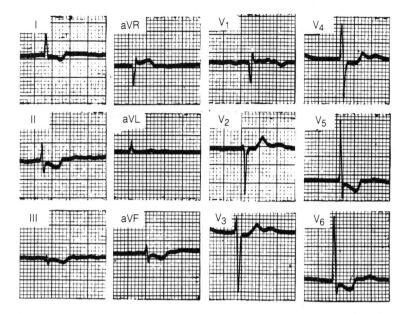

Figure 16-2. Digitalis effect. The rhythm is atrial fibrillation. The ST segment depression produces an oblique downward ST segment in leads I, II, III, aVF, and V_{5-6}. The T waves are dragged downward. Prominent U waves are best seen in V_{2-4}; U waves are not indicative of digitalis effect, although digitalis may enhance their amplitude.

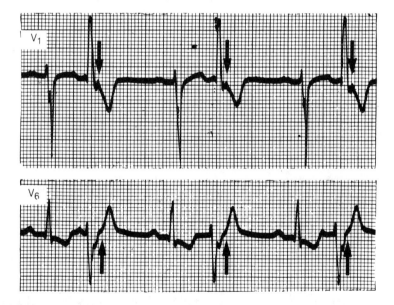

Figure 16-3. Sinus rhythm with ventricular bigeminy due to digitalis toxicity. Ventricular premature complexes follow each sinus-conducted QRS at a fixed coupling interval. ST segment depression and T wave inversion in the sinus-conducted beats is seen in V_6; however, since each sinus-conducted beat is a postextrasystolic one, correct interpretation of ST–T abnormalities is difficult. The sinus rate is not measurable when ventricular bigeminy is present since consecutive sinus complexes are not present. Although ventricular bigeminy in this patient was associated with a toxic serum level of digoxin, this arrhythmia is not specific for digitalis intoxication. If a ventricular arrhythmia is due to digitalis toxicity, it is expected to disappear as the serum level of digitalis is lowered. Note the presence of P waves deforming the ST segments of the premature ventricular depolarizations (arrows); since the intervals between them and the preceding sinus P waves is not half the measured sinus cycle length, they are probably retrogradely conducted.

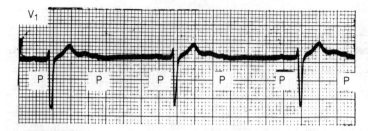

Figure 16-4. Second-degree AV block due to digitalis toxicity. The AV conduction ratio is 2:1, the sinus rate is 86/min, and the ventricular rate is 43/min. The PR interval of the conducted P waves is within normal limits. The QRS complexes are narrow. Since bundle branch block is not present, the conduction block is probably occurring within the AV node.

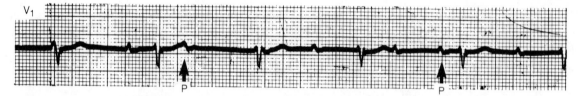

Figure 16-5. Complete AV block due to digitalis toxicity. The atrial rate is 66/min (nonconducted atrial premature beats [P] are also present) and the ventricular rate is 52/min. The QRS complexes are narrow, suggesting that the focus of origin of the QRS rhythm is in the AV junction or His bundle.

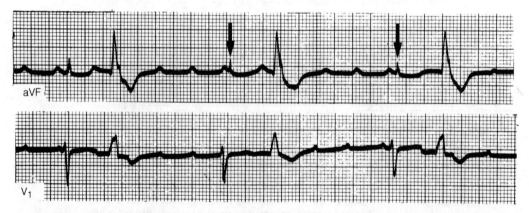

Figure 16-6. Atrial tachycardia with AV block and ventricular bigeminy, resulting from digitalis toxicity. The atrial rate is 164/min and is independent of the QRS rhythm. The QRS complexes are narrow, suggesting an AV junctional origin. Following each narrow QRS complex, a ventricular premature complex occurs (ventricular bigeminy). Because the intervals between the premature ventricular complexes and the normal-appearing complexes are regular, and because the premature complexes occur at fixed coupling intervals to the normal complexes, the QRS rhythm is presumed to be regular. Note that some junctional QRS complexes (arrows) appear to be deformed by portions of the superimposed P waves (such deformities can be mistaken for artifacts).

block is not expected with digitalis use. Sinus bradycardia due to sinus arrest or SA exit block may occur in patients taking digitalis who have high vagal tone or those in whom sympathetic tone is diminished. Atrial flutter and fibrillation are uncommon manifestations of digitalis toxicity. When the underlying atrial rhythm is filbrillation, the diagnosis of digitalis toxicity can be made from the recognition of high-degree AV block, with a *regular* QRS rhythm originating in junctional or ventricular tissue. **Exit block** of both type I and type II varieties (see Chapter 11) from the focus of origin of the QRS rhythm is also seen. Ventricular ectopic impulses may occur. Table 16–2 lists the manifestations of digitalis intoxication in patients with atrial fibrillation.

Table 16–2. Electrocardiographic manifestations of digitalis toxicity in the presence of atrial fibrillation.

Regular QRS rhythm (reflecting AV block and a subsidiary pacemaker with origin in the AV junction, bundle branches, or distal Purkinje tissue)
QRS rhythm with episodic type II (2:1, 3:1) exit block (occurring in any portion of the AV node–His-Purkinje system)
QRS rhythm with periodicity suggesting type I (Wenckebach) exit block (occurring in any portion of the AV node–His-Purkinje system)
Ventricular arrhythmias

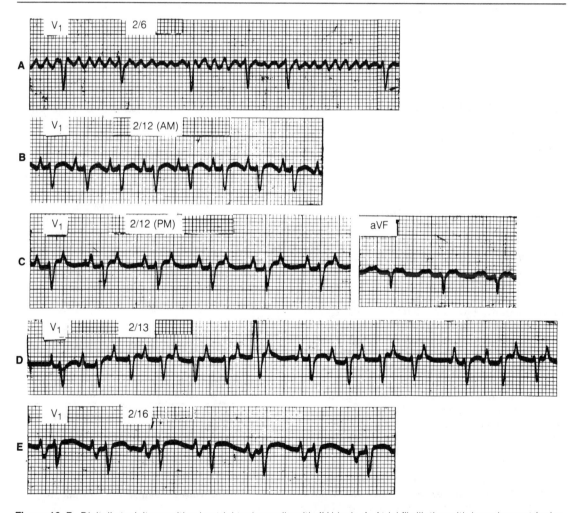

Figure 16–7. Digitalis toxicity resulting in atrial tachycardia with AV block. *A:* Atrial fibrillation with irregular ventricular rate is present. *B:* Atrial tachycardia at a rate of 160/min with 1:1 AV conduction is now present..The sudden appearance of atrial tachycardia during treatment of atrial fibrillation with digitalis should raise the suspicion of digitalis intoxication. *C:* After additional digitalis, AV block has occurred, resulting in an atrial tachycardia with 2:1 AV conduction; an increase in the atrial rate has also occurred. *D:* Atrial tachycardia remains when the digitalis is discontinued, but the 2:1 AV block has been replaced by type I (Wenckebach) second-degree AV block, and more 1:1 AV conduction of atrial impulses is present. *E:* Resumption of sinus rhythm.

Table 16-3. Classification of antiarrhythmic drugs.

Class		Examples	Depress (fast phase 0 Sodium channel blockade)	Prolong action potential duration	Depress calcium (slow) channel response	Depress phase 4 depolarization
IA	(membrane anesthetics)	Quinidine Procainamide Disopyramide	+ +	+	0	+
IB	(membrane anesthetics)	Lidocaine Tocainide Mexiletine	+ +	−	0	−
IC	(membrane anesthetics)	Flecainide Encainide	+ +	0/ −	0/ +	+
II	(beta blockers)	Propranolol Timolol Nadolol	0/ +	0/ −	0	+
III	—	Bretylium Amiodarone	+	+ +	0	+
IV	(calcium blockers)	Verapamil Diltiazem	0	+	+ +	+

+ + Major effect; + minor effect; 0 = no effect, − = shortens

ANTIARRHYTHMIC DRUGS

Antiarrhythmic agents have been classified into 4 types, based upon their predominant cellular electrophysiologic effects (Table 16-3).

TYPE I ANTIARRHYTHMIC DRUGS

While all type I antiarrhythmic agents are capable of producing similar electrocardiographic abnormalities, the drug most commonly associated with such changes is quinidine. Quinidine can produce ST segment depression, and flattening and inversion of the T waves in left ventricular epicardial leads, in a fashion similar to digitalis (Fig 16-8). However, prolongation of the QTU interval because of the development of a prominent U wave is the most commonly observed electrocardiographic change (Fig 16-9).

Toxic electrocardiographic manifestations of quinidine therapy (as well as all type I antiarrhythmic agents in certain patients) are as follows: (1) **prolongation of the QRS duration,** reflecting the effect of quinidine on the conduction velocity in the bundle branches and Purkinje system; (2) **ventricular arrhythmias,** including ventricular tachycardia (often polymorphic) and fibrillation (Fig 16-10); (3) **ventricular standstill** (Fig 16-11); (4) **sinus bradycardia** due to SA exit block or slowing of impulse formation (or both); (5) **atrial standstill;** (6) first-, second-, and third-degree **AV block;** and (7) **AV dissociation.** The toxic manifestations of quinidine are an extension of its therapeutic effects of slowing the rate of discharge of

an ectopic focus and producing local conduction block.

A particular type of ventricular tachycardia, termed **torsades de pointes,** can occur in patients receiving type I antiarrhythmic agents (see Chapter 13). This is a *polymorphic,* irregular, usually nonsustained ventricular tachycardia, in which the QRS complexes appear to twist about an isoelectric baseline (Fig 16-12). While not entirely specific for type I antiarrhythmic therapy (this tachycardia has been seen during amiodarone treatment and as a result of a long QT interval due to hypokalemia or congenital QT prolongation), its occurrence generally constitutes a contraindication to the further use of these medications.

The electrocardiographic manifestations of type I antiarrhythmic agents are listed in Table 16-4.

Table 16-4. Electrocardiographic manifestations of type I antiarrhythmic agent therapy.

USUAL EFFECTS (often unrelated to serum drug levels)
  Prolonged QTU interval
  Prominent U wave
  ST segment depression
  Decreased T wave amplitude
  T wave inversion
  Increased P wave duration
TOXIC EFFECTS (serum drug levels often, but not always, in the "toxic" range)
  Prolonged QRS duration
  Polymorphic ventricular tachycardia (torsades de pointes)
  Sinus bradycardia
  Sinus arrest
  Sinoatrial block
  AV block

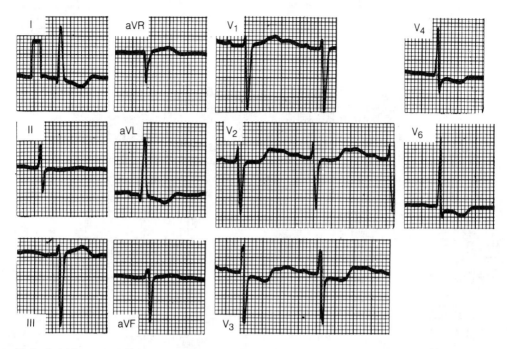

Figure 16-8. Quinidine effect. The rhythm is sinus; the PR interval is 0.2 s. The pattern of left ventricular hypertrophy with associated ST–T wave changes is present. The ST–T abnormalities in V_{2-3} may be contributed to by quinidine, since they are not expected to result from the ventricular hypertrophy alone. The QTU interval is prolonged to 0.6 s and represents an effect of quinidine. Since the QTU interval does not correlate directly with the serum level of the drug, prolongation of this interval does not predict the presence of quinidine toxicity.

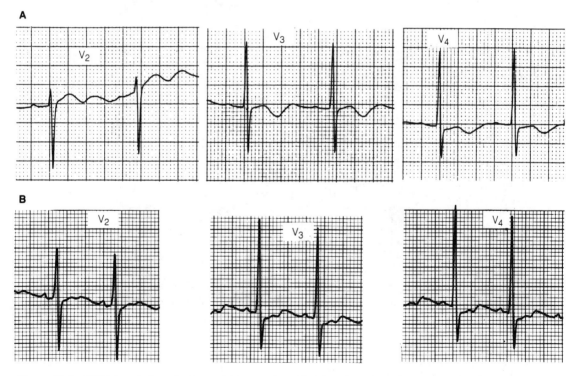

Figure 16-9. QTU intervals in patients receiving procainamide (A) and quinidine (B). In addition to prolongation of the QTU interval, a very prominent U wave may be inscribed. The serum potassium levels in both instances were normal. Patient B was also receiving digoxin.

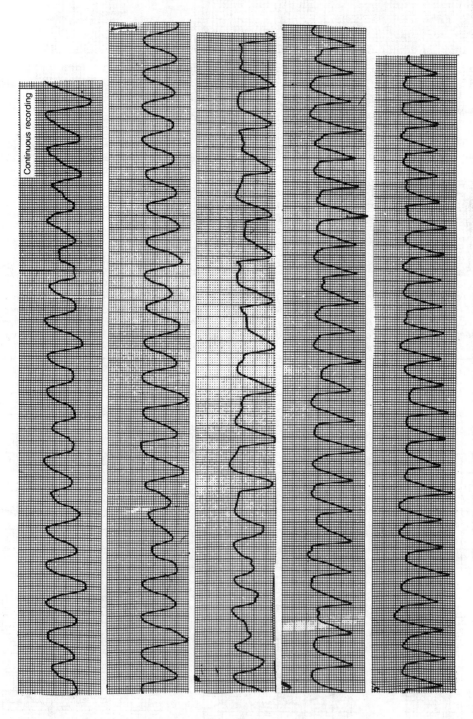

Continuous recording

Figure 16–10. Procainamide toxicity (level = 28 mg/dL) in a patient with renal failure. A markedly broad and bizarre QRS rhythm resembling a sine wave is present initially. The QRS complex duration spontaneously shortens and T waves become discernible. Atrial activity is not identified. The tachycardia is presumably ventricular in origin, although this cannot be known with absolute certainty in the presence of toxic levels of procainamide. The patient later developed the rhythm shown in Fig 16–11 and expired.

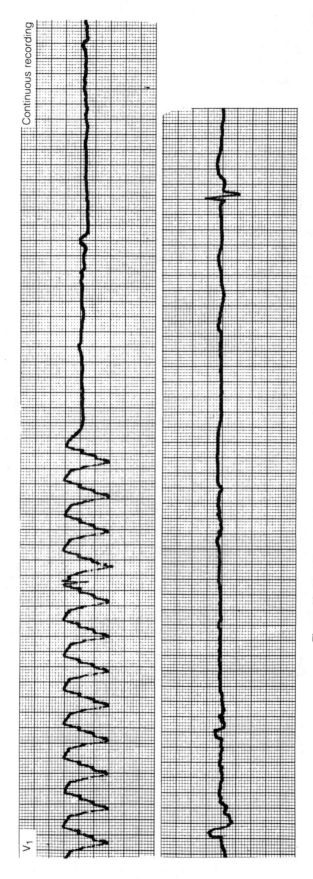

Figure 16–11. Monomorphic ventricular tachycardia leading to ventricular standstill in a patient with renal failure and serum procainamide level of 28 mg/dL. The patient could not be resuscitated.

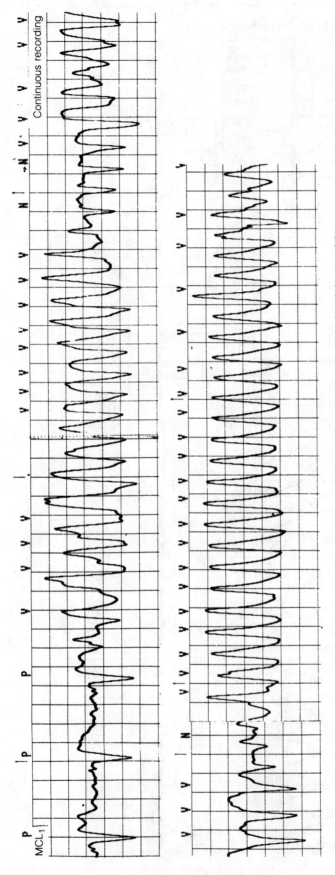

Figure 16-12. Polymorphic ventricular tachycardia (torsades de pointes) due to quinidine toxicity. The QRS configurations change from upright to inverted in this MCL$_1$ monitor lead. The polymorphic tachycardia is initiated by an R-on-T premature ventricular depolarization. The tachycardia becomes monomorphic as it continues; this is a relatively unusual sequence of events.

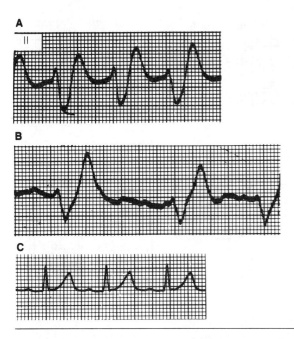

A

B

C

Figure 16-13. Amitriptyline toxicity due to an overdose in a suicide attempt. *A:* A wide complex QRS rhythm without discernible atrial activity is present. This could represent sinus rhythm with sinoventricular conduction (due to atrial arrest), junctional rhythm with intraventricular aberration, or ventricular rhythm. *B:* With supportive treatment, the atrial rhythm is now fibrillation. The QRS rhythm is irregular and is thus responding to the fibrillatory impulses. The QRS complexes are less broad and bizarre than in (A). *C:* Normal sinus rhythm restored, with prolongation of the QT interval to 0.46 s. The QRS configuration is normal.

PHENOTHIAZINES & RELATED DRUGS

The phenothiazines and the antidepressant agents imipramine, amitriptyline, and related compounds are myocardial depressants that impair AV and intraventricular conduction (Fig 16-13). With excessive doses, ST segment depression, T wave flattening and inversion, and prolongation of the QT interval with prominent U waves occur. Eventually, both AV and intraventricular conduction disturbances arise, similar to type I antiarrhythmic drug toxicity. Ventricular tachycardia also not uncommonly occurs.

HYPERKALEMIA

Although a reasonably good correlation between serum potassium level and the ECG exists, the ECG actually reflects the *gradient* between myocardial intracellular and extracellular potassium ions.

The initial electrocardiographic evidence of elevated extracellular potassium level is the appearance of *slender, narrow-based, tented* T waves, often best seen in the precordial leads. The peaked T waves are often, but not always, tall. Therefore, although tall T waves might suggest hyperkalemia, they are by no means diagnostic of it, since normal individuals and patients with posterior wall myocardial infarction may show a similar pattern. However, *peaking* of the T waves should raise a suspicion of hyperkalemia (Figs 16–14 and 16–15).

With further elevation of serum potassium, the P waves disappear, and the QRS complexes become broad and bizarre in configuration, sometimes resembling a **sine wave** (Fig 16-16). While the QRS rhythm might suggest a ventricular focus of origin, intracardiac electrographic studies indicate that it might arise from the bundle of His, with marked intraventricular conduction delay, or from the sinus node. The latter rhythm is termed **sinoventricular conduction** and represents sinus rhythm, with the sinus impulses being transmitted via intra-atrial conduction tissue to the AV node and thence to the ventricles. Despite transmission of the sinus impulse through the atria, the atrial muscle fails to be depolarized because of the hyperkalemia. Because atrial depolarization does not occur, P waves are not inscribed on the surface ECG. The diagnosis is confirmed when, upon treatment of the hyperkalemia, P waves appear that have the same rate as the prior QRS rhythm (Fig 10-9).

ST segment elevation is occasionally seen with severe hyperkalemia (Fig 16-17), possibly representing local hyperkalemia associated with myocardial necrosis. The pattern may be confused with acute myocardial infarction due to coronary artery disease.

HYPOKALEMIA

The typical electrocardiographic features of hypokalemia are inscription of a **prominent U wave,** PR interval prolongation, ST segment depression in left ventricular epicardial leads, and low T wave

Figure 16-14. Hyperkalemia. Tall, slender, tented T waves are seen in I, II, III, aVF, and V_{2-6}. The T wave amplitude is a much less specific criterion for hyperkalemia than is its peaked configuration.

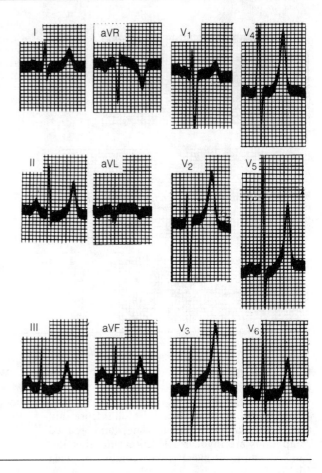

Figure 16-15. Normal ECG which might suggest hyperkalemia. The T waves in leads I, II, aVF, and V_{2-6} are tall and somewhat peaked, but they do not have a narrow base and thus are not "tented." Tall T waves do not themselves indicate hyperkalemia.

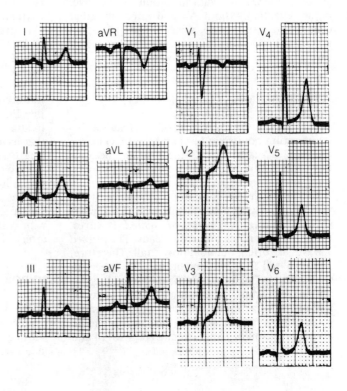

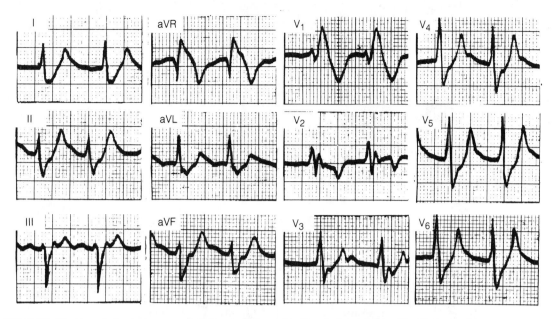

Figure 16–16. Hyperkalemia (serum potassium = 8.9 meq/L). The rhythm is sinus. The PR interval is prolonged, but the exact PR interval cannot be determined since the P waves interrupt the T waves of the preceding QRS complexes. The QRS complexes are broad (0.16 s) and have a right bundle branch block pattern. Tented, peaked T waves are present in the lateral precordial leads. Unless prior tracings are available which document the existence of established first-degree and right bundle branch block, these findings should be presumed to be due to the hyperkalemia until proved otherwise.

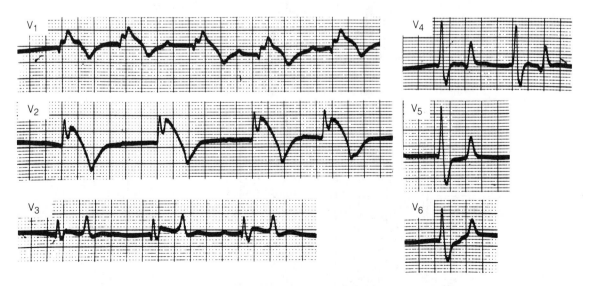

Figure 16–17. ST segment elevation, especially noteworthy in leads V_{1-2}, due to hyperkalemia (serum potassium = 9.3 meq/L). Tented T waves are seen in V_{3-6}. Note that they are peaked, although not tall. Tall T waves are not diagnostic of hyperkalemia, whereas tented T waves strongly suggest this diagnosis.

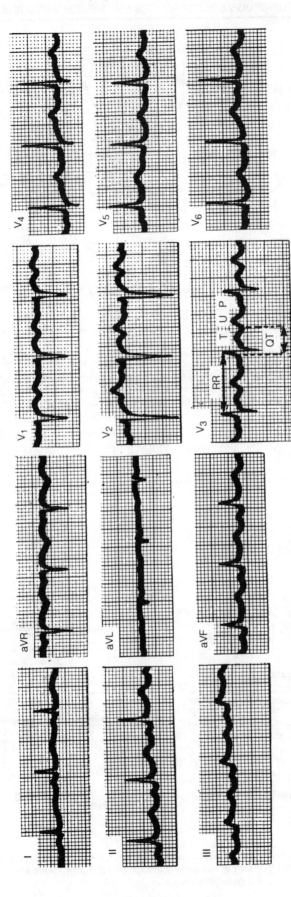

Figure 16–18. Hypokalemia (serum potassium = 2.3 meq/L). An apparently upright T wave is seen in leads II, III, aVF, and V$_{5-6}$. If this deflection were the T wave, the QT interval would be 0.4 s (corrected for the RR interval of 0.66 s, the QT$_c$ = 0.5 s) and therefore prolonged. In leads V$_{1-4}$ separate T and U waves are clearly evident. The true QT interval in V$_3$ is 0.29 s (QT$_c$ = 0.36 s), which is normal. Whereas a prominent U wave has many causes, a **giant U wave,** which exceeds the height of the T wave in the same lead, should raise the suspicion of hypokalemia.

amplitude. The prominent U wave may be due to prolonged Purkinje system repolarization. The U wave is often superimposed upon the T wave of the preceding QRS complex and is not always readily distinguished from it. Thus, a long "QT" interval may in fact represent a long QTU interval, the actual QT interval being normal (Fig 16–18). Hypomagnesemia may produce similar electrocardiographic abnormalities to hypokalemia; they are often, but not always, present together. If potassium replacement fails to normalize the QTU interval, hypomagnesemia should be suspected.

Prominent U waves are not diagnostic of hypokalemia, as they also occur in the course of therapy with type I antiarrhythmic drugs, amiodarone, phenothiazines, or tricyclic antidepressants, and in the hereditary long QT interval syndromes. U waves may also be seen in sinus bradycardia, left ventricular hypertrophy, and in acute and chronic ischemic heart disease. However, a **giant U wave** that exceeds the T wave in amplitude in a given ECG lead is strongly suggestive of electrolyte imbalance. (Figs 16–18 and 16–19).

A **postextrasystolic U wave** is a term applied to the appearance of a prominent U wave in a postextrasystolic P–QRST complex, where it was not present in the basic complexes (Fig 16–20). While this phenomenon might suggest the diagnosis of hypokalemia, it is not specific for it, because postextrasystolic T and U wave changes may occur in various clinical conditions.

HYPERCALCEMIA

Elevation of serum calcium levels to above 12 mg/dL results in shortening of the QT interval because of shortening of the **QT segment** (the interval between the beginning of the QRS complex and the beginning of the T wave) (Fig 16–21). The QT segment may be obliterated in severe hypercalcemia. A **J wave** has also been described as occurring rarely. Arrhythmias are uncommon.

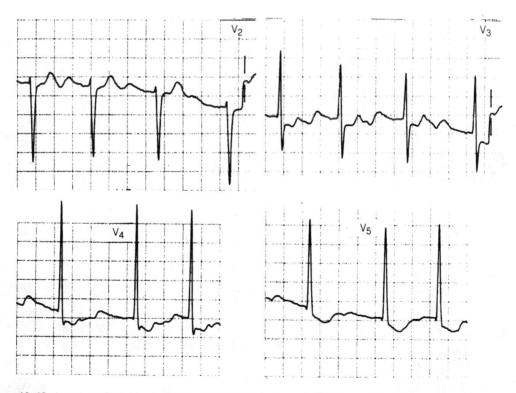

Figure 16–19. Hypokalemia in a patient with atrial fibrillation. The atrial fibrillation with its attendant irregular QRS rate can sometimes make the QT and QTU intervals difficult to measure; in addition, the fibrillatory waves can alter the morphology of a U wave of low amplitude. In this example, a giant U wave, exceeding the T wave amplitude in V$_{3-4}$, is easily seen. The QT interval (best seen in V$_{2-3}$) is 0.36 s; the QU interval is about 0.58 s.

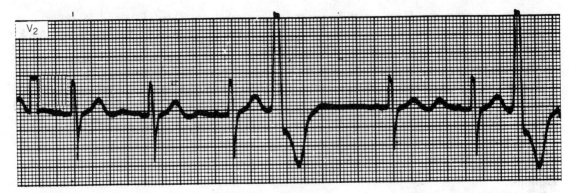

Figure 16-20. Postextrasystolic U wave accentuation. The rhythm is sinus. U waves can be seen throughout the rhythm strip; however, the U wave of the sinus best following the premature ventricular complex is markedly accentuated in amplitude. Although the diagnosis of hypokalemia should be considered, postextrasystolic U wave accentuation is a nonspecific finding.

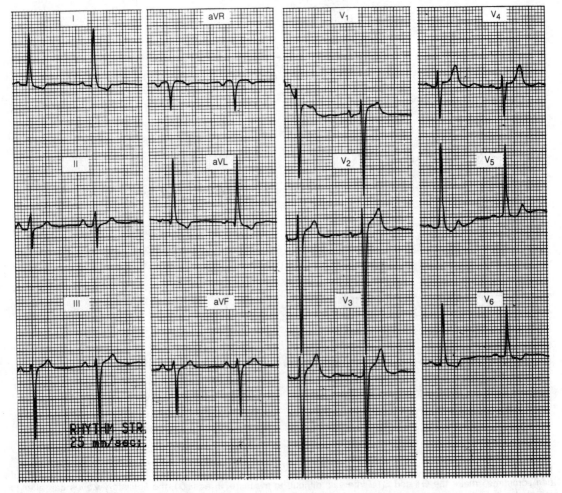

Figure 16-21. Hypercalcemia in a patient with carcinoma. The QT interval is only 0.28–0.3, due to virtual absence of the QT segment. This degree of QT interval shortening is not seen during digitalis treatment.

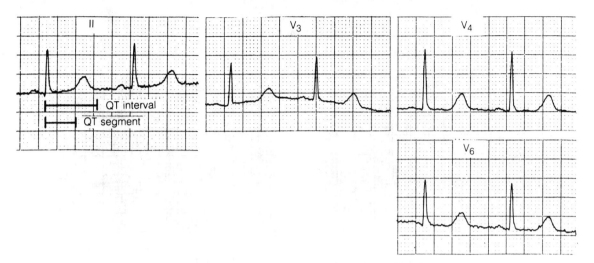

Figure 16-22. Hypocalcemia. The QT interval is prolonged to 0.56 s. The lengthening of the QT interval is due to a prolongation of the QT segment (to 0.34 s) and not to any abnormality of the T wave itself.

HYPOCALCEMIA

Low levels of serum calcium produce a lengthening of the QT interval that is due to prolongation of the QT segment (the interval between the onset of the QRS complex and the beginning of the T wave) (Fig 16-22). It is important to distinguish lengthening of the QT interval due to inscription of a U wave from that due to prolongation of the QT segment. In the former, the electrolyte disturbance is hypokalemia, whereas in the latter it is hypocalcemia. As with hypercalcemia, arrhythmias are uncommon.

REFERENCES

Bashour T et al: Atrioventricular and intraventricular conduction in hyperkalemia. *Am J Cardiol* 1975;**35**:199.

Elkayam U, Frishman W: Cardiovascular effects of phenothiazines. *Am Heart J* 1980;**100**:397.

Ettinger PO et al: Ventricular conduction delay and asystole during systemic hyperkalemia. *Am J Cardiol* 1974;**33**:876.

Helfant RH: Hypokalemia and arrhythmias. *Am J Med* 1986;**80**:13.

Khardori R et al: Electrocardiographic finding simulating acute myocardial infarction in a compound metabolic aberration. *Am J Med* 1985;**78**:529.

O'Neil JP, Chung EK: Unusual electrocardiographic finding: Bifascicular block due to hyperkalemia. *Am J Med* 1976;**61**:537.

Sherf LM, James TN: A new electrocardiographic concept: Synchronized sinoventricular conduction. *Dis Chest* 1969;**55**:127.

Surawicz B, Lasseter KC: Effect of drugs on the electrocardiogram. *Prog Cardiovasc Dis* 1970;**13**:26.

Figure 16–T1.
TEST TRACINGS

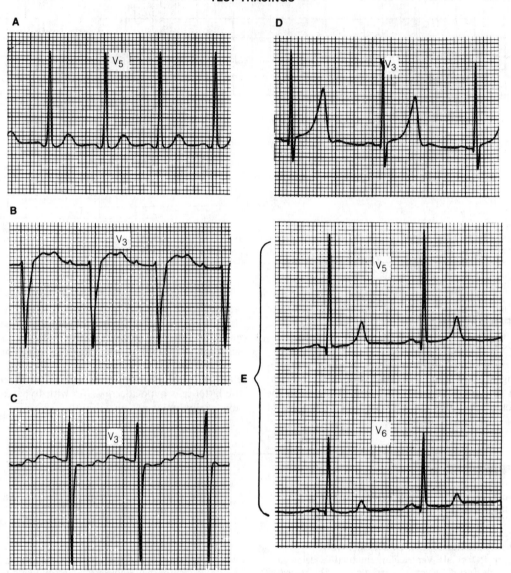

Which of the tracings suggest one or more of the following?

Hypokalemia	B, C
Hypocalcemia	E
Normal	D
Hypomagnesemia	B, C
Hyperkalemia	E
Hypercalcemia	A

Figure 16-T2.
TEST TRACINGS

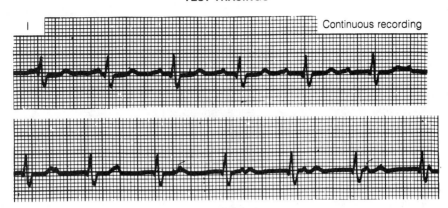

What is the atrial rhythm and rate?	Sinus, rate 83/min.
What is the QRS rate?	80/min.
Are the P waves and QRS complexes associated or dissociated?	Dissociated.
Is complete AV block present?	Since capture is not seen, AV block is possible but not likely.
What is the probable origin of the QRS rhythm? Why?	The origin is probably junctional, since the QRS complexes are narrow and normal-appearing.
Is the QRS rhythm an accelerated one or an escape one? Why?	Accelerated, since it exceeds the atrial rate.
Could digitalis cause this rhythm disturbance?	Yes; the patient's serum digoxin level was in the toxic range.

Figure 16-T3.
TEST TRACINGS

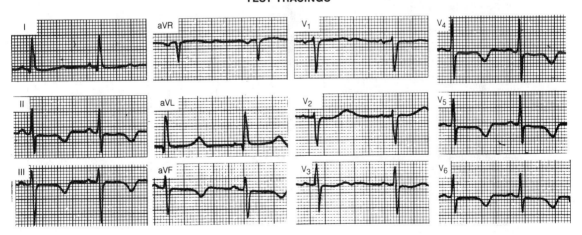

What is the atrial rate and rhythm?	Sinus, rate 67/min.
What is the QRS duration?	0.08 s.
What is the QT interval?	0.58 s.
In which leads is a U wave visible?	V_2, V_3.
What is the QT segment interval?	0.3 s.
Name 3 possible causes for this tracing.	Hypokalemia, type I antiarrhythmic drug toxicity, congenital QT interval prolongation. This patient had the last diagnosis.

Figure 16–T4.
TEST TRACINGS

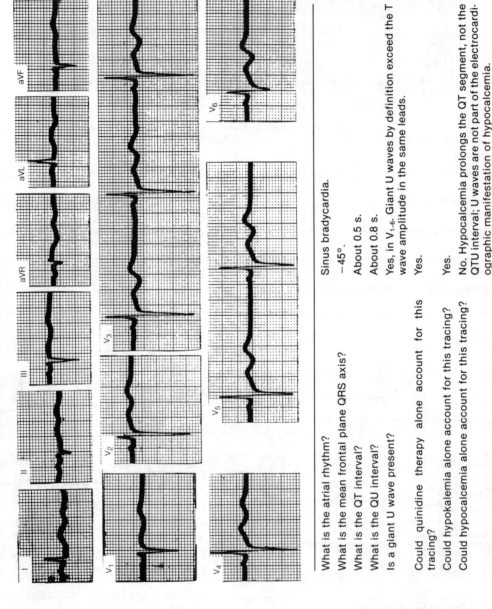

What is the atrial rhythm? — Sinus bradycardia.

What is the mean frontal plane QRS axis? — −45°.

What is the QT interval? — About 0.5 s.

What is the QU interval? — About 0.8 s.

Is a giant U wave present? — Yes, in V_{1-6}. Giant U waves by definition exceed the T wave amplitude in the same leads.

Could quinidine therapy alone account for this tracing? — Yes.

Could hypokalemia alone account for this tracing? — Yes.

Could hypocalcemia alone account for this tracing? — No. Hypocalcemia prolongs the QT segment, not the QTU interval; U waves are not part of the electrocardiographic manifestation of hypocalcemia.

The patient was receiving both digitalis and quinidine; in addition, he was hypokalemic.

Figure 16-T5.
TEST TRACINGS

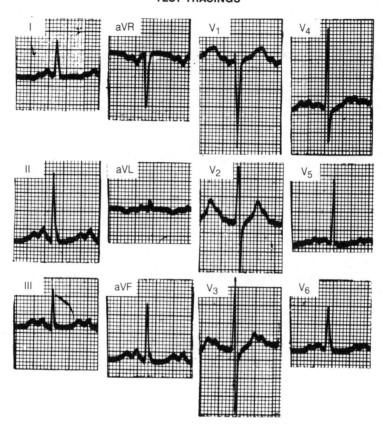

What is the PR interval?	0.16 s (best seen in aVF).
Do the P waves suggest atrial abnormality?	No. They are normal. The notching results from the end of the U wave of the preceding QRST complex encroaching on the P wave.
Is the QT interval normal?	Yes, measured in the precordial leads, which clearly show a U wave superimposed on the T wave; this superimposition is not distinguished in the limb leads.

Figure 16-T6.
TEST TRACINGS

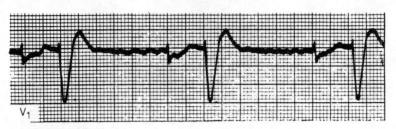

V_1

What is the rhythm?

Atrial fibrillation, ventricular bigeminy.

Is there evidence of high-degree AV block?

Yes. The coupling intervals between the narrow QRS complexes and the premature ventricular complexes are fixed; and the intervals between the premature ventricular complexes and the subsequent QRS complexes are also fixed. This suggests underlying regularization of the ventricular rhythm, compatible with AV block.

Of the following, which could likely cause this rhythm? Procainamide, quinidine, digitalis, propranolol (a beta blocker), verapamil (a calcium channel blocker), lithium.

Digitalis.

Figure 16-T7.
TEST TRACINGS

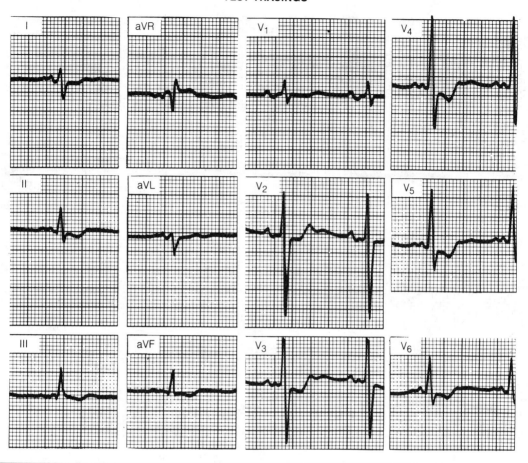

What is the rhythm?	Sinus.
What is the mean frontal plane QRS axis?	+105°.
Are criteria for right ventricular hypertrophy met? Which?	Yes. The mean QRS axis is shifted rightward, and an Rs complex is present in V_1.
Are criteria for atrial abnormality met? What are the criteria and which atrium is "abnormal"?	Yes. The P waves are broad and notched in leads II and aVF, and there is a prominent (but not abnormally so) negative component in V_1.
This patient has mitral valve stenosis. Which medications is she likely to be receiving? Why?	Digitalis (note the digitalis effect on the ST segments) and quinidine (note the long QTU interval with prominent U waves).

Figure 16–T8.
TEST TRACINGS

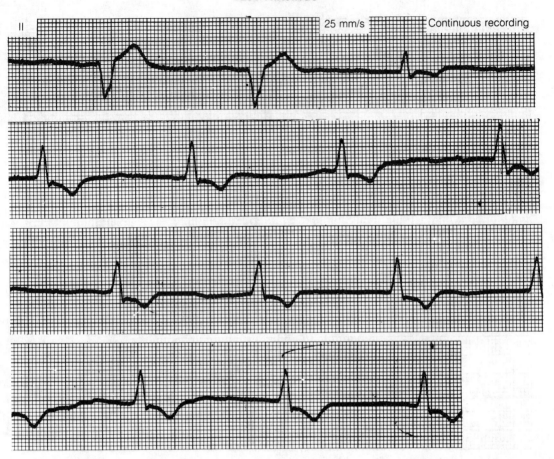

This continuous recording was obtained in a patient with renal failure, normal serum electrolytes, and a serum level of procainamide that was in the toxic range.

What is the atrial rhythm and rate?

Atrial activity cannot be discerned.

What characterizes the ventricular rhythm?

It is irregular, and the QRS complex morphology is variable (at least 3 types of QRS complexes are seen, one of which—the third complex in the top strip—may be a fusion complex).

What is the likely focus of origin of the rhythm? Why?

Because of the slow rate of 37/min and the broad, bizarre QRS complexes, the rhythm may be originating in ventricular tissue. However, in the presence of procainamide toxicity the focus of origin is not certain, since one effect of this drug is to prolong the QRS duration.

Figure 16–T9.
TEST TRACINGS

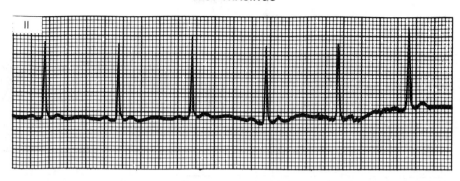

| What electrolyte abnormality does this tracing suggest? Why? | Hypercalcemia, in view of the markedly short QR interval (0.25 s), due to virtual absence of the QT segment. The serum calcium was 21 mg/dL. |

Figure 16–T10.
TEST TRACINGS

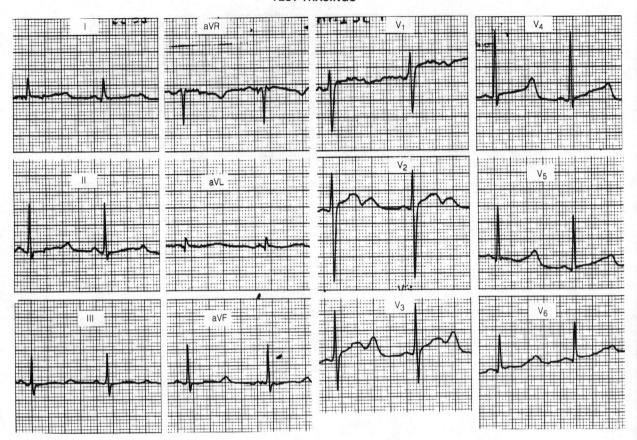

Is QT interval prolongation present?

Yes.

Is this due to prolongation of the QT segment or the superimposition of a U wave?

Although the limb leads might suggest that the QT interval prolongation is due to prolongation of the QT segment, inspection of the precordial leads supplies evidence that the QT segment is normal and a U wave is responsible for the findings in the limb leads.

What is the QT interval?

0.4 s (measured from V_{2-3}).

What is the QU interval?

0.6 s.

The patient was receiving procainamide therapy. The serum potassium was normal.

Figure 16-T11.
TEST TRACINGS

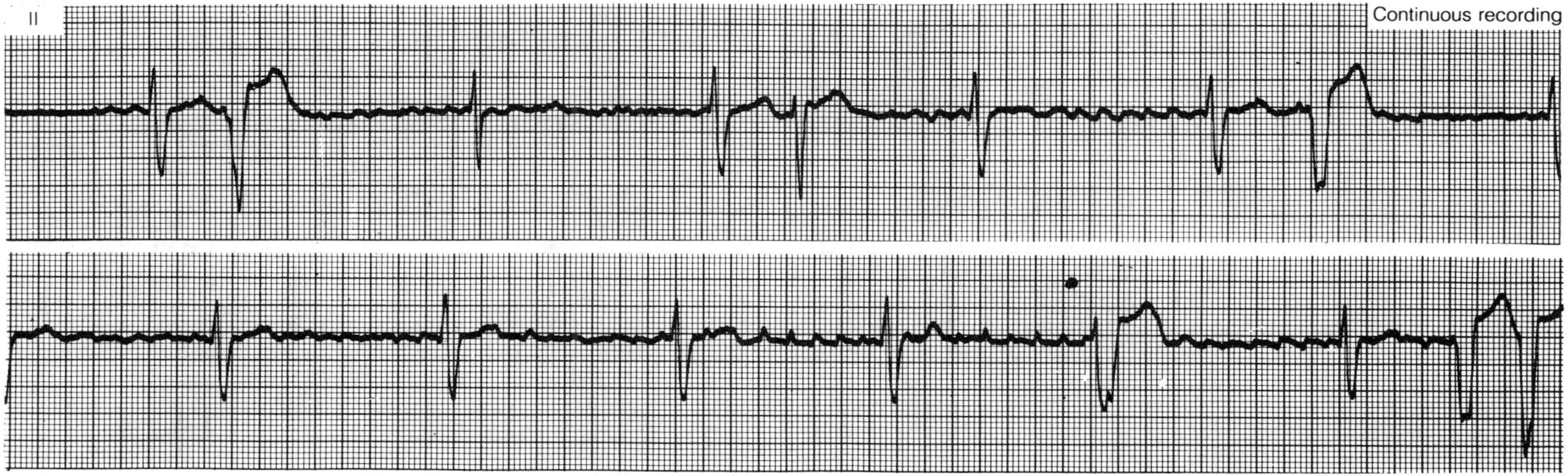

Continuous recording

This continuously recorded lead II rhythm strip was obtained from a patient whose serum digoxin level was 3.9 ng/dL.

Which features are compatible with an electrocardiographic diagnosis of digitalis toxicity?

Slow ventricular response in atrial fibrillation, regularization of ventricular rate (at times quite regular), ventricular premature depolarizations, ventricular couplets.

Figure 16–T12.
TEST TRACINGS

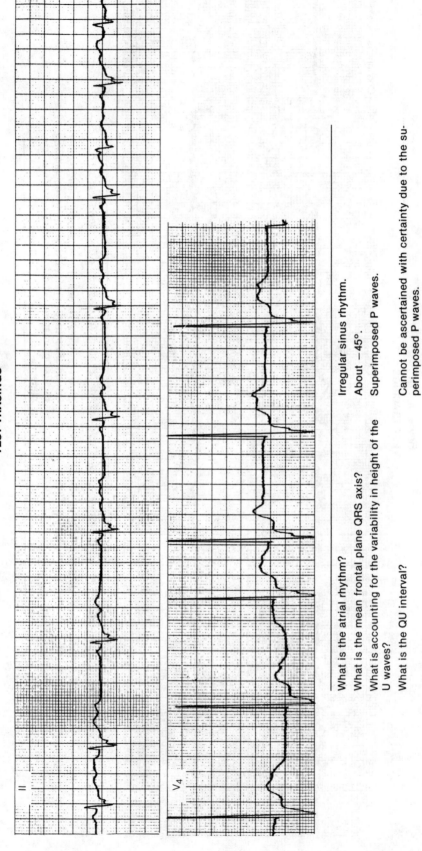

What is the atrial rhythm?   Irregular sinus rhythm.

What is the mean frontal plane QRS axis?   About −45°.

What is accounting for the variability in height of the U waves?   Superimposed P waves.

What is the QU interval?   Cannot be ascertained with certainty due to the superimposed P waves.

What is the diagnosis?   Irregular sinus rhythm with episodic 2:1 AV conduction.

Cardiac Pacing

17

Temporary or permanent cardiac pacing, in which an electrical stimulus results in depolarization of cardiac tissue, is indicated in any situation in which bradycardia results in sysmptoms of cerebral hypoperfusion or hemodynamic decompensation. Temporary cardiac pacing is usually accomplished by transvenous insertion of electrodes into the right atrium or right ventricle (or both). Permanent pacing is effected by the same transvenous route and, in some circumstances, by epicardial placement of electrodes via thoracotomy or a subxiphoid approach. Most pacing systems today are placed transvenously.

The Pacemaker Identification Code

Because of the complexity of pacing system design, an identification code describing the function of the available pacemaker generators has been developed. The code consists of 5 letters. The first letter stands for the chamber paced (atrium [A], ventricle [V], or both or double [D]). The second letter stands for the chamber in which sensing the electrical signal occurs (atrium [A], ventricle [V], both [D], or neither [O]). The third letter refers to the **mode of response** of the generator to a sensed signal (inhibited output [I], triggered output [T] in which an output pulse is delivered upon sensing an electrical signal, and not applicable [O]). The fourth letter stands for the type of changes that can be made noninvasively and reversibly in most currently available pacemaker generators, called **programmability** (rate or energy output only [or both] [S], or multiple functions including rate, energy output, ability to sense an electrical signal of varying magnitude, refractory period after a sensed or paced beat, and other more complex variables [M]). The fifth letter stands for the response of the pulse generator to sensing tachycardias and reflects the antitachycardia function available in some pacemaker generators.

TYPES OF CARDIAC PACING

Asynchronous Pacing (VOO, AOO, & DOO)

Asynchronous pacemakers do not sense any electrical signals. Thus, they deliver output pulses without regard to any spontaneous electrical activity occurring within the heart. Because spontaneous cardiac activity is not sensed, competitive rhythms may result. Whereas asynchronous pacemaker generators were the first devices available and are no longer manufactured, asynchronous pacing occurs whenever a magnet is placed over an implanted generator in order to evaluate pacing function. With a magnet in place, asynchronous pacing and concomitant occurrence of the patient's spontaneous rhythm result in iatrogenic parasystole (Fig 17-1). At the energy output of today's generators (2.5–7.5 V) repetitive ventricular or atrial rhythms are usually not observed, although this possibility exists.

Demand Single Chamber Pacing VVI, AAI, VVT, & AAT)

Both sensing and pacing circuits are present in these units. Upon sensing a spontaneous intracardiac signal, some generators (VVI and AAI) will have inhibition of their output pulses, and no pacemaker artifact will appear (Fig 17-2). Other generators are designed to deliver an output pulse when an electrical event is sensed; this is termed a **triggered response** (VVT and AAT). The triggered output pulse is delivered at the precise **time of sensing** the intracardiac signal, and thus falls *within* the sensed complex and does not contribute to activation of the cardiac chamber (Fig 17-3).

Electrical signals sensed by demand pacemaker generators may originate not from the heart but from the environment (electrocautery, diathermy units, or microwave ovens) or from the patient (muscle potentials). Such sensed signals may cause inhibition of certain units, leading to pauses in paced rhythm. Triggered pulse generators are designed to emit output pulses upon sensing of signals, whatever their origin; thus, pauses in paced rhythm do not occur. Newer generator design and programmability have helped to reduce these "oversensing" problems.

The pacing function of a demand pulse generator cannot be evaluated if the patient's spontaneous rhythm exceeds the programmed rate of the generator, since the pulse generator output will be inhibited. Application of a magnet over the generator converts it to asynchronous mode of function, and capture (stimulation) of the atria or ventricles by the pacemaker can be confirmed, provided that the pacing stimuli fall outside the refractory period of the cardiac tissue (Fig 17-1). Conversely, if the patient is continually paced, the sensing function of the generator cannot be evaluated, since no spontaneous complexes, which would be sensed, occur. **Rate programming**, in

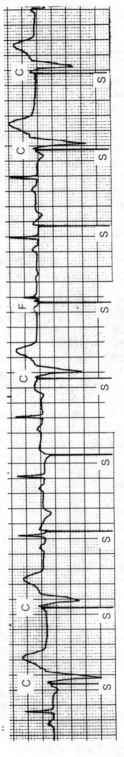

Figure 17–1. Asynchronous ventricular pacing (VOO) produced by placing a magnet over the implanted pulse generator. Pacing stimuli (S) are delivered to the ventricles at the **magnet rate** of 60/min. Sensing of spontaneous QRS complexes does not occur, and the pacing stimuli are therefore delivered at regular intervals. Pacing of the ventricles (C) occurs when ventricular tissue is not refractory. A fusion complex, in which ventricular activation occurs via both the pacing stimulus and transmission of the sinus impulse over the normal AV–node-His-Purkinje system is seen (F).

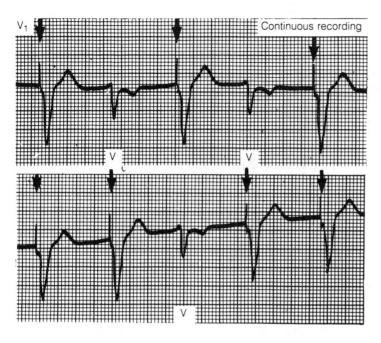

Figure 17-2. Ventricular-inhibited pacing (VVI). The generator has been programmed to pace at a rate of 75/min (interstimulus interval = 0.8 s), and output pulses are delivered 0.8 s after sensed spontaneous QRS complexes (V). When no spontaneous QRS complexes are sensed, ventricular pacing at the programmed rate occurs (arrows).

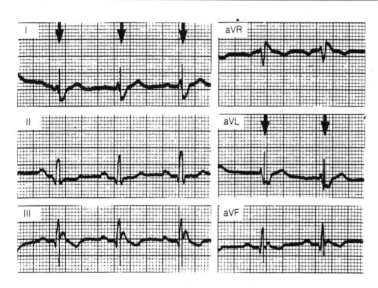

Figure 17-3. Triggered ventricular pacing (VVT). The QRS complexes are spontaneous and stimulated by the sinus P waves that precede them. Within each QRS complex, occurring about 40 ms after the onset of its inscription, is a pacing artifact (arrows), indicating that the complexes were sensed. The pacing artifacts do not contribute to ventricular activation. Triggered pacing might be confused with failure to sense unless the precise mode of function of the implanted generator is known.

which the rate of the pulse generator is noninvasively and reversibly lowered, may allow a spontaneous cardiac rhythm to emerge, which should then be sensed.

P-Synchronous Pacing (VAT & VDD)

P-synchronous pacing systems are dual-chamber systems, in which electrodes are placed in both the atrium and the ventricle. When the atrial electrode senses an electrical signal, a ventricular pacing stimulus is delivered after a programmable **AV delay**, which corresponds roughly to the PR interval (Fig 17-4). Whereas earlier, now obsolete, units (VAT) did not sense ventricular activity, thus resulting in the potential for competitive ventricular rhythms, newer devices (VDD) sense ventricular as well as atrial activity. Since sensing of atrial activity occurs with these devices, **tracking** of the atrial rhythm in a 1:1 ratio occurs, allowing for an increase in the ventricular paced rate concomitant with the increase in sinus rate. The pulse generator is designed so as not to allow rapid ventricular paced rates to occur should the atrial rate become too fast. If no atrial activity is sensed, these pulse generators pace the ventricles on demand, at the programmed **backup rate.**

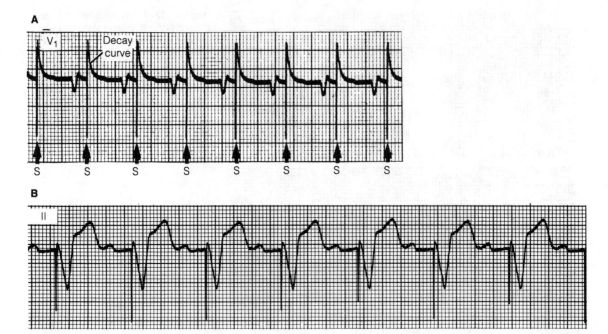

Figure 17-4. P-synchronous pacing (VDD). *A:* The atrial rhythm is sinus. After the (programmed) AV delay, a ventricular stimulus (S) is delivered. Thus, the ventricular paced rate is the same as the sinus rate. Should the atrial rate become very rapid, specific pacemaker design features disallow 1:1 AV pacing in order to protect the ventricles from a rapid paced rate. If spontaneous P wave activity does not occur, the generator paces the ventricles on demand at its programmed rate. In this tracing, a prominent **decay curve** artifact (arrow) follows the delivery of the pacing stimulus, obscuring the QRST complex. Another lead should be employed to accurately assess pacing function. *B:* In this tracing, the paced QRST complexes are clearly seen. Although the *backup rate* of this pulse generator was set at 50/min, the pacing rate is *tracking* the sensed atrial activity, which is occurring at a rate of about 72/min. The **AV delay** has been set at 250 ms in this patient. The P-to-stimulus interval is measured to be 0.28 s, indicating that the P wave was not sensed at its precise onset of inscription in the surface ECG, but about 30 ms after this (0.28–0.25 s). The precise time of sensing a P wave or QRS complex depends upon impulse conduction time within the cardiac chamber, quality of the intracardiac signal, and location of the atrial or ventricular electrode(s).

AV Pacing (DVI)

DVI pacemaker generators have the capability of pacing both the atrium and the ventricle, but they sense only ventricular electrical activity. Since atrial sensing does not occur, the atrial stimulus is always emitted; thus, the possibility of competitive atrial rhythms exists if an atrial pacing stimulus falls in the atrial vulnerable period. With these units, the ventricles will be paced at the programmed AV interval after an atrial pacing stimulus has been delivered. Should a sinus P wave occur and stimulate a spontaneous QRS complex, some generators respond by inhibition of ventricular output, others by delivery of an output pulse at the end of the programmed AV delay, into the refractory period of ventricular tissue, and still others by delivery of an output pulse within the AV interval.

"Universal" Pacing (DDD)

DDD generators are capable of sensing and pacing the atrium and of sensing and pacing the ventricle on demand (Fig 17-5). They thus approach the physiology of normal AV conduction in many patients who require cardiac pacing. Problems associated with the use of DDD devices, as well as VDD devices, relate to their ability to sense retrograde atrial activity and stimulate the ventricles in response, thus creating an artificial extra–AV nodal bypass tract and causing a **pacemaker-mediated reentry tachycardia.** Newer design features are expected to obviate these difficulties.

All dual-chamber devices depend upon a stable atrial rhythm for proper function. If the atrial rhythm is fibrillation, flutter, multifocal tachycardia, or frequent episodes of automatic tachycardia, these generators should not be implanted, and single-chamber ventricular-inhibited or rate-adaptive devices implanted instead.

In patients with atrial arrhythmias who are not candidates for VDD and DDD pacemaker generators, and in patients in whom sinus node dysfunction prevents acceleration of rate, yet would benefit from an increase in paced atrial and/or ventricular rates in response to increases in metabolic demand, generators employing **biosensors** are being evaluated. Some biosensors currently being investigated include right ventricular temperature, right ventricular pH, QT interval, and muscular activity. Changes in these parameters which reflect physiologic needs result in changes in paced rates. Thus, these pacing systems have been termed **rate-adaptive.**

UNIPOLAR & BIPOLAR PACING

Unipolar pacing systems have one electrode in the heart (the cathode) and the other electrode at the generator (the anode). The large distance between the cathode and anode in these systems results in large pacing artifacts whose direction in the frontal plane points toward the anode (generator) (Fig 17–6).

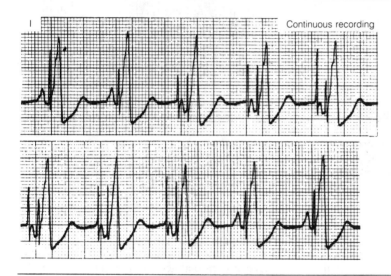

Figure 17–5. Atrial and ventricular pacing in DDD pacing. The first two P waves are sinus and inhibit the atrial pacing output circuit. The atrial rate then slows slightly, and the remaining P waves are paced at the programmed rate of 72/min. All QRS complexes are paced, since no spontaneous QRS complexes occur within the programmed AV interval of 0.14 s. Had a spontaneous QRS complex been stimulated by either a sinus or paced P wave, the ventricular output would have been inhibited.

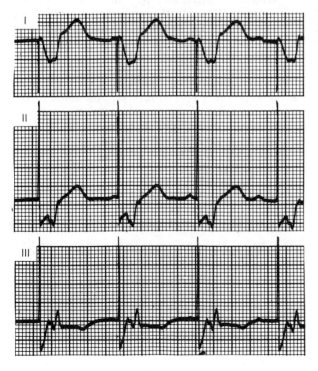

Figure 17–6. Unipolar ventricular pacing system implanted on the left ventricular epicardial surface during cardiac surgery. The large amplitude of the pacing stimuli indicates that this is a unipolar system. The axis of the pacing artifacts is inferiorly directed, indicating that the generator lies inferior to the heart (it was in the upper abdominal wall). The paced QRS complexes have a right bundle branch block pattern, consistent with left ventricular activation occurring earlier than right ventricular activation.

Bipolar pacing systems have both electrodes within the heart, usually 1–2 cm apart. Either the distal (tip) electrode or the proximal (ring) electrode may serve as the cathode. Because of the small interelectrode distance, the pacing artifact is small and its direction in the frontal plane reflects the direction of current flow (Fig 17–7).

ECGs recorded on **digital ECG machines,** rather than on analog ones, can show marked variation in the amplitude and polarity of the pacing impulse. This is because the digital equipment samples the pacing stimulus at specific temporal intervals, and then recreates it on paper. Thus, the inscribed stimulus artifact is not seen in real time. In some instances, the pacing stimulus is entirely invisible, raising the question of failure of generator output. Recognition of this artifact of recording in patients with pacemakers is important in order to avoid erroneous diagnoses of pacemaker malfunction (Fig 17–8).

ELECTROCARDIOGRAPHIC PATTERNS OF PACED COMPLEXES

The configurations of paced complexes will depend upon how the myocardium is depolarized. Paced atrial complexes will reflect the sequence of atrial activation initiated by the pacing impulse and thus, in part, the site of the pacing electrode. Since the atrial electrodes may be located in the atrial appendage or screwed into any portion of atrial tissue, paced P waves will have variable contours (Figs 17–5 and 17–9).

Pacing from the right ventricular endocardial or epicardial apical area will produce QRS complexes that have a *left* bundle branch block configuration (since the right ventricular myocardium is depolarized in advance of the left ventricular myocardium), and a *superior* mean frontal plane axis (since the apex of the heart is depolarized before the base) (Fig 17–10A and B). Paced QRS complexes usually have a duration of 0.12–0.18 s; if they are substantially longer, intrinsic myocardial disease should be suspected.

Pacing from the right ventricular outflow tract results in QRS complexes that have a *left* bundle branch block pattern (since the right ventricular myocardium is depolarized in advance of the left ventricular myocardium) and an *inferiorly directed* mean frontal plane axis (since the base of the heart is depolarized before the apex) (Fig 17–10C). Occasionally, pacing from a site high on the interventricular septum can result in paced QRS complexes that show an indeterminate conduction delay pattern or ones that appear narrow and relatively normal. This reflects activation of both the right and left sides of the interventricular septum nearly simultaneously.

Pacing from the left ventricular epicardium will

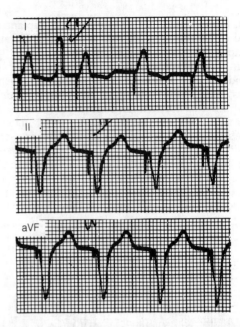

Figure 17–7. Bipolar ventricular pacing. The pacing artifacts have a small amplitude, indicating a small interelectrode distance. They are negatively directed in leads II and III, reflecting an inferior to superior direction of current flow. Thus, the distal (tip) electrode has been made negative and the proximal (ring) electrode has been made positive, with current traveling from tip to ring.

produce paced QRS complexes that have a *right* bundle branch block pattern, reflecting left ventricular myocardial activation in advance of right ventricular activation (Fig 17–6). The mean frontal plane QRS axis will depend upon the location of the epicardial electrodes relative to each other (bipolar system) or to the pulse generator (unipolar system).

Spontaneous QRS complexes occurring in patients with pacemakers often show marked T wave inversion (Fig 17–11). Although the cause of the T wave inversion is not understood, it should not be interpreted to indicate myocardial disease. Simiar T wave abnormalities may be seen in patients with intermittent intraventricular conduction delays and in patients with rapid supraventricular tachyarrhythmias.

PACEMAKER MALFUNCTION

The general categories of pacemaker malfunction are **failure to sense** and **failure to capture.** Sensing of unwanted electrical signals (such as T waves, myopotentials, and environmental signals such as electrocautery) does *not* represent failure to sense and is termed **oversensing.** Programming the pulse generator to "see" electrical signals of

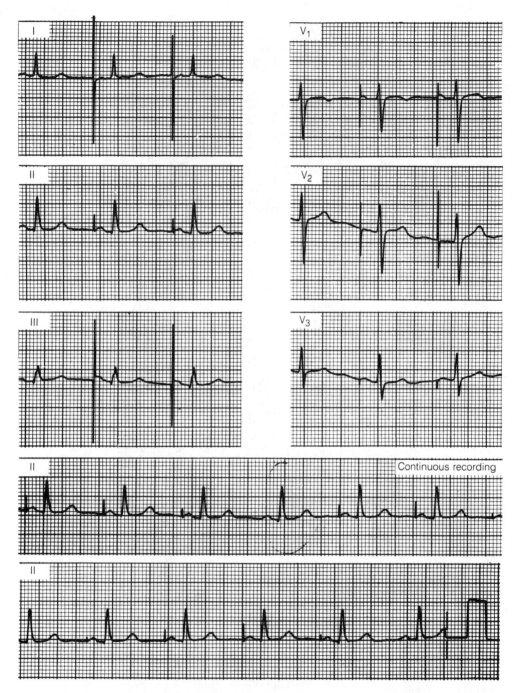

Figure 17-8. DDD pacing in which atrial pacing is followed by normally conducted QRS complexes, inhibiting ventricular output. Note the variation in amplitude of the output pulses, mimicking electrode fracture. Recording the ECG using analog equipment will clarify the issue.

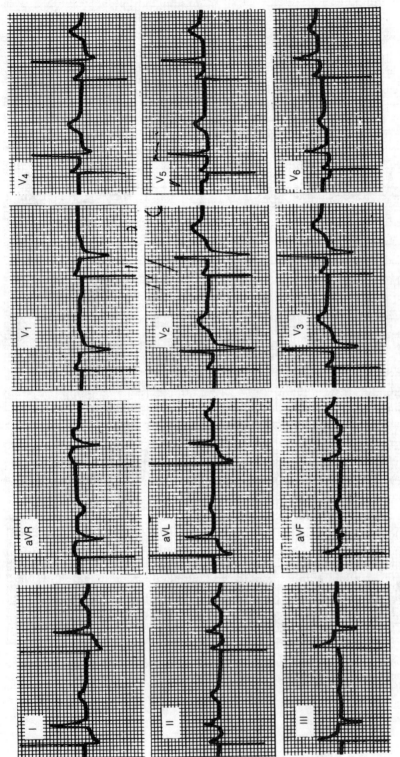

Figure 17–9. Transvenous atrial pacing with intact AV conduction. The atrial electrode is unipolar, accounting for the large pacing artifacts. The large artifact and its associated **decay curve** often obscure the contour of the paced P waves. In this tracing, the paced P waves are upright in II, III, and aVF and negative in I and aVL. Since the P wave vector is directed inferiorly and rightward, the atrial electrode is located in the high right atrium.

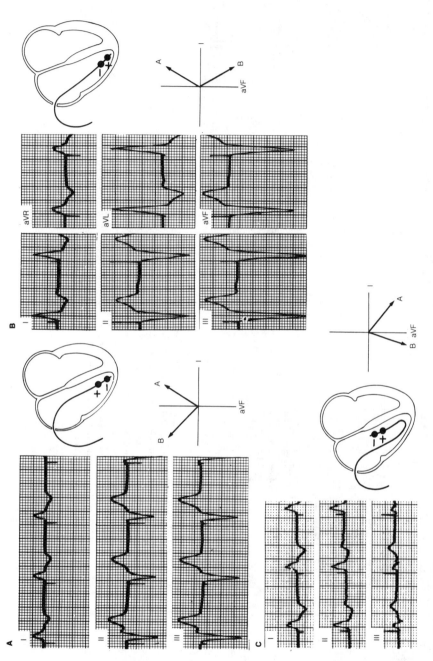

Figure 17–10. Diagrammatic illustrations of bipolar pacing systems. *A:* The pacing catheter is located in the right ventricular apical area. The distal (tip) electrode is the cathode and the proximal (ring) electrode is the anode. The pacing artifact is small because of the small interelectrode distance. Since current flows from cathode to anode, the pacing artifact axis is oriented rightward and superiorly (arrow B), producing small negative deflections in I, II, and III. The myocardium is depolarized leftward and superiorly (arrow A), resulting in upright QRS complexes in lead I and negative QRS complexes in II and III. *B:* The distal (tip) electrode is the anode and the proximal (ring) electrode is the cathode. The pacing artifact is oriented leftward and inferiorly (arrow B), resulting in upright deflections in II, III, and aVF. The myocardium is depolarized leftward and superiorly (arrow A), resulting in upright QRS complexes in leads I and aVL and negative complexes in II, III, and aVF. *C:* The pacing catheter is located in the outflow tract of the right ventricle. Current flows from cathode to anode (tip to ring), and thus the pacing artifacts are directed inferiorly, resulting in upright deflections in II and III. Since current is also flowing from left to right in this diagram, the pacing artifact is negative in lead I. The myocardium is depolarized from base to apex, resulting in upright QRS complexes in II and III.

291

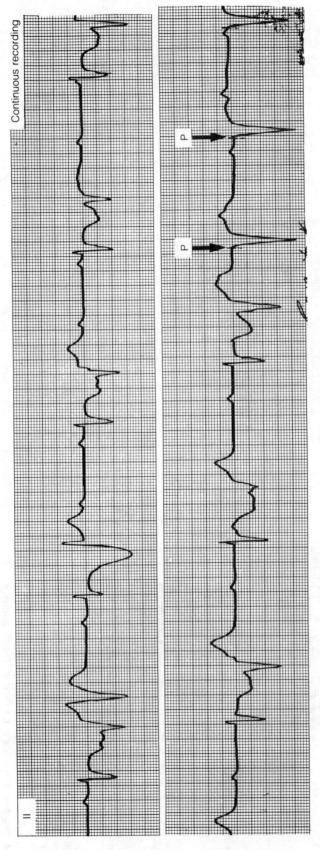

Continuous recording

Figure 17–11. Noninvasive programming of the pacemaker rate to below that of the patient's spontaneous rhythm and rate. Sinus rhythm with high-degree AV block is present. Ventricular premature complexes and couplets are seen, which are probably bradycardia-dependent since they were not observed at faster QRS rates. There is marked QT interval prolongation with diffusely abnormal ST–T waves. This patient was receiving no cardiac medications and her electrolytes were normal. The ST–T wave abnormalities are not specific for any diagnosis, and are commonly observed in patients with pacemakers during normal spontaneous rhythm. At the end of the strip, the pacemaker rate has been increased and the last 3 QRS complexes are paced.

larger magnitude will often solve the problem. Conversely, **undersensing** or cardiac electrical signals due to poor signal quality may represent not sensing failure but rather reflects the suboptimal nature of the signal itself. Undersensed QRS complexes are not rare and tend to originate in ventricular tissue (premature ventricular depolarizations) or occur during acute myocardial infarction or because of drug toxicity and electrolyte imbalance (Fig 17–12).

Failure to sense spontaneous complexes results in the delivery of a pacing stimulus earlier than expected (Fig 17–12). This may cause competitive atrial or ventricular rhythms, which may on occasion be life-threatening.

Occasionally, in patients with transvenous right ventricular VVI pacing systems, pacing artifacts occur within spontaneous QRS complexes having a right bundle branch block configuration (Fig 17–13). Failure to sense QRS complexes having a right bundle branch block pattern indicates that, because of the delay in conduction in the right bundle branch, the wave of ventricular depolarization did not reach the area of the pacing catheter in the right ventricular apex before the pacing stimulus was due to arrive. This phenomenon may also be observed in patients with inferior and right ventricular myocardial infarction and is probably due to the conduction delay resulting from ventricular scarring. Because failure to "see" the

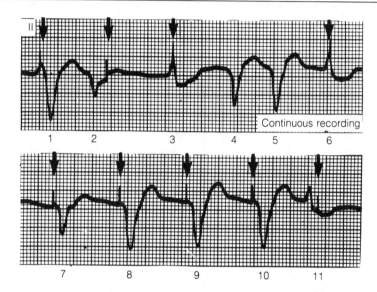

Figure 17–12. Intermittent "failure" to sense. Pacing stimuli are delivered earlier than expected (QRS complexes 2, 3, 6, and 11), indicating failure to sense those complexes, which is probably due to their poor signal quality. The delivery of pacing stimuli in the ventricular vulnerable period could result in repetitive ventricular rhythms.

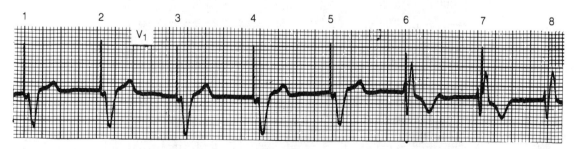

Figure 17–13. Transvenous right ventricular demand pacing system with electrode catheter located in the right ventricular apex. QRS complexes 6, 7, and 8 are spontaneous and show a right bundle branch block configuration. The first 2 of these have pacing artifacts within them, indicating that they were not sensed. This is due to the right ventricular conduction delay, with consequent late arrival at the electrode of the ventricular activation wave front. This does not represent sensing failure. As the differential diagnosis of this rhythm strip includes **triggered pacing** with episodic failure to sense those QRS complexes not containing a pacing artifact within them, knowledge of the mode of function of the implanted device is mandatory.

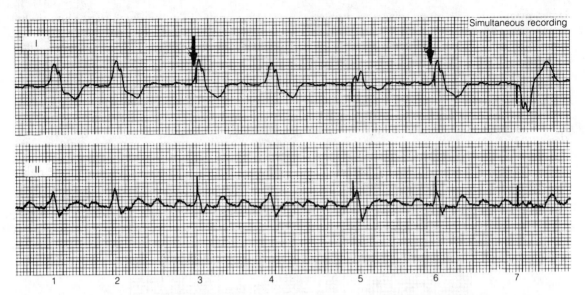

Figure 17-14. Left ventricular epicardial VVI pacing system in a patient with underlying left bundle branch block. The last QRS complex in the tracing is the only purely paced complex. QRS complexes 1 through 6 are spontaneous complexes, and the fifth is a fusion complex. Pacing artifacts (arrows) appear within 2 of the spontaneous QRS complexes, indicating that they were not sensed. Sensing function was normal in this patient: this rhythm strip illustrates that the conduction delay over the left ventricle caused by the underlying left bundle branch block delayed the depolarization wave front from reaching the epicardical electrodes in time to inhibit the output of the pulse generator (programmed at 60/min).

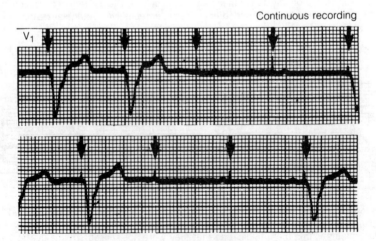

Figure 17-15. Intermittent failure to capture. Pacing artifacts are indicated by the arrows. Long pauses in paced rhythm, during which pacing artifacts occur but do not stimulate QRS complexes, indicate failure to pace. The problem could be due to generator failure or an increase in the myocardial stimulation threshold.

wave front of ventricular activation is due to intrinsic conduction system disease, true failure to sense is not present. The same principles apply to patients with left ventricular epicardial electrodes who have underlying left bundle branch block (Fig 17–14).

Failure to pace is present when pacing stimuli do not depolarize myocardium (Fig 17–15). This may result from poor electrode position, from pulse generator output reduction (battery end-of-life), or from an increase in myocardial stimulation threshold due to acute myocardial infarction, drug toxicity, electrolyte imbalance, cardiopulmonary resuscitation, or fibrosis at the pacing catheter tip. Pacing failure can be managed acutely by noninvasive programming of the energy output of the genrator to its maximum, but lead repositioning or implantation of a new generator (or both) may be required, depending upon the underlying problem.

REFERENCES

Chung EK: *Artificial Cardiac Pacing; Practical Approach.* Williams & Wilkins, 1979.

Furman S, Hayes DL, Holmes DR Jr: *A Practice of Cardiac Pacing.* Futura, 1986.

Goldschlager N (editor): Cardiac Pacemakers. *Cardiol Clin* 1985;**3**:1.

Mond HG: *Cardiac Pacemaker: Function and Malfunction.* Grune & Stratton, 1983.

Figure 17-T1.
TEST TRACINGS

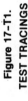

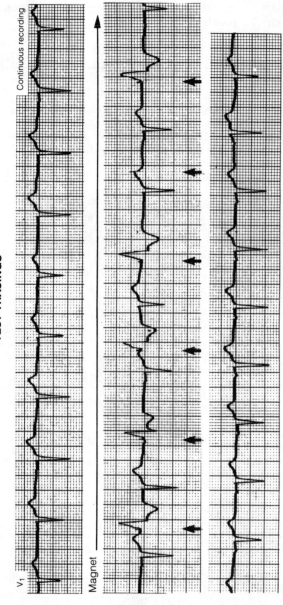

The patient has a VVI pacing system in place.

Is sensing function normal? How do you know?

Yes, since no output pulses are delivered during normal sinus rhythm (top and bottom strips).

Is pacing function normal? How do you know?

Pacing function can be assessed in this patient only by slowing his intrinsic rate below that of the pacemaker, or by applying a magnet over the pulse generator, thus converting it to VOO function in which spontaneous QRS complexes will not be sensed. Capture is demonstrated in the middle strip, during application of the magnet.

The fifth pacing output pulse in the middle strip fails to capture the ventricles. Does this indicate failure to pace? Explain the finding.

The ventricles are refractory during delivery of this pacing stimulus, having just been depolarized by the preceding beat. Pacing will occur only at those times during which ventricular tissue is not refractory.

Which type of pacemaker malfunction would have been diagnosed had it not been known that a magnet had been applied?

Failure to sense.

Figure 17-T2.
TEST TRACINGS

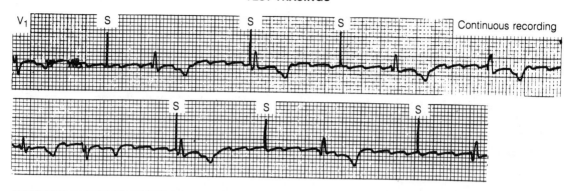

The patient has a VII pacing system in place.

Is sensing function intact? How do you know?

Yes. Spontaneous QRS complexes inhibit the pacemaker output.

Is pacing function intact? How do you know?

No. Pacing stimuli are delivered (S) which fail to produce a QRS complex.

What is the programmed rate of the pacemaker? How is this measured?

Two consecutive output pulses must be present for rate to be determined. In this patient, the programmed rate is 60/min.

What is the escape interval of the pacemaker? How is it measured?

About 1000 ms, measured from a spontaneous QRS complex to the first paced complex which follows it. This is usually (but not always) the same as the programmed interstimulus interval.

Figure 17-T3.
TEST TRACINGS

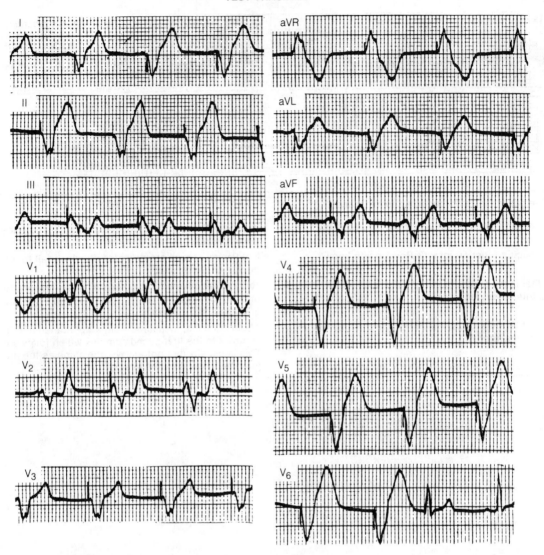

Describe the features of this ventricular pacing system.

Is the system unipolar or bipolar? Why?

Bipolar, since the amplitude of the pacing artifacts is small.

What is the morphology of the paced QRS complexes?

Right bundle branch block configuration.

Where are the electrodes located?

Left ventricle (epicardial surface).

Is pacing function intact? How is this known?

Yes. Output stimuli are always followed by QRS complexes.

Is sensing function normal? How is this known?

Yes. The spontaneous QRS complexes in V_6 inhibit the generator output.

Is acute anterior wall myocardial infarction present?

Cannot tell, since ventricular depolarization is abnormal, and repolarization changes cannot be interpreted.

Figure 17-T4.
TEST TRACINGS

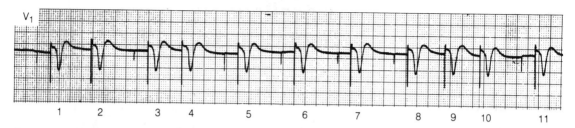

A DDD pacing system is in place.

Is atrial sensing intact? How do you know?

Cannot tell with certainty, since no spontaneous P waves are seen. However, the earlier-than-expected paced QRS complexes (2,4,9,10) suggest that they have been triggered by sensing of some atrial electrical activity by the atrial electrode.

Is atrial pacing intact? How do you know?

No. Atrial output pulses are not followed by paced P waves.

Is ventricular sensing intact? How do you know?

Cannot tell, since there are no spontaneous QRS complexes.

Is ventricular pacing intact? How do you know?

Yes. All ventricular output pulses are followed by paced QRS complexes.

This patient had severe hyperkalemia which resulted in atrial arrest despite the delivery of electrical pacing stimuli. Since atrial muscle is not depolarized, a P wave is not generated.

18 Miscellaneous Abnormal Electrocardiographic Patterns

PERICARDITIS

The earliest electrocardiographic evidence of pericarditis is ST segment elevation in those leads overlying the involved area, reflecting **epicardial injury current.** The ST segment elevation may be diffuse or localized. The ST segment elevation is typically *concave* upward, in contrast to that of acute myocardial infarction, which is convex upward (Fig 18-1). Lead aVR or V_1 (or both) may show (reciprocal) ST segment depression (Fig 18-1). After days or weeks, depending upon the clinical course of the pericarditis, the ST segments become isoelectric and the T waves inverted (Figs 18-1, 18-2 and 18-3). Occasionally, the ST elevation resolves without T wave inversion, or T wave inversion may occur and persist for months. Abnormal Q waves are not present in pericarditis.

In pericarditis with effusion, *serial* ECGs may show a decrease in voltage of P waves and QRS complexes. Low voltage per se, however, is not specific for pericardial effusion (Table 18-1). **Electrical alternans** may occur (Figs 18-4 and 18-5). Electrical alternans, in which the height of the complexes alternates, can involve the QRS complexes, P waves, T waves, U waves, and even the ST segments. Its genesis is poorly understood. Electrical alternans is seen in severe heart disease due to any cause as well as in large pericardial effusion and is therefore not specific for this diagnosis. Electrical alternans should not be confused with **mechanical (pulsus) alternans,** in which ventricular contractions of alternating force produce blood pressures of alternating magnitude.

PR segment depression is commonly seen in pericarditis (Fig 18-1). This represents prominence of the atrial repolarization (T_a) wave and may reflect atrial involvement in the pericardial process. Because PR segment depression is also seen in atrial infarction and during exercise, it is not specific for the diagnosis of pericarditis. However, if pericarditis is the cause, the PR segment depression is usually present in both limb and precordial leads.

Atrial arrhythmias are frequent in pericarditis.

The ST segment elevation of pericarditis may be confused with early repolarization changes in normal individuals (see Chapter 5). However, ST segment depression in lead aVR and V_1 is not a usual feature of normal variant ECGs; and PR segment depression, if it is present, tends to be

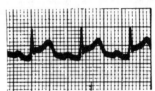
Concave ST elevation in pericarditis

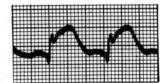
Convex ST elevation in myocardial infarction

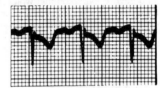
Cavity complex; pericarditis

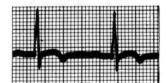
Late pattern; pericarditis

Figure 18-1. Electrocardiographic patterns in pericarditis and myocardial infarction.

Table 18-1. Causes of low voltage in the electrocardiogram.

Pericardial effusion (any etiology)
Chronic obstructive pulmonary disease
Obesity
Myxedema
Infiltrative heart disease
   Scleroderma
   Amyloidosis
   Tumor
Anasarca
Pericardial constriction
Cardiomyopathy (any etiology)
Pleural effusion
Pneumothorax

less widespread than in pericarditis. Finally, the serial electrocardiographic changes that accompany resolving pericarditis are not a feature of the normal variant ECG, in which the ST elevations are stable over time.

MYOCARDITIS

Any acute or chronic disease can involve the myocardium and thereby result in electrocardiographic abnormalities that are not specific for a particular diagnosis. These abnormalities include the following: (1) prolongation of the PR interval; (2) arrhythmias, (3) ST segment abnormalities; (4) isolated T wave abnormalities; (5) prolongation of the QT interval; and (6) changes in the QRS con-

figuration, which may mimic myocardial infarction (Fig 18–6). Since the electrocardiographic changes are nondiagnostic, clinical correlation is mandatory.

HYPERTHYROIDISM

The usual electrocardiographic findings in hyperthyroidism are sinus tachycardia and nonspecific ST and T wave abnormalities (Fig 18–7). Atrial fibrillation with a very rapid ventricular rate (due to enhanced AV nodal conduction of the fibrillatory impulses) may also be seen. The abnormalities are expected to resolve with treatment of the hyperthyroidism, but normalization of the ECG may take weeks to months.

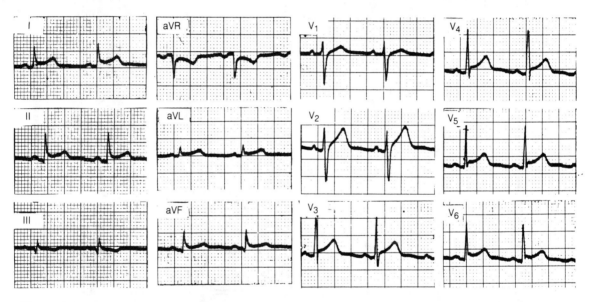

Figure 18–2. Acute pericarditis. ST segment elevation with concave upward curvature is seen in leads I, II, aVL, aVF, and V$_{2-6}$. Reciprocal ST segment depression is seen in lead aVR.

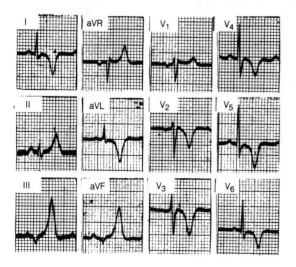

Figure 18–3. Pericarditis (late pattern). Deep, symmetrically inverted T waves in I, aVL, and V$_{2-6}$. The marked T wave abnormalities, unusual in pericarditis, may indicate concomitant myocarditis.

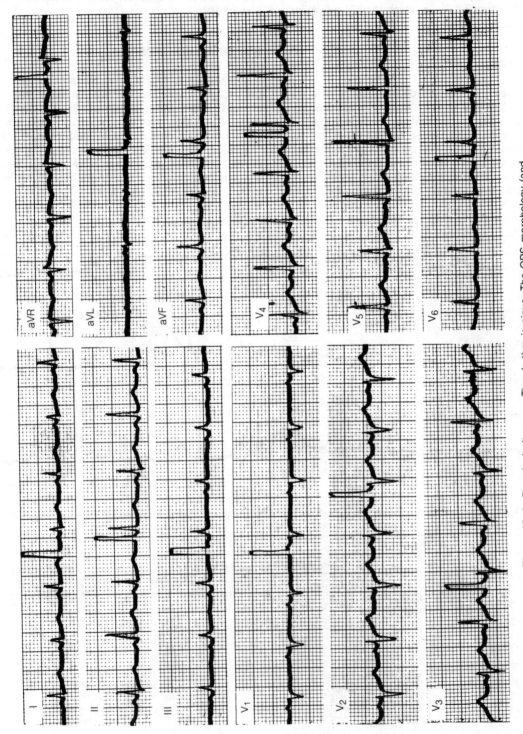

Figure 18–4. Electrical alternans. The rhythm is sinus. The QRS morphology (and polarity in some leads) alternates in an absolutely regular fashion.

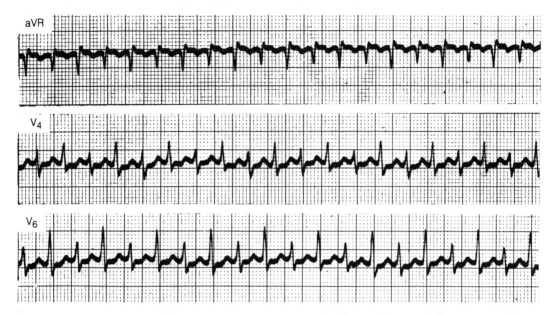

Figure 18-5. Apparent electrical alternans. The rhythm is a reentry supraventricular tachycardia with a rate of 200/min. The alternation of the QRS amplitude in the presence of reentry tachycardia does not represent electrical alternans but rather reflects antegrade conduction to the ventricles over 2 pathways in alternating fashion.

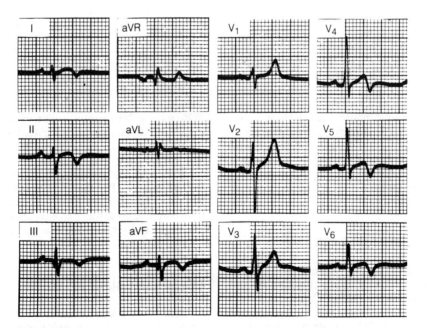

Figure 18-6. Abnormal ECG with nondiagnostic ST–T wave abnormalities. The T waves are deeply and symmetrically inverted in I, II, III, and V_{4-6}, suggesting a diffuse myocardial process. The clinical diagnosis was acute viral myocarditis in a 22-year-old-man.

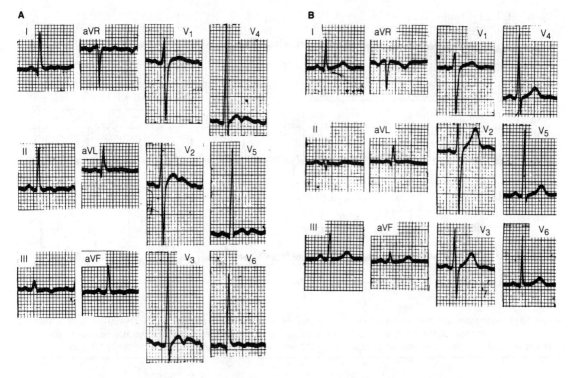

Figure 18-7. Hyperthyroidism. *A:* Taken prior to therapy for hyperthyroidism. Rate = 110/min. The T waves are inverted in I, II, III, aVF, and V_6, flat in aVL, and diphasic in V_{2-5}. These changes are nonspecific. $RV_5 + SV_1 = 40$ mm. Ordinarily, this would be suggestive of left ventricular hypertrophy, but these voltage criteria are invalid in the presence of hyperthyroidism. *B:* ECG recorded when patient was euthyroid.

MYXEDEMA

Electrocardiograpic features suggesting myxedema include sinus bradycardia, prolongation of the PR interval, low QRS and P wave voltages, and flat T waves (Fig 18–8). As with hyperthyroidism, these abnormalities regress with treatment of the myxedema, but the resolution may take weeks to months.

TRAUMATIC HEART DISEASE

Trauma to the heart can produce coronary artery laceration, coronary artery thrombosis, and myocardial contusion. The ECG may therefore reflect abnormalities of acute myocardial necrosis and may mimic completely acute myocardial infarction due to coronary artery disease. Electrocardiographic patterns of pericarditis are common (Fig 18–9). Supraventricular and ventricular arrhythmias may occur and may be life-threatening.

TUMOR

Primary or metastatic tumor of the heart produces electrocardiographic patterns compatible with infiltration of the myocardial tissue. Thus, low voltage, q waves suggesting myocardial infarction, and intraventricular conduction delays may all be seen (Fig 18–10). The low voltage may be due to replacement of the myocardium by tumor tissue or to associated malignant pericardial effusion. Arrhythmias are also seen.

NEUROMUSCULAR DISEASES

Friedreich's ataxia, progressive muscular dystrophy (Duchenne or pseudohypertrophic), and myotonia dystrophica are neuromuscular diseases commonly associated with electrocardiographic abnormalities. PR interval prolongation, arrhythmias, and nonspecific ST and T wave abnormali-

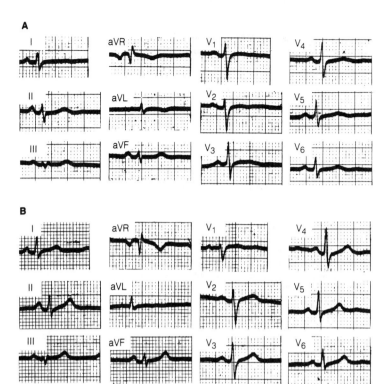

Figure 18-8. Myxedema. *A:* The QRS complexes are of low voltage and the T waves of low amplitude in all leads. *B:* Three weeks after thyroid therapy: The T waves are now of normal amplitude, and there is a slight increase in the QRS voltage.

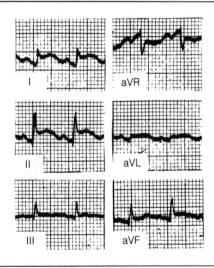

Figure 18-9. Cardiac trauma due to gunshot wound to the chest. ST segment elevation is present in all leads except aVR, which shows ST depression. PR segment depression is seen in I, II, and aVF. These diffuse changes could reflect pericarditis and myocarditis or myocardial necrosis; serial ECGs are required for correct interpretation.

ties are the changes most commonly observed, but hypertrophy patterns and deviation of the mean frontal plane QRS axis also occur.

HYPOTHERMIA

The electrocardiographic manifestations of hypothermia include sinus bradycardia (often extreme), atrial fibrillation, escape rhythms, prolongation of the QT interval, and **Osborne ("J")** waves. The J waves are waves inscribed at the terminal portion of the QRS complexes, before the ST segment and T wave (Fig 18-11). Although their genesis is incompletely understood, they likely reflect the different sensitivity to temperature of the cellular NA^+ and Ca^{2+} depolarizing currents. J waves should not be mistaken for portions of QRS complexes or for ST segment elevation. J waves, atrial fibrillation, and ventricular fibrillation reflect severe hypothermia (25°C or less).

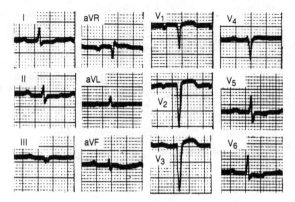

Figure 18-10. Metastatic bronchogenic carcinoma involving the heart. The QRS complexes have low voltage in the limb leads. QRS complexes are present in V_{1-2}, and ST segment elevation is seen in V_{2-3}. Although these findings might suggest anterior wall myocardial infarction due to coronary disease, in this case they are due to replacement of the myocardium by tumor tissue. The ECG records the electrically "dead" or "silent" area of tissue but cannot, of course, distinguish its cause.

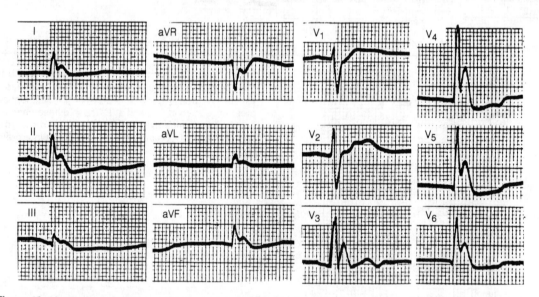

Figure 18-11. Hypothermia. The ventricular rate is 50/min. Atrial activity is not seen. The QRS complexes are narrow and are deformed at their terminal portions by a slurred wave occurring prior to the inscription of the ST–T waves; this is the J wave. The QT interval is prolonged. (Courtesy of R Brindis, MD.)

REFERENCES

Karjalainen J: Functional and myocarditis-induced T-wave abnormalities: Effect of orthostasis, beta-blockade, and epinephrine. *Chest* 1983;**83**:868.

Spodick DH: Differential characteristics of the electrocardiogram in early repolarization and acute pericarditis. *N Engl J Med* 1976;**295**:523.

Stolar I et al: P wave changes in intracerebral hemorrhage: Clinical, echocardiographic, and CT scan correlation. *Am Heart J* 1984;**107**:784.

Yamour BJ et al: Electrocardiographic changes in cerebrovascular hemorrhage. *Am Heart J* 1980;**99**:294.

Figure 18-T1.
TEST TRACINGS

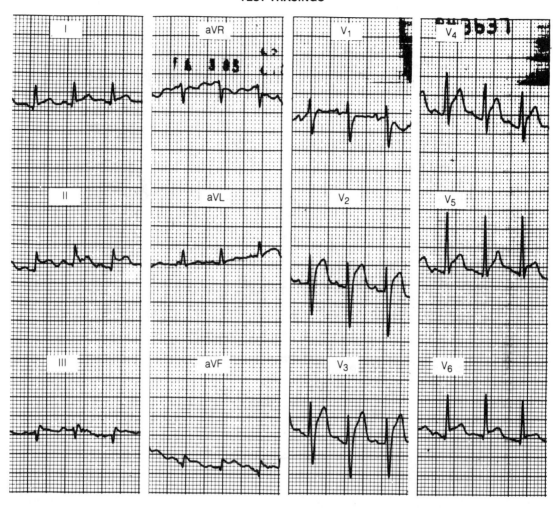

What features of this ECG are compatible with pericarditis?

Diffuse ST segment elevation except in aVR, in which ST segment depression is present.

Is PR segment depression present?

The PR segment cannot be identified with certainty since, due to the sinus tachycardia, there is no isoelectric baseline visible.

Is acute myocardial infarction probable or not? Why or why not?

The ST segment elevation is too diffuse to suggest acute myocardial infarction in a particular region of myocardium.

Is pericardial effusion likely to be present? Why or why not?

Cannot tell from a single ECG; serial ECGs, which show a decrease in voltage, are required for this diagnosis.

Is electrical alternans present?

No: there is baseline movement (which was in fact due to respiration) but no alternation in amplitude of the P–QRST complexes.

Figure 18–T2.
TEST TRACINGS

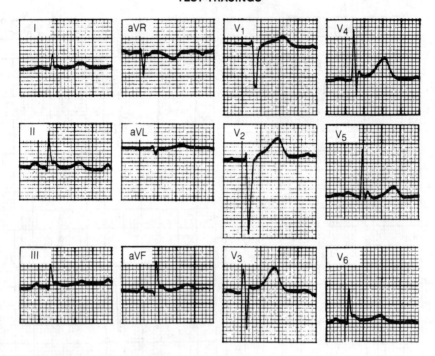

Does this tracing represent early repolarization?	No.
Does this tracing represent ST segment elevation?	No.
Is intraventricular conduction delay present?	No.
What is the wave at the terminal portion of the QRS complexes?	The J wave (best seen in II, III, aVF, and V_{4-6}).
What is the diagnosis?	Hypothermia.

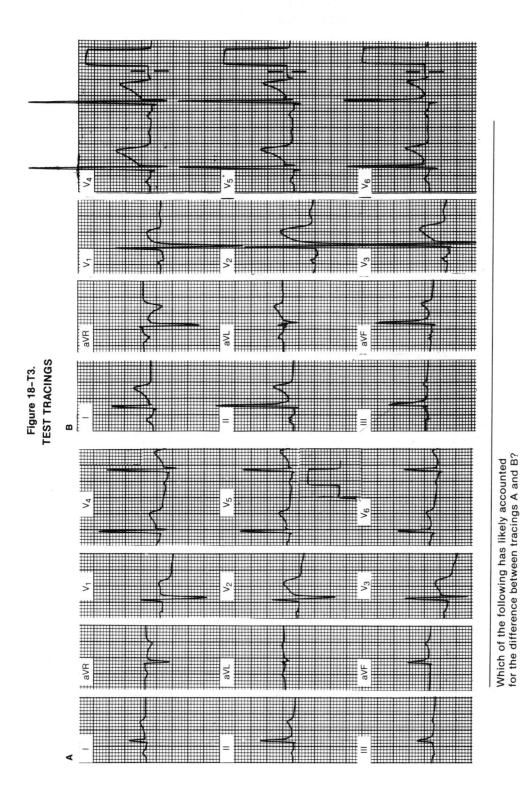

Figure 18–T3.
TEST TRACINGS

Which of the following has likely accounted
for the difference between tracings A and B?

Acute myocardial infarction

Acute pericarditis

Acute myocarditis

Artifact of recording

Artifact. Note the double standard in tracing B.

Figure 18-T4.
TEST TRACINGS

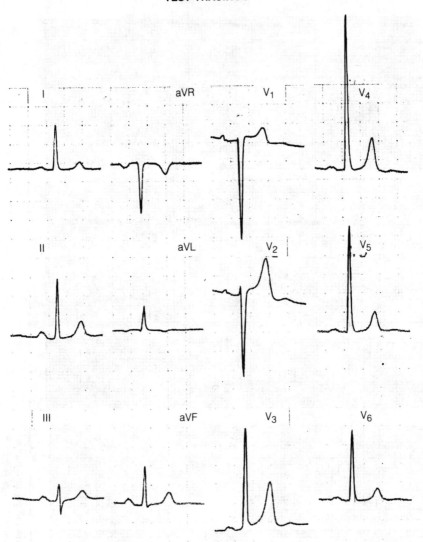

What features might suggest pericarditis?	The ST elevation in V_{2-3}.
What features suggest that pericarditis is not present?	Neither diffuse ST elevation nor PR segment depression are present.
What features suggest acute myocardial infarction?	The ST elevation in V_{2-3} and the peaked T waves in V_{2-5}.
Is hyperkalemia suggested?	Possibly, in view of the tented T waves in V_{2-5}.
What is the diagnosis?	Clinical correlation is mandatory. The patient was a normal healthy individual.

Figure 18-T5.
TEST TRACINGS

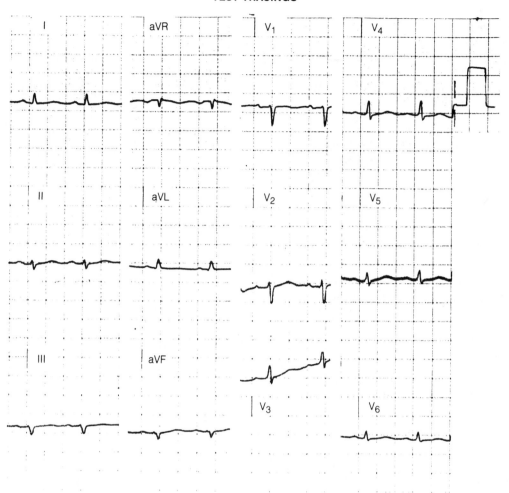

What is the mean frontal plane QRS axis?	−30°.
What is the P wave axis?	+30°.
Are the ST segments elevated, depressed, or normal-appearing?	Normal-appearing.
Is the ECG understandardized?	No; the calibration is indicated at the right of the tracing.
What is the abnormality in this tracing?	Diffuse low voltage.
List some causes of this finding.	See Table 18-1.

The patient had biventricular congestive heart failure with anasarca. With diuresis, the electrocardiographic voltage increased somewhat.

19

Exercise Electrocardiography

Since the resting ECG is normal in 25–40% of patients with angina due to coronary artery disease, exercise tests have been developed to provoke myocardial ischemia. Exercise test protocols are designed to impose **incremental work loads** on the patient, with a resulting increase in heart rate and blood pressure. The tests are performed either by walking on a motorized treadmill, or by pedaling a bicycle while sitting upright or lying supine. Continuous electrocardiographic monitoring is performed throughout the test, and a 12-lead ECG is recorded every 90 seconds during exercise and every minute in the post-exercise recovery period, unless the clinical circumstances warrant other approaches. Since the limb leads are applied to the torso in the exercising patient (rather than on the upper and lower extremities themselves), some differences in QRS axis, morphology, and voltage from those usually recorded might be observed.

The product of the heart rate and systolic blood pressure (the **double product**) is an index of myocardial oxygen consumption; the exercise-induced increase in double product should be met by an increase in myocardial blood flow unless this is limited by obstructive coronary artery disease or an increase in coronary artery vasomotor tone, or spasm. If coronary artery blood flow is insufficient to meet the metabolic demands of the myocardium, myocardial ischemia develops, with its attendant effects on the ECG.

Indications for Exercise Testing

The usual indications for exercise testing are the evaluation of chest pain syndromes (Table 19–1). The clinical history serves to help classify the patient into groups in which the chest pain is felt to be of ischemic or nonischemic origin. The prevalence of atherosclerotic coronary artery disease demonstrated by coronary arteriography will vary according to the clinical presentation (Table 19–2), as well as according to the patient's age, sex, and presence or absence of risk factors for coronary disease (such as hypertension, smoking, hypercholesterolemia, and diabetes). Since the accuracy of the interpretation of the exercise ECG for the disease being diagnosed depends upon the prevalence of the disease (Table 19–3), careful clinical evaluation of the patient prior to the exercise test is most important. For example, patients with a history highly suggestive of typical effort angina are *likely* to have underlying coronary disease, so an exercise ECG suggesting myocardial ischemia is likely to be a true result (**true-positive**

Table 19-1. Indications for exercise testing.

I. Evaluation of chest pain syndromes
   A. Typical angina of effort
   B. Atypical chest pain considered to be of cardiac origin
   C. Atypical chest pain not considered to be of cardiac origin
II. Evaluation of effort tolerance
   A. Postmyocardial infarction
   B. Postmyocardial revascularization
   C. Valvular heart disease
   D. Disability assessment
III. Arrhythmia detection
IV. Evaluation of the effect of therapy
   A. Exercise BP in hypertensive patients
   B. Antianginal medications
   C. Antiarrhythmic medication or myocardial revascularization (or both) procedures for exercise-related rhythm disturbances.

Table 19-2. Prevalences of Angiographically documented coronary artery disease in patients undergoing exercise tests for the evaluation of chest pain.

	Age less than 50		Age greater than 50	
	Men	Women	Men	Women
Nonspecific chest pain	10%	5%	20%	7%
Chest pain of probable cardiac origin	55%	30%	70%	35%
Chest pain of definite cardiac origin	85%	60%	95%	75%

Table 19-3. Predictive accuracy of exercise electrocardiography for the diagnosis of coronary artery disease.

	+ test		− test	
	Men	Women	Men	Women
Angina pectoris				
Typical	100%	83%	55%	45%
Probable	82%	45%	70%	71%
Chest pain, non-cardiac origin	45%	0%	83%	97%

Table 19-4. Causes of 'false-negative' exercise ECGs.

1. Angiographically demonstrated lesions do not produce functional myocardial ischemia
2. Use of a single monitoring electrocardiographic lead
3. Past myocardial infarction which obscures ischemic electrocardiographic abnormalities

ECG result) (Table 19–3). In contrast, patients with nonspecific chest pain not reminiscent of angina are *unlikely* to have coronary disease, so an abnormal exercise ECG is likely to represent a false result (**false-positive** ECG result).

Patients with typical angina who have a normal exercise test but who have coronary artery disease documented angiographically should be considered to have anatomic coronary disease which either is unassociated with demonstrable myocardial ischemia, or does not produce ECG abnormalities for other physiologic or technical reasons (a **false-negative** ECG result, Table 19–4).

Definitions of Test Functions

The definitions of the function of a given test, such as the exercise test, are given in Table 5–1.

For treadmill exercise testing, the *overall* test sensitivity should be in the range of about 65% (sensitivity increases with increasing extent and severity of coronary artery disease), and the specificity 90–95%. The post-test risk of disease will reflect the pre-test risk for the disease together with the added information provided by the test itself.

Exercise tests are terminated when the patient develops symptoms or signs of myocardial ischemia, when the ECG indicates the probability of severe multivessel coronary disease, or when maximum (exhaustive) exercise has been performed (Table 19–5, page 316).

ELECTROCARDIOGRAPHIC ABNORMALITIES

The ST segment and T wave abnormalities which are indicative of myocardial ischemia are: ST segment *elevation,* which reflects transmural ischemic injury (unless past Q wave infarction is represented in the same ECG leads that show ST elevation), and ST segment *depression,* which reflects nontransmural ischemic injury. ST segment depression is further characterized as *downsloping, horizontal,* and *slowly upsloping* (Fig 19–1); in all cases, the J point must be depressed at *least 1 mm* below the isoelectric baseline for the diagnosis of myocardial ischemia to be considered. J point depression with a rapidly upsloping ST segment is a normal response to exercise.

Exercise responses other than ECG abnormalities are often helpful in suggesting the presence of severe coronary disease (Table 19–6, page 316), and in assessing prognosis.

Downsloping ST depression (Fig 19–2 on pages 314–315) is the most specific electrocardiographic abnormality for the diagnosis of fixed obstructive coronary artery disease based on the coronary arteriogram (exceeding 95%) and usually indicates severe multivessel disease. Horizontal ST depression is slightly less specific (about 85%), followed by slowly upsloping ST depression, defined as at least 2 mm of ST depression below the baseline 80 ms after the J point (75–80%). ST segment

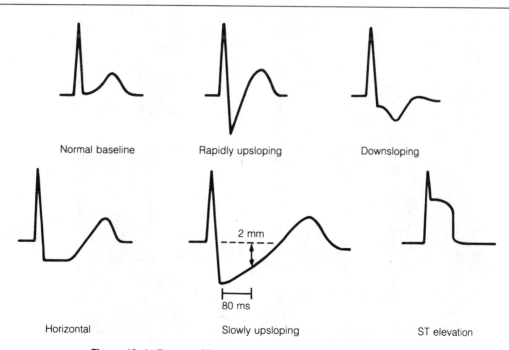

Figure 19–1. Types of ST segment and T wave responses to exercise.

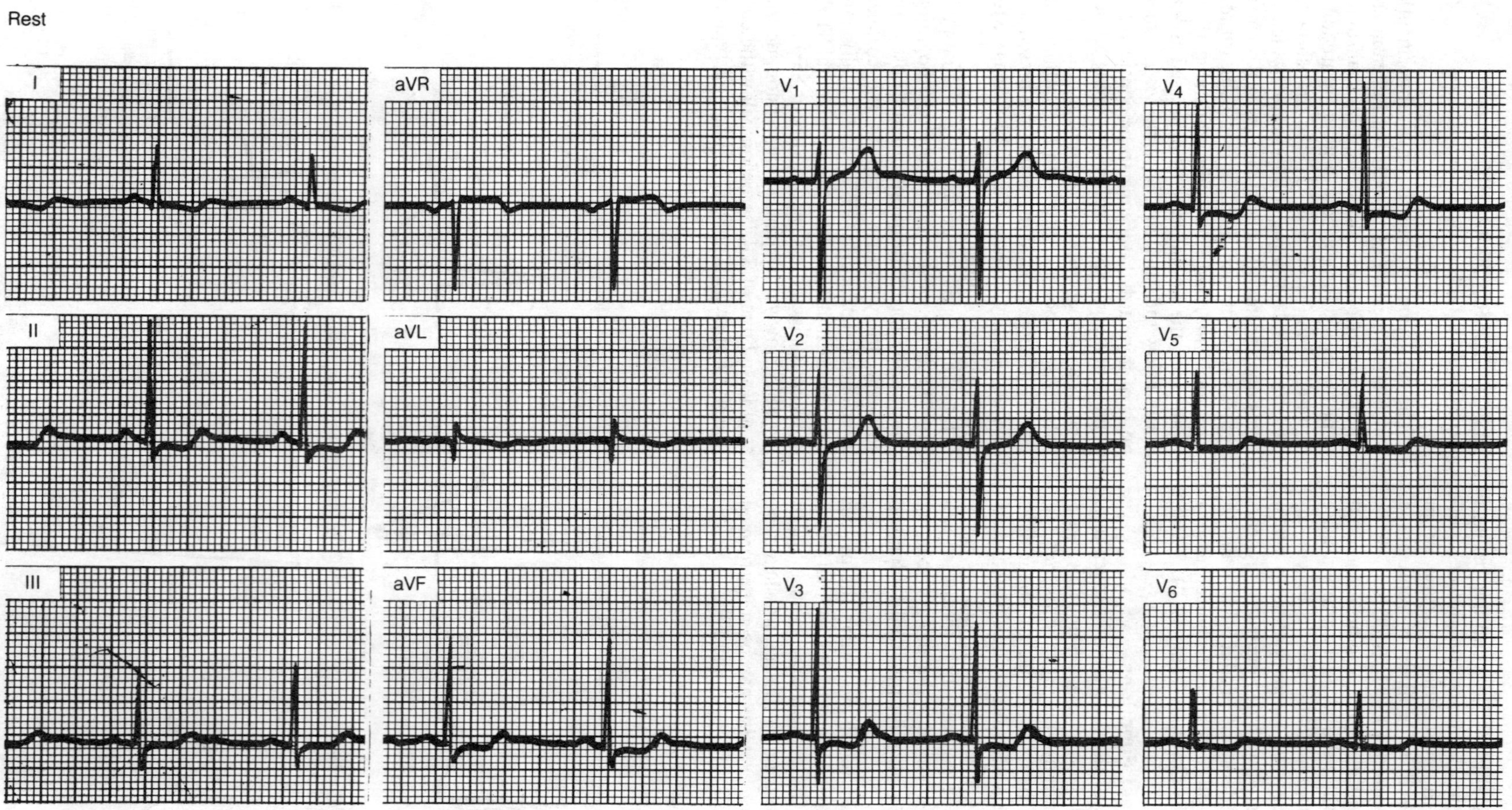

Figure 19-2. Abnormal exercise ECG in a patient with severe 3-vessel coronary artery disease and chest pain. The resting ECG shows horizontal ST depression in leads II, aVF, and V₃, and downsloping ST depression in lead V₁. After exercise, downsloping ST depression is present in leads II, aVF, and V₂₋₅. The additional 1 or more mm of J point depression as well as the changes in ST segment configuration constitute an ischemic response, despite the baseline electrocardiographic abnormalities.

Postexercise recovery, 1 min

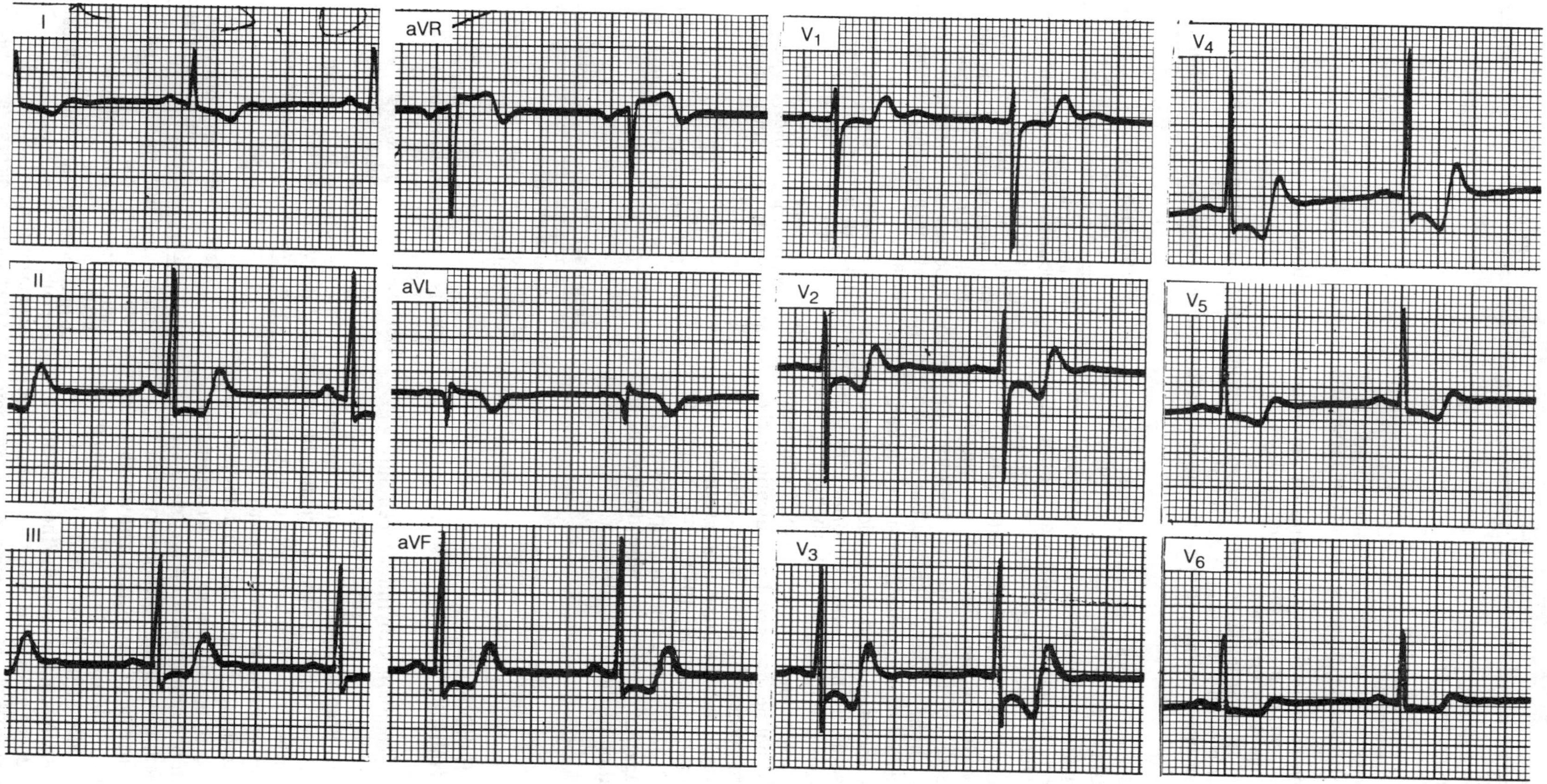

Figure 19-2. (continued)

315

Table 19-5. Indications for terminating exercise tests.

I. Symptoms
    A. Anginal pain
    B. Shortness of breath
    C. Dizziness
    D. Unsteady gait
II. Signs of ischemia
    A. Abnormal ST segment depression or elevation
    B. Hypotension in presence of chest pain and/or abnormal ECG
III. Arrhythmia
    A. Three or more consecutive premature ventricular depolarizations
    B. Multiform premature ventricular complexes
    C. Abrupt bradyarrhythmias
IV. Blood pressure abnormalities not necessarily indicating myocardial ischemia
    A. Systolic pressure exceeding 250 mm Hg
    B. Hypotension (10 mm Hg or greater fall in systolic pressure relative to the prior determination)

elevation indicates severe occlusive disease or coronary spasm (Fig 19–3, on pages 317–319) unless underlying Q wave infarction is present, in which case it represents left ventricular wall motion abnormality (Fig 19–4, on page 320). **ST segment alternans** (Fig 19–5, on page 321), and exercise induced **U wave inversion** (Fig 19–6, on page 322) are considered to represent specific responses for advanced coronary artery stenosis, but they are rarely observed, and are thus insensitive markers.

Certain conditions and medications can produce ST segment and T wave abnormalities that mimic myocardial ischemia (Table 19–7); thus, the electrocardiographic response to exercise in these patients cannot be interpreted as indicating ischemia due to coronary artery disease, although ischemia may in fact be present on grounds other than coronary disease (Fig 19–7, 19–8, and 19–9, pages 323–324). PR segment depression (Fig 19–10, page 325) does not cause difficulties in interpretation of the ST segment.

EXERCISE-INDUCED ARRHYTHMIAS

The most common arrhythmias seen during exercise are ventricular and supraventricular tachyarrhythmias. Bradyarrhythmias due to sinus node dysfunction, sinoatrial or atrioventricular block, or vagal mechanisms are much more unusual. The mechanisms of exercise-induced arrhythmias are enhanced automaticity, conduction delay, and abnormal triggering, similar to all arrhythmogenesis; which one or combination are operative in a given patient is often not precisely known.

The occurrence of ventricular arrhythmias during exercise is related to age as well as to the presence or absence of structural heart disease (Table 19–8). In asymptomatic subjects, the incidence of exercise-induced ventricular arrhythmias increases with age; about 50% of persons over age 50 may have these arrhythmias, usually at rapid heart

Table 19-6. Exercise responses indicating severe coronary artery disease.

(1) ST segment response
    downsloping depression
    elevation
(2) Early onset of ischemic abnormalities
(3) Prolonged duration of ischemic abnormalities in postexercise recovery period
(4) Hypotension associated with chest pain or electrocardiographic evidence ischemia (or of both)

ABNORMAL EXERCISE RESPONSES
NOT HELPFUL IN PREDICTING DEGREE OF SEVERITY
OF CORONARY ARTERY DISEASE

(1) Appearance of ischemic ECG during exercise versus during recovery period
(2) Ventricular arrhythmias at rapid heart rate
(3) Atrial arrhythmias
(4) Bradyarrhythmias
(5) Blood pressure abnormalities
    a. Blunted rise in systolic blood pressure
    b. Failure of diastolic pressure to fall

Table 19-7. Causes of false-positive exercise ECGs.

(1) Hyperventilation
(2) Abnormal left ventricular depolarization and repolarization
    a. Left bundle branch block
    b. Wolff-Parkinson-White conduction
(3) Left ventricular hypertrophy
(4) Digitalis preparations
(5) Baseline abnormalities
    a. Nondiagnostic ST–T wave abnormalities
    b. Hypokalemia
    c. Positional ST–T abnormalities
    d. Mitral valve prolapse
    e. Vasoregulatory abnormalities

Table 19-8. Conditions associated with exercise-induced arrhythmias.

Normal subjects without structural heart disease
Coronary artery disease
Cardiomyopathy (obstructive, hypertrophic, congestive)
Mitral valve prolapse
Long QT interval (drug-related, idiopathic, hereditary)
Digitalis
Pulmonary disease
Congenital heart disease (atrial septal defect, tetralogy of Fallot)

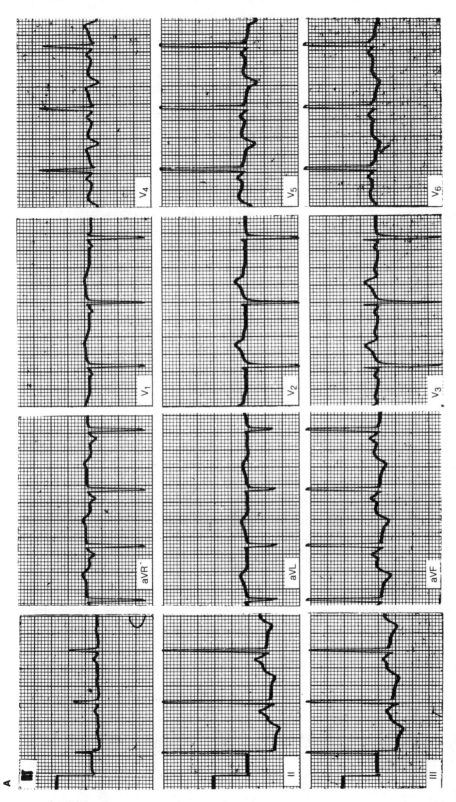

Figure 19-3. Exercise ECG in a 38-year-old hypertensive woman. The ECG recorded at rest (A) indicates left ventricular hypertrophy. At 4.5 min of treadmill exercise (B), and QRS duration has widened to 0.16 s; a wide S wave is present in leads I, aVL, and V$_6$ and an rSR' is present in leads aVR and V$_{1-2}$ indicating right bundle branch block; a Q wave is present in leads V$_{3-4}$; and marked ST segment elevation is present in leads V$_{2-6}$. All these abnormalities have reversed by 3 min in the postexercise recovery period (C). In the recovery tracings the T wave amplitude is markedly increased ("hyperacute" T wave, see Chapter 9). All abnormalities resolved by 10 min.

This series of tracings indicates exercise-induced severe transmural ischemic injury to the anterior wall and interventricular septum, to include fibers of the right bundle branch, producing the right bundle branch block. Transient Q waves may be seen in transmural ischemic injury. The patient had a single 50% lesion in the left anterior descending coronary artery, with provokable spasm at the time of coronary arteriography. *(continued)*

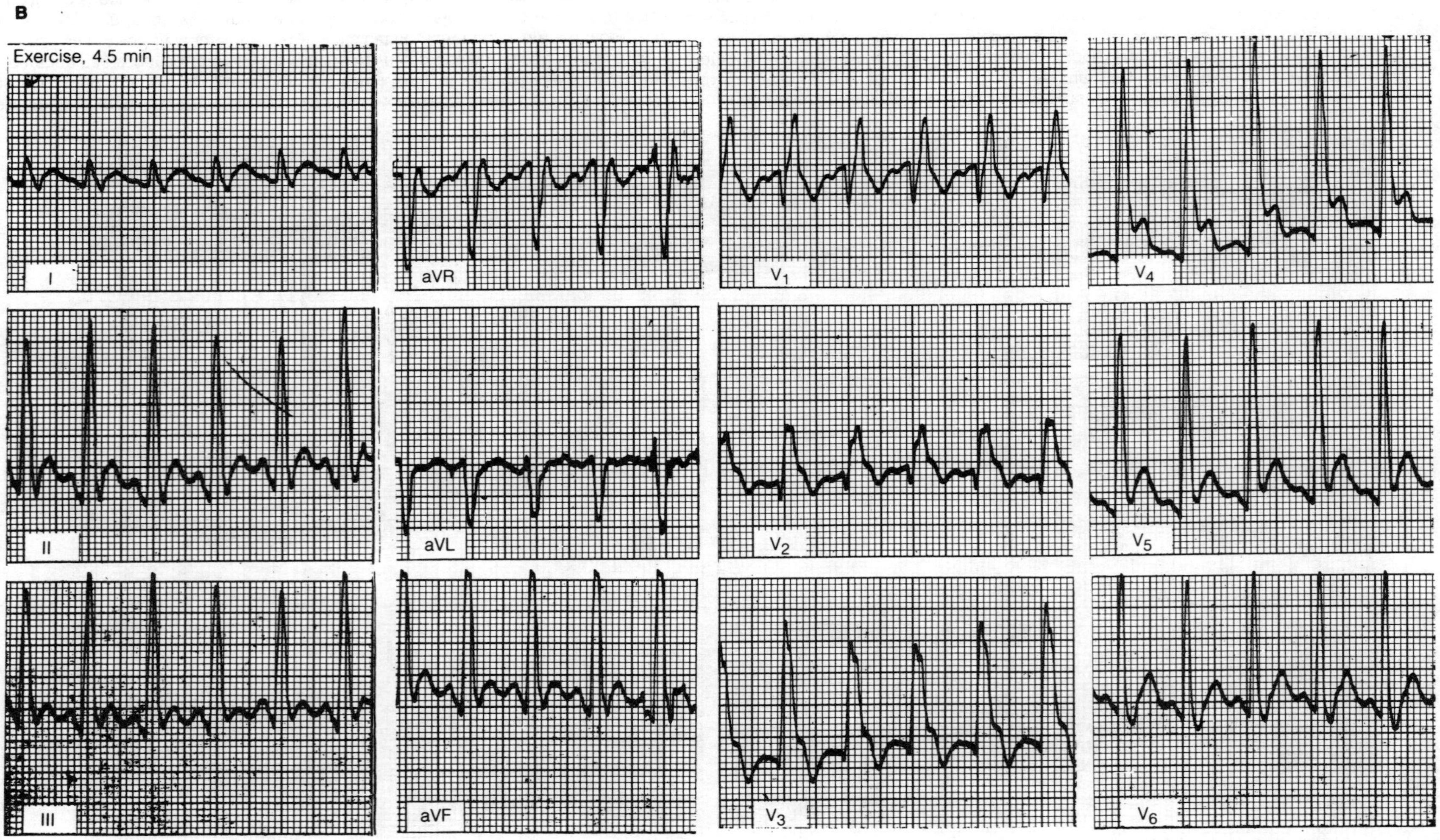

B

Exercise, 4.5 min

I aVR V1 V4

II aVL V2 V5

III aVF V3 V6

Figure 19-3. (continued)

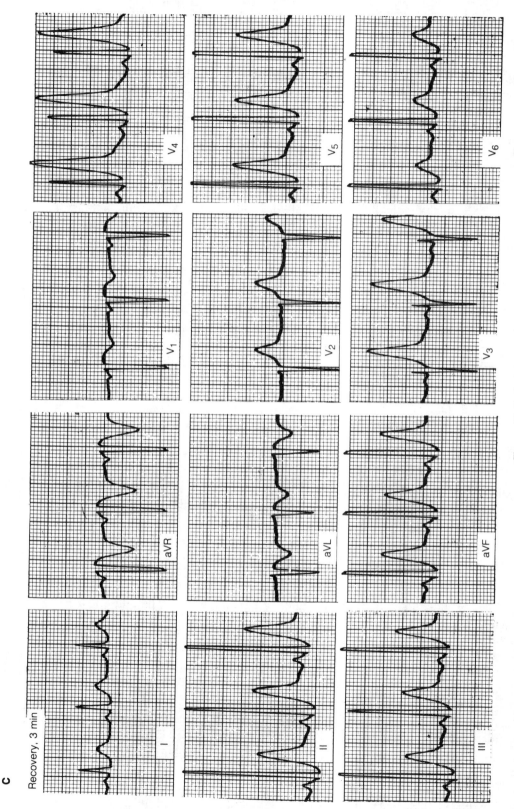

Recovery, 3 min

I, II, III, aVR, aVL, aVF, V₁, V₂, V₃, V₄, V₅, V₆

Figure 19–3. *(continued)*

c

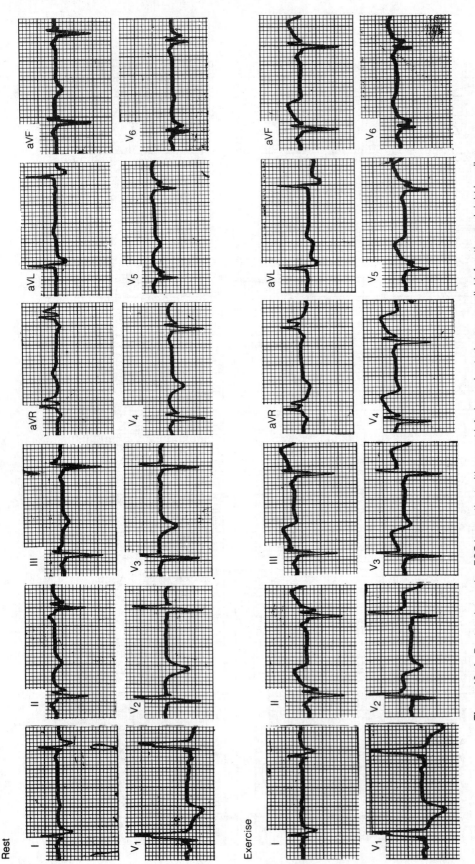

Figure 19–4. Rest and exercise ECG in a patient with recent inferior and anterior myocardial infarction and right bundle branch block. At rest Q waves and T wave inversions are present in leads II, III, and aVF, and leads V$_{2-6}$, indicating the myocardial infarction. There is mild ST segment elevation in leads II, III, and V$_{2-5}$, and the ST segments have a cove-plane configuration, compatible with underlying ventricular wall motion disorder. During exercise, the ST segment elevation is more pronounced, and the T waves are now upright in leads II, III, aVF, and V$_{4-6}$. Downsloping ST segment depression is present in lead aVL. The augmentation in ST segment elevation during exercise in leads showing a Q wave does not indicate myocardial ischemia, but is considered to represent the underlying ventricular wall motion abnormality. The meaning of the change from inverted to upright T waves during exercise is not understood. Myocardial ischemia is suggested in these tracings by the occurrence of ST segment depression in lead aVL, although a reciprocal phenomenon cannot be excluded with certainty.

320

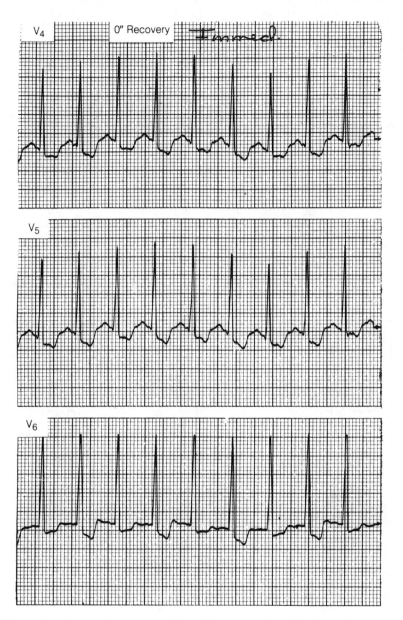

Figure 19–5. Simultaneously recorded leads V_{4-6} in a patient with a 3-vessel coronary disease and a 95% proximal lesion in the left anterior descending coronary artery. Alternation in both depth and configuration of the ST segments is seen. While insensitive, this observation seems to be specific for severe, multivessel coronary disease. (Tracing courtesy of C Quock, MD.)

Rest   Exercise

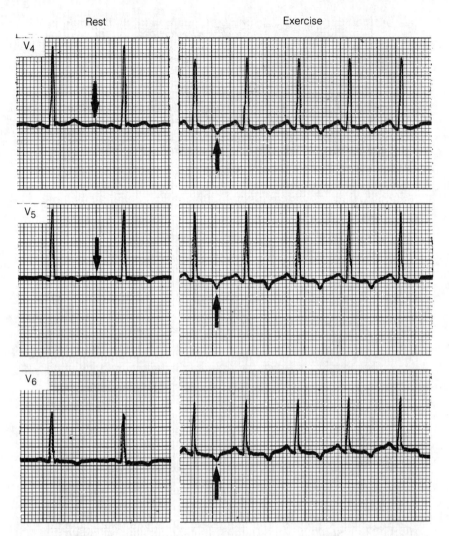

Figure 19-6. U wave inversion with exercise. The simultaneously recorded leads V_{4-6} at rest show nonspecific T wave abnormalities; the U waves are upright (arrows above the complexes). During exercise, the QT interval shortens and the U waves are now inverted (arrows below the complexes). This is an insensitive highly specific finding for disease in the left anterior descending coronary artery.

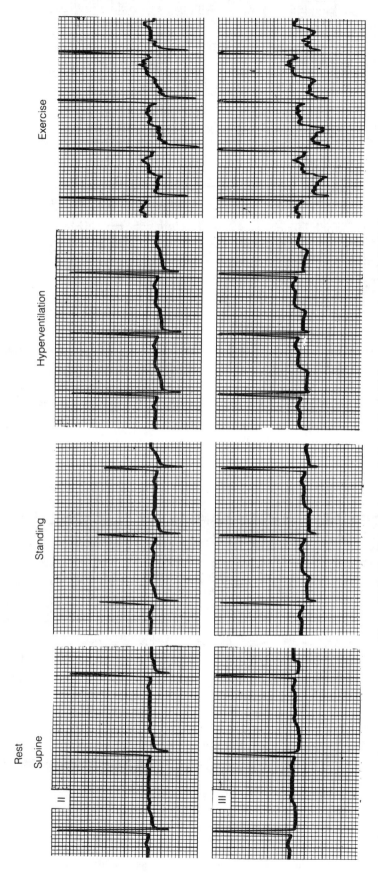

Figure 19-7. Simultaneously recorded leads II and III demonstrate nonspecific ST–T abnormalities at rest, both in the supine and standing positions. The ST segment is scooped in the supine lead III tracing but becomes horizontal with terminal T wave inversion in the standing position. Vigorous hyperventilation accentuates the abnormalities in both leads. During exercise, the ST segment becomes further depressed, is horizontal to slowly upsloping in lead II and downsloping in lead III. Because of the hyperventilation-induced ST–T abnormalities, the additional abnormalities induced by exercise should not be interpreted as indicating myocardial ischemia. This patient had normal coronary arteries.

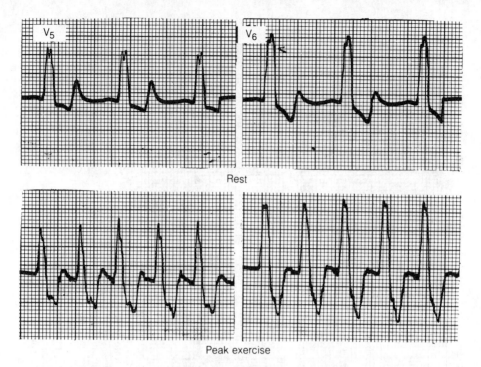

Rest

Peak exercise

Figure 19-8. Exercise ECG in a patient with left bundle branch block, indicated by the prolonged QRS duration and notched R waves in leads V_{5-6}. Secondary ST–T wave abnormalities due to the left bundle branch block are present. With exercise, the ST segment becomes markedly depressed to 6 mm below the baseline. Because of the underlying abnormality in left ventricular depolarization and repolarization, however, such changes cannot be interpreted as indicating myocardial ischemia. The patient had a normal thallium-201 perfusion study and normal coronary arteries at angiography.

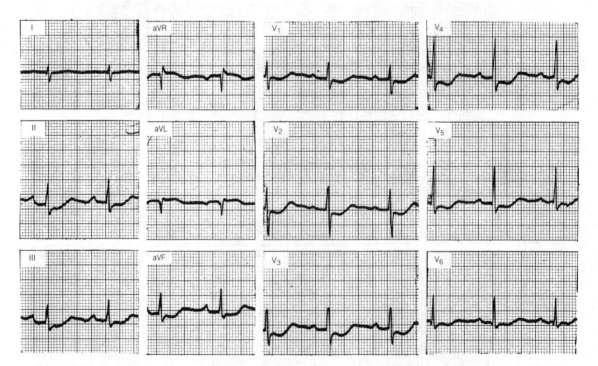

Figure 19-9. The preexercise 12-lead ECG shows a small Q wave in lead I, a notched Q wave in aVL, and a tall R wave in lead V_1, indicating posterolateral myocardial infarction, (see Chapter 9). There is J point depresson in leads II, III, aVF, and V_{2-5}. While these could be considered to be related to the recent myocardial infarction, or due to nonspecific causes, they were due to hypokalemia (serum K^+ = 2.6 meq/L), and were totally reversed after potassium replacement. In view of the electrolyte abnormality and abnormal baseline ECG, the exercise test was postponed.

Rest   Exercise

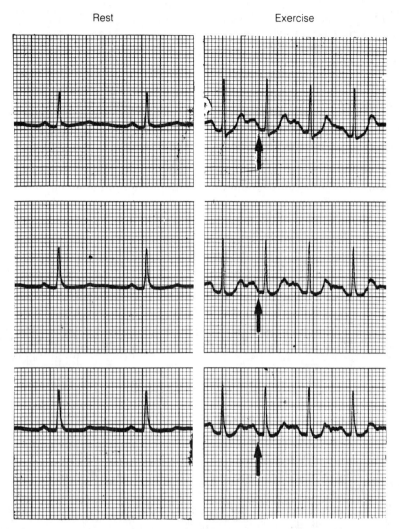

Figure 19-10. The effect of PR segment depression on the exercise ECG. The simultaneously recorded baseline leads I, II, and III show mild T wave flattening. With exercise, the PR segment (arrows) is depressed 1 mm below the end of the P wave, and 2 mm below the TP segment. At this heart rate the TP segment cannot be considered to represent the isoelectric baseline; the onset of the QRS complex should be taken to represent this baseline. The PR segment depression does not deform the ST segment significantly.

rates, exceeding 130/min. In patients with structural heart disease, ventricular arrhythmias tend to occur at lower heart rates (below 130/min) and, in patients with coronary artery disease, often together with electrocardiographic evidence of myocardial ischemia. The ventricular arrhythmias may consist of uniform or multiform premature complexes, couplets or bursts (Fig 19–11), or sustained tachycardia which may be monomorphic or polymorphic (Fig 19–12). Ventricular fibrillation is decidedly rare, and is therefore not accurately predicted by the prevaililng heart rate, or frequency or complexity of ventricular extrasystoles.

Sustained supraventricular tachyarrhythmias are seen in only about 1% of patients undergoing exercise testing. The usual rhythm is atrial fibrillation or ectopic atrial tachycardia, although atrial flutter is occasionally encountered. Paroxysmal supraventricular reentrant tachycardia is distinctly unusual. These arrhythmias are almost always self-terminating. Exercise can normalize intraventricular conduction in patients with accessory AV conduction of the Wolff-Parkinson-White type, due to both the vagolysis and the sympathetic stimulation associated with exercise. These alterations in autonomic tone can result in

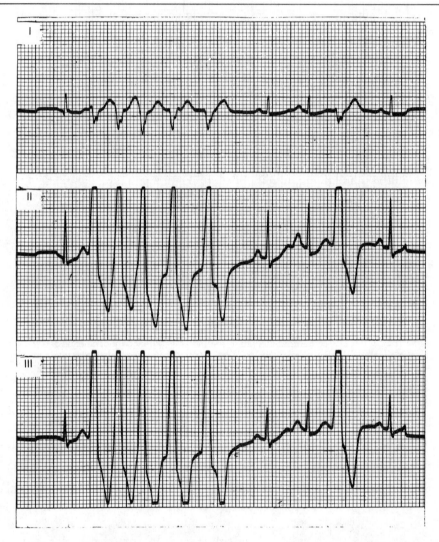

Figure 19-11. Simultaneously recorded leads I, II, and III in a patient during treadmill exercise. A burst of nonsustained ventricular tachycardia occurs at a heart rate of about 136/min. There is no electrocardiographic evidence of myocardial ischemia. The right axis deviation suggests that the origin of the tachycardia is near the base of the heart, with superoinferior activation of the myocardium. Such tachycardias are often found during electrophysiologic study to originate in the outflow tract of the right ventricle.

facilitation of conduction over the normal AV node–His-Purkinje system, with consequent normalization of the PR interval and disappearance or attenuation of the delta wave (Fig 19–13).

Bradyarrhythmias are uncommonly seen with exercise since sympathetic tone is high. The overall incidence is about 1%. Abrupt and unexpected sinus bradycardia may result from excessive blood pressure increases or from reflex mechanisms associated with elevated left ventricular intracavitary pressures; hypotension often accompanies the bradycardia. Pauses in sinus rhythm may result from sinoatrial block due to rapid sinus rates with fatigue of the sinoatrial conduction path-

ways. Similarly, AV block can occur if the sinus rate is sufficiently rapid as to find the His-Purkinje system refractory. AV block occurring during exercise usually results from conduction delays in the His bundle or fascicular system (or both); pacemaker therapy is generally warranted in such patients.

Rate-dependent intraventricular conduction delays occur infrequently, with an incidence of less than 1%. It is important to recognize such conduction delays in order to avoid erroneous interpretation of the findings as ventricular tachycardia or myocardial ischemia (or both) (Fig 19–14, page 329).

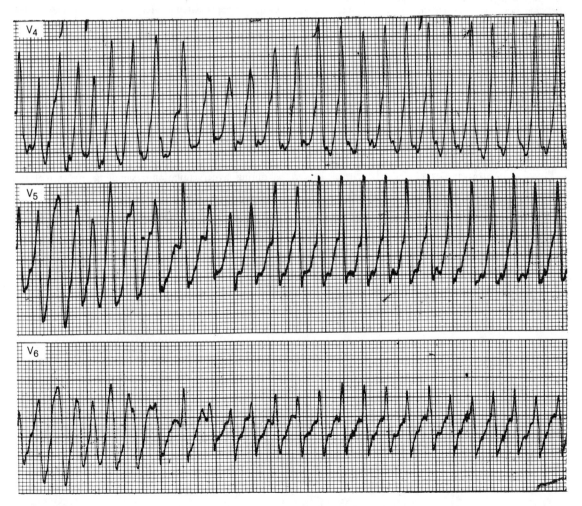

Figure 19-12. Sustained monomorphic ventricular tachycardia with slightly irregular rate occurring 2 min into the postexercise recovery period in a patient with documented coronary artery disease and evidence of myocardial ischemia. The rhythm required DC cardioversion for termination.

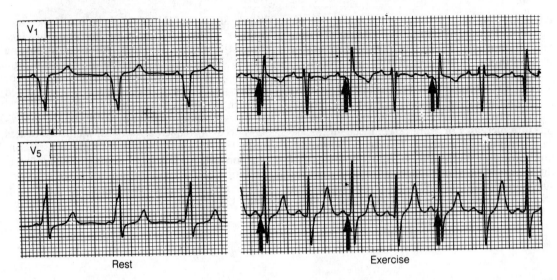

Figure 19-13. Simultaneously recorded leads V_1 and V_5 at rest and after 6 min of treadmill exercise. The resting tracing indicates accessory AV conduction of the Wolff-Parkinson-White type, with a short PR interval and a broad delta wave which is negative in lead V_1 and positive in lead V_5. During exercise, the PR interval normalizes and the QRS complexes become more narrow and normal-appearing. A small delta wave can be appreciated in alternate QRS complexes; these complexes also have a slightly shorter PR interval, indicating some degree of conduction over the accessory pathway (fusion complexes, arrows). These findings illustrate enhancement of AV conduction over the normal AV node–His-Purkinje pathways, probably resulting from the high sympathetic tone associated with exercise.

REFERENCES

Borer JS et al: Sensitivity, specificity, and predictive accuracy of radionuclide cineangiography during exercise in patients with coronary artery disease: Comparison with exercise electrocardiography. *Circulation* 1979;**60**:572.

Chaitman BR et al: The importance of clinical subsets in interpreting maximal treadmill exercise test results: The role of multiple-lead ECG systems. *Circulation* 1979;**59**:560.

Freisinger GC et al: Exercise electrocardiography and vasoregulatory abnormalities. *Am J Cardiol* 1972;**30**:733.

Goldschlager N, Selzer A, Cohn K: Treadmill stress tests as indicators of presence and severity of coronary artery disease. *Ann Intern Med* 1976;**85**:277.

Lary D, Goldschlager N: Electrocardiographic changes during hyperventilation resembling myocardial ischemia in patients with normal coronary arteriograms. *Am Heart J* 1974;**87**:383.

Sox HC Jr: Exercise testing in suspected coronary artery disease. *DM* 1985;**31**:1.

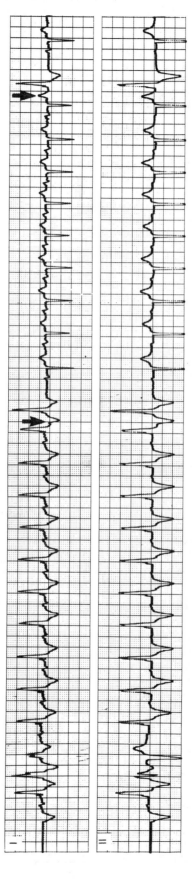

Figure 19–14. Simultaneously recorded leads V_1 and V_2 during recovery from maximum exercise. The first 7 QRS complexes have a right bundle branch block pattern; the seventh QRS complex is premature, and is preceded by an atrial premature complex which deforms the preceding T wave (first arrow). The postextrasystolic pause allows recovery of the right bundle branch, resulting in normal intraventricular conduction of the next 9 sinus impulses. The next-to-last QRS complex is preceded by a premature atrial complex (second arrow), and is conducted to the ventricles with a right bundle branch block pattern; following the postextrasystolic pause intraventricular conduction is again normal. The sinus rate appears to be regular throughout the rhythm strips although small changes which cannot be precisely measured can account for rate-dependent phenomena. The aberrant intraventricular conduction, once established by a premature supraventricular impulse, can be maintained by continued **concealed conduction** of the supraventricular or transseptally conducted impulses into the right bundle branch, maintaining it in a refractory state until recovery is allowed.

20   Ambulatory Electrocardiographic Monitoring

Dynamic ambulatory electrocardiographic monitoring is a technique by which cardiac rhythm, rate, and QRST morphology can be evaluated during a patient's usual daily activities. A precordial lead system is connected to a portable electrocardiographic monitoring device which records the electrocardiographic signal on magnetic tape; the magnetic tape is later played back on a scanner incorporating a time clock and oscilloscope. By this means, the cardiac rate and rhythm, as well as displacement of the ST segment, can be analyzed visually and by computer techniques. Recognition of premature depolarizations and their presumed supraventricular or ventricular origin by means of analysis of QRS complex duration and polarity allows the counting of premature complexes. Computer analysis allows the construction of temporally sequenced histograms of heart rate, extrasystolic activity, and ST segment deviation (Fig 20-1). Newer scanners can display pacing stimuli so that their actual delivery can be known with certainty, thus aiding in the evaluation of normal and abnormal pacemaker function.

THE ELECTRODE SYSTEM

The bipolar electrode system employs 3 electrodes to record a single electrocardiographic lead and 5 electrodes to record 2 leads simultaneously. Two exploring electrodes are usually placed over bone (to minimize motion artifact) near the V_1 and V_5 positions (over the fourth or fifth rib to the right of the sternum and over the fifth rib at the left midaxillary line, respectively), two indifferent electrodes over the manubrium, and one ground electrode over the ninth or tenth rib at the right midaxillary line (Fig 20-2, page 334). This configuration yields bipolar leads termed CM_1 (or MCL_1) and CM_5 (or MCL_5), respectively. Similar bipolar electrode systems are employed for bedside electrocardiographic monitoring in critical care units and telemetry facilities.

The V_1 lead is especially useful in rhythm analysis since P waves are usually well seen in this lead. However, the simultaneous recording of two electrocardiographic channels is preferred whenever feasible, in order to avoid erroneous diagnoses based on low voltage signals (Fig 20-3, page 335) or artifacts. Substantial variation in QRST mor-

phology with body position can occur (Fig 20-4, page 336); therefore, prior to beginning the ambulatory recording, the electrocardiographic tracings should be performed with the patient sitting, lying, and standing in order to identify these positional changes upon playback of the tape.

THE PATIENT DIARY

The patient is instructed to maintain a detailed activity diary during the monitoring period so that clinical correlation may be made between symptoms and recorded electrocardiographic events. An *event marker* on the recording can be activated by the patient when symptoms occur; some scanners are automatically activated by the event marker to write out the electrocardiogram in real time for later analysis by the physician.

INDICATIONS FOR DYNAMIC ELECTROCARDIOGRAPHY

The indications for ambulatory electrocardiographic monitoring are listed in Table 20-1. Some individuals have symptoms so infrequently that

Table 20-1. Indications for dynamic ambulatory electrocardiographic monitoring.

(1) Evaluation of symptoms suggesting underlying cardiac arrhythmia
Dizziness
Presyncope
Syncope
Palpitations
Episodic breathlessness
(2) Evaluation of baseline ectopy
Patients with known ectopy prior to beginning treatment
Postmyocardial infarction patients
(3) Arrhythmia analysis
Type (supraventricular, ventricular)
Frequency (number of ectopic complexes per hour)
Grade of severity
Uniform or multiform configuration
Doublets, triplets, bursts
Nonsustained, sustained tachycardias
(4) Evaluation of response to antiarrhythmic treatment
(5) Documentation of myocardial ischemia
(6) Evaluation of pacemaker function
(7) Evaluation of ventricular rate in atrial fibrillation

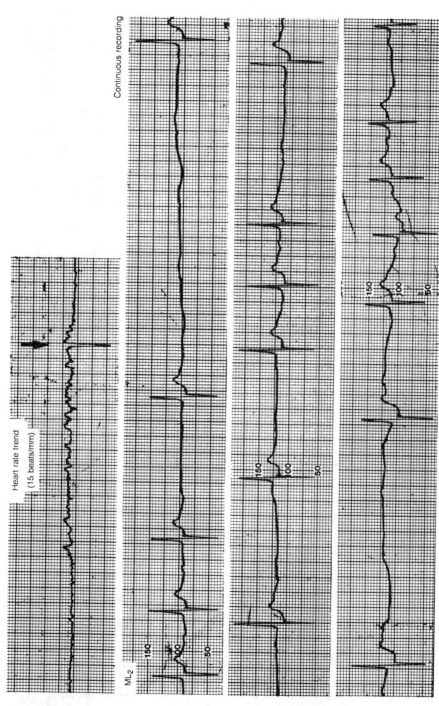

Figure 20–1. Trends of heart rate (A and B) and ST segment deviation (C) graphed over time. *A:* The heart rate, displayed at a speed of 15 complexes per millimeter, shows an abrupt fall (arrow), which is due to episodic bradycardias displayed below at a normal speed of 25 mm/s. *B:* The heart rate trend (top) shows abrupt episodic increases in rate (arrows), which correspond to bursts of ventricular tachycardia, one episode of which is displayed below, printed out at 25 mm/s. The ST segment trend (bottom) shows that the increases in heart rate are accompanied by varying degrees of deviation (de-pression) of the ST segment from the baseline (arrow). The ST segment deviation recorded in the trend represents the abnormal ST–T waves of the tachycardia complexes. *C:* Heart rate and ST segment trends recorded at 15 complexes/mm. Two episodes of marked ST elevation are recorded; the first is preceded by a less prominent ST segment deviation and accompanying increase in heart rate. The actual events occurring during these times are seen in Fig. 20–5. *(continued)*

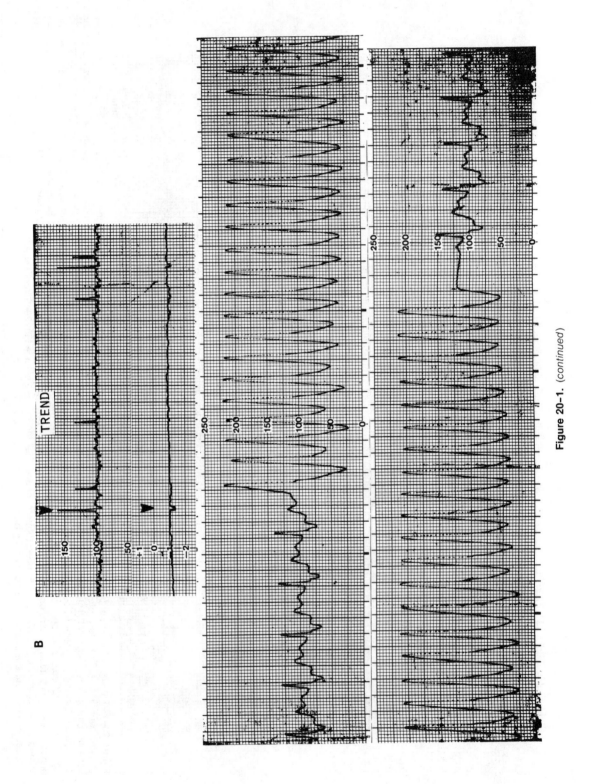

Figure 20-1. (continued)

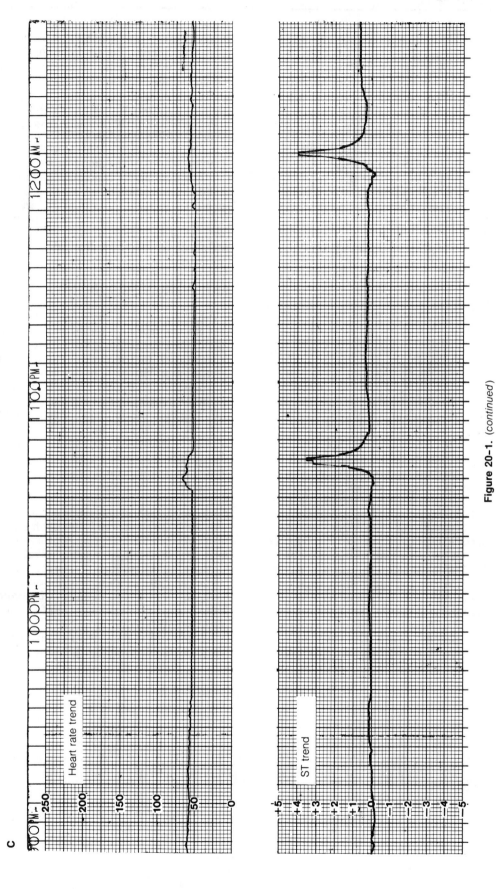

Figure 20-1. (continued)

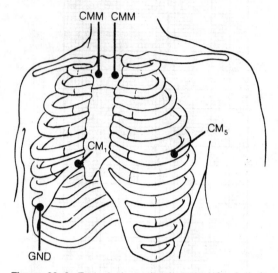

Figure 20-2. Typical electrode placement for ambulatory (or bedside) ECG recording. Two bipolar electricardiographic leads are recorded simultaneously by placing the exploring electrodes over the selected areas (usually over the V_1 [CM_1] and V_5 [CM_5] positions), the indifferent electrodes over the manubrium (CMM), and the ground electrode (GND) over the right lower ribs.

wearing a 24-hour monitor yields little useful data. These patients are candidates for an **event recorder.** The event recorder is a small hand-held device that is carried in the patient's pocket or purse. It is switched on only at the time the patient is actually having the symptom, and placed on the anterior chest wall. The ECG is recorded from the body surface on magnetic tape or computer chip and later scanned in similar fashion to a 24-hour monitor. The taped recording can also be transmitted via telephone to a receiving station for immediate display and interpretation. Since the event recorder is used only during the occurrence of symptoms, it may be carried by the patient for prolonged periods of time. The advantage of the event recorder is its use only during symptoms; the disadvantage is that electrocardiographic events

unaccompanied by symptoms will *not* be recorded. In contrast, the advantage of the 24-hour monitor is its recording of *all* electrocardiographic events, including those *unaccompanied* by symptoms; thus, potentially serious rhythm disturbances and silent ischemia can be detected.

In contrast to rhythm disturbances that are unaccompanied by symptoms, ST segment displacement indicating myocardial ischemia is clinically silent two-thirds of the time (Fig 20-5, page 337); thus, the dynamic ECG becomes an essential tool in the documentation of silent ischemia and its response to therapy. Abnormal ST segment displacement has been found to be relatively specific for myocardial ischemia, occurring in less than 5% of normal healthy individuals.

ARTIFACTS OF RECORDING

Recording artifacts may result from **incomplete tape erasure, tape drag** within the recording apparatus, **loose connections, battery depletion,** and **movement of the electrodes** (Figs 20-6 through 20-10, pages 338–342). Incomplete tape erasure can result in the display of electrocardiographic tracings belonging to two different patients, confounding both the automatic scanner and the interpreter (Fig 20-6). Tape drag results in the recording of spuriously rapid cardiac rhythms. The clue to this diagnosis is a narrowing of *all* ECG complexes and intervals (Fig 20-7); however; depending upon the amount of tape drag, tachycardias can be mimicked quite well. Movement of the electrode(s), such as may occur during rubbing or scratching the chest, can cause rhythmic artifacts that can resemble malignant ventricular arrhythmias (Fig 20-9 and 20-10); the correct diagnosis is made by identifying the underlying cardiac rhythm and rate which remain undisturbed by the "pseudo"-arrhythmia. Simultaneous recording of 2 ECG channels is extremely helpful in assessing recording artifacts.

An approach to the analysis of ambulatory electrocardiographic monitoring is offered in Table 20-2.

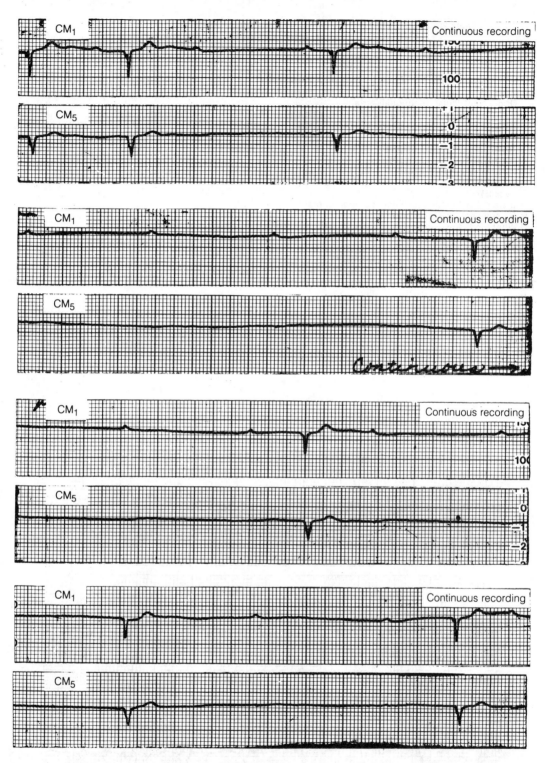

Figure 20-3. Simultaneously recorded bipolar ECG leads CM_1 and CM_5 in a patient complaining of syncopal spells. Marked slowing of the narrow complex QRS rate occurs. Analysis of the CM_5 lead alone would suggest that the slowing of rate is due to sinus arrest, causing the emergence of a slow junctional escape rhythm. The CM_1 lead, however, clearly shows the presence of continuing sinus rhythm. Thus, the correct diagnosis is paroxysmal complete AV block. The long PR interval of the single conducted sinus impulse and the slowing of sinus rate suggests the possibilty of a vagal component to the bradycardia.

Table 20-2. Guidelines for interpretation of dynamic electrocardiographic recordings
(Clinical correlation is required for all recorded events.)

1. What is the underlying cardiac rhythm and rate?
2. Are premature depolarizations present?
     What is their origin? Frequency? Degree of complexity?
3. Are sustained or nonsustained tachycardias present?
     Origin (ventricular, junctional, atrial)?
     What is their minimum and maximum duration?
     What is their method of onset and termination?
     Is there a relationship to time of day? To prevailing heart rate? To dosing of medications?
     To accompanying ST segment changes? To taking of medication?
4. Are bradyarrhythmias present?
     What kind (sinus, supraventricular, ventricular)?
     What is the mechanism (sinus slowing, sinus pauses, AV block, postextrasystolic pauses, post-tachycardia
     pauses)?
5. Is pacemaker function (sensing, pacing) normal?
6. Is ST segment deviation present?
     What kind (downsloping depression, horizontal depression, elevation)?
     What is the frequency?
     What is the minimum and maximum duration?
     Is there an accompanying arrhythmia?
     Is there a relationship to time of day? To heart rate? To activity?

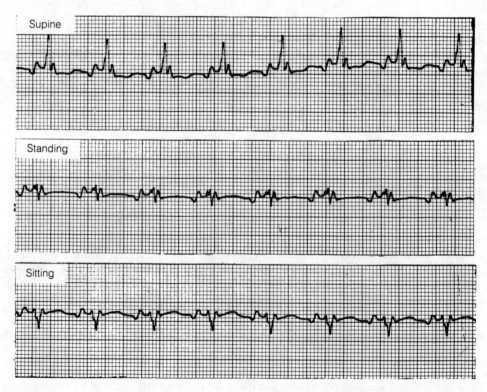

Figure 20-4. Changes in QRST morphology associated with changing body position. Identification of positional alterations in morphology prior to beginning the recording will avoid erroneous interpretation of these alterations as conduction delays or arrhythmias.

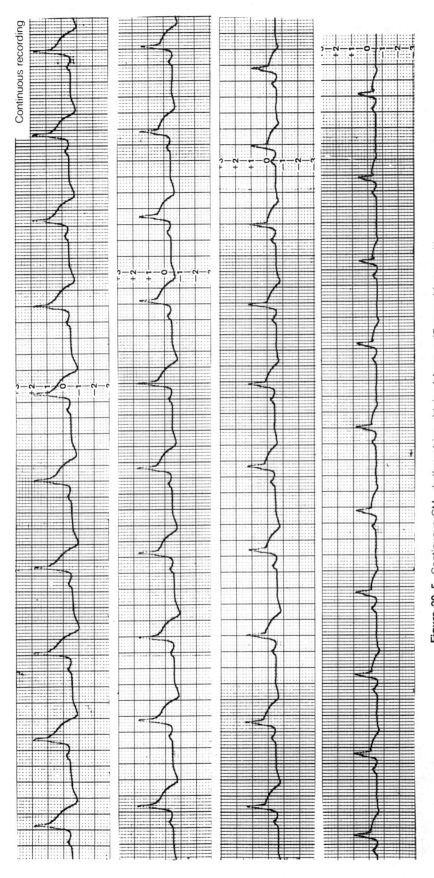

Figure 20-5. Continuous CM5 rhythm strips obtained from a 47-year-old man with documented coronary artery disease and episodic pain at rest. These and many other recordings were unaccompanied by clinical symptoms and were unrelated to increases in heart rate; a typical episode lasted for 40 s with a range of 15 to 90 s. Marked ST segment elevation (13 mm) is present in this tracing; the ST segment elevation is accompanied by an increase in R wave amplitude. Documentation of clinically silent myocardial ischemic episodes such as these aids in patient management and is an important means of follow-up.

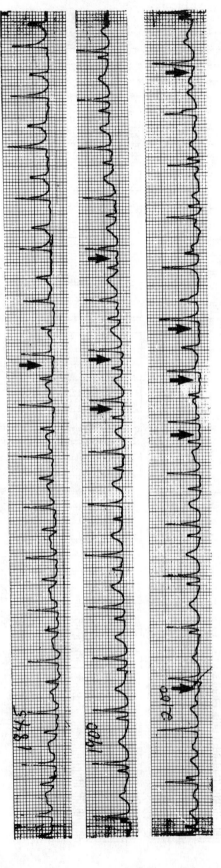

Figure 20-6. Continuous recording from a 64-year-old woman with spells of light-headedness. A regular QRS rhythm at a rate of 94/min is present; the QT interval is 0.32 s. Each QRS complex is preceded by a low-voltage P wave at 0.11 s (arrows mark some of these). Other upright deflections are occurring at a regular rate of 100/min; these deflections are smaller than the QRS complexes and are dissociated from them. These smaller upright deflections are also QRS complexes, themselves preceded by low voltage P waves at intervals of 0.19 s (closed circles); these P waves deform the T waves of the large QRS complexes. This rhythm strip illustrates the technical problem of **incomplete tape erasure,** resulting in the display of a rhythm strip containing electrocardiographic data from 2 different patients. This tracing was initially misinterpreted as atrial parasystole, the smaller upright complexes being mistaken for tall, peaked P waves. Identification of 2 distinct cardiac rhythms dissociated from each other will serve to avoid this error.

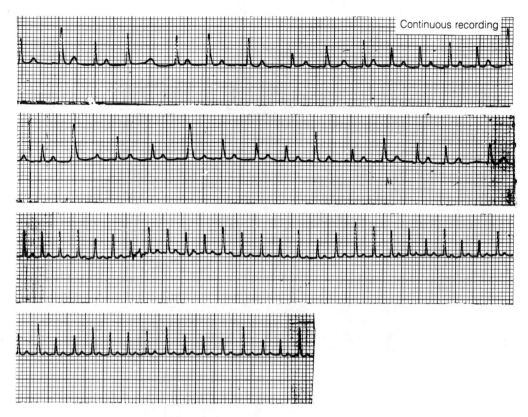

Continuous recording

Figure 20-7. Noncontinuous rhythm strips illustrating a **pseudotachycardia** due to **tape drag.** Episodic slowing of tape speed, a not infrequent occurrence, results in more P-QRST complexes being recorded per segment of tape. On playback, a tachycardia is simulated. In the top strip, episodic, momentary tape drag is occurring; it becomes sustained in the bottom strip. The diagnosis is made by identifying a simultaneously shortening of all prevailing P wave and QRS durations, and PR, QT, and TP intervals.

In this example, battery depletion in the recording device was also present, and probably accounts for the varying QRS amplitude.

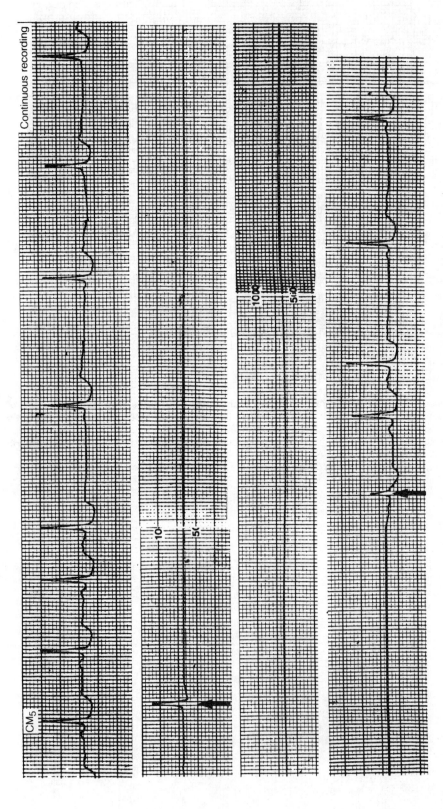

Figure 20–8. Continuous CM_5 recording from an 82-year-old woman with documented bradycardia-tachycardia syndrome; the possibility of a prolonged pause in cardiac rhythm was therefore real. In this example, however, the apparent pause was caused by an intermittently loose connection between the electrodes and their insertion into the recording device, resulting in absence of recording of all electrocardiographic signals. The clue to the artifactual nature of this tracing lies in the attenuated QRST morphology of the complexes beginning and ending the "pause" in rhythm (arrows).

340

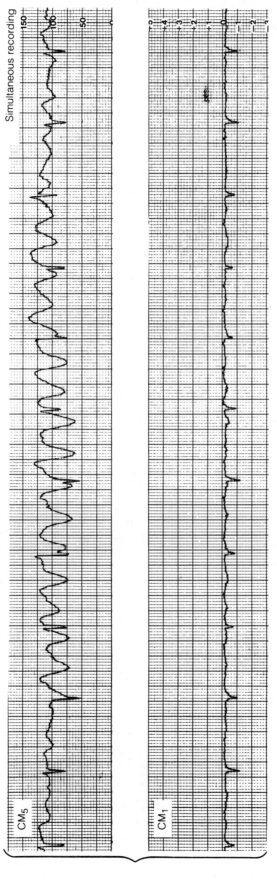

Figure 20-9. Simultaneously recorded CM₅ and CM₁ leads illustrating motion artifact caused by scratching the skin near the exploring electrode on the left anterior chest wall. A wide complex, somewhat irregular, polymorphic ventricular tachycardia is simulated. The simultaneously displayed CM₁ channel clearly shows sinus rhythm continuing undisturbed. On careful inspection of the CM₅ rhythm strip, rS deflections of brief duration and regular rate can be identified through the artifactual undulations. Simultaneously recorded electrocardiographic leads and discernment of an undisturbed underlying rhythm can confirm the diagnosis of motion artifact, and avoid erroneous rhythm interpretations.

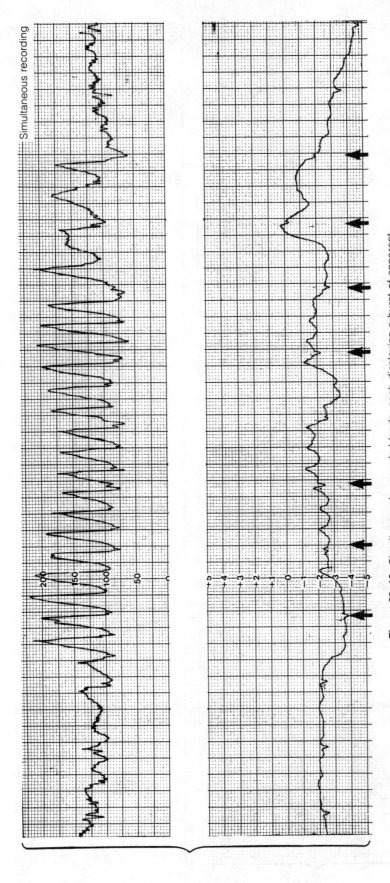

Figure 20-10. Simultaneously recorded leads, each displaying a burst of apparent wide complex QRS rhythm. Careful measurement of the QRS rate prior to its onset and after its termination reveals it to be regular and undisturbed. Close inspection of the bottom strip reveals the underlying QRS complexes (arrow). Since the underlying rhythm and rate are not affected, the apparent wide complex rhythm, simulating monomorphic ventricular tachycardia, is artifact, probably caused by motion of the electrodes. Recording of this motion artifact in both electrocardiographic channels could easily confuse the interpreter unless such tracings are subject to critical analysis.

Figure 20-T1.
TEST TRACINGS

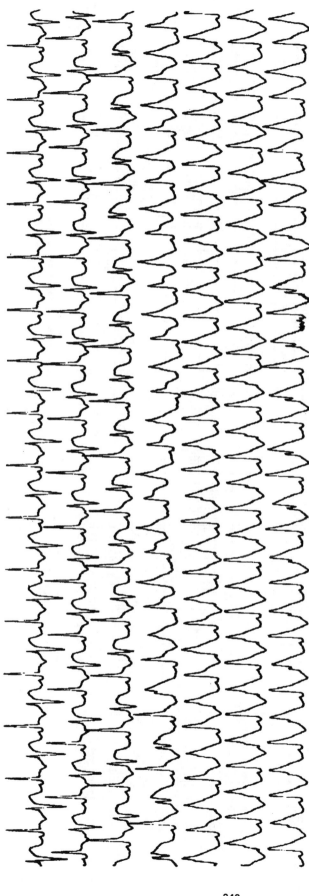

What is the predominant rhythm?

What is the rate?

What is the wide QRS complex rhythm?

Sinus with ventricular bigeminy.

Not known since it is bigeminal and consecutive sinus complexes are not seen.

Sinus rhythm with ventricular bigeminy. The appearance of an apparent wide complex rhythm is caused by marked ST segment elevation which deforms the descending portion of the R waves of both the sinus-generated and premature ventricular complexes. Ventricular tachycardia may be mimicked by ST segment elevation.

Figure 20–T2.
TEST TRACINGS

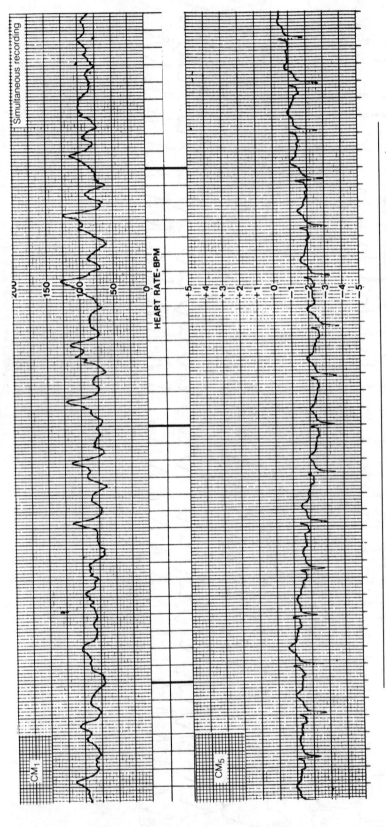

What is the predominant rhythm?

What is probably indicated by the CM₅ tracing?

Sinus, seen only in the CM₁ lead. A bizarre polymorphic ventricular tachycardia is mimicked by artifact in CM₅.

Motion artifact causing movement of the electrode, and totally obscuring the underlying cardiac rhythm.

Figure 20-T3.
TEST TRACINGS

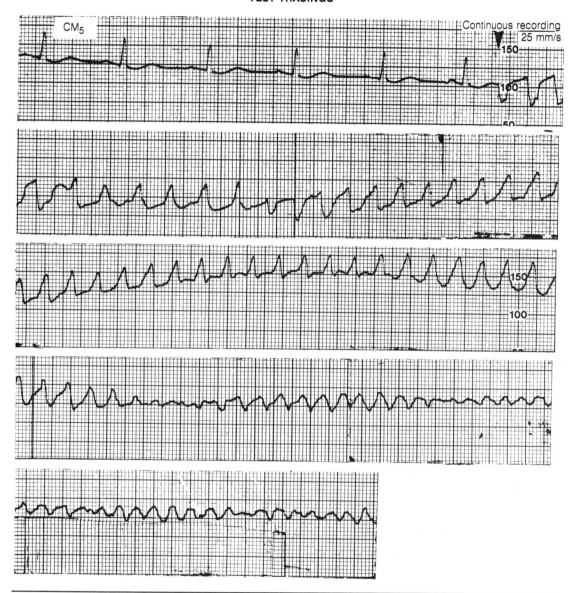

The rate trend depicts an abrupt fall in heart rate at the arrow. What could this be caused by?

Loose connections or a cardiac arrhythmia whose QRS signals are of insufficient magnitude to be recorded on the magnetic tape.

What is the rhythm?

Initially sinus, with an R-on-T premature ventricular depolarization which initiates a polymorphic ventricular tachycardia, subsequently degenerating into ventricular fibrillation. The arrow on the rate trend coincides with the onset of the ventricular tachycardia; the later disturbance in the trend represents closed chest compression during attempted cardiopulmonary resuscitation.

21

Analysis & Interpretation of the Electrocardiogram: Guidelines

The present chapter summarizes the steps required in the interpretation and analysis of ECGs. It thus also functions as a quick review of and handy reference to the information contained in earlier chapters.

Interpretation of the ECG involves analysis of both the cardiac rhythm and the morphology of the complexes. The steps required in such an analysis are described in Table 21-1.

Guidelines to Interpreting the ECG

It should be borne in mind that the ECG conveys information which must always be correlated with the clinical condition of the patient in order to be meaningful. With this in mind, and knowing the meaning of the various waves, complexes, and intervals and the range for normal for each, one is now prepared to analyze an ECG in the following manner.

I. DETERMINE RATE (see Chapter 4)

A. Ventricular Rate: Measure the interval between 2 R waves and correct for rate per minute by dividing into 60.

B. Atrial Rate: If sinus rhythm with normal AV conduction, the atrial rate will be the same as the ventricular rate. If the rhythm is not normal sinus and regular atrial activity is evident, measure the PP interval and determine the atrial rate per minute by dividing into 60.

II. DETERMINE RHYTHM.

A. Sinus Rhythm: Regular and equal atrial and ventricular rates; P waves have normal morphology; the PR interval is normal (see Chapter 4).

1. Sinus bradycardia—Sinus rhythm, rate less than 60/min.

2. Sinus tachycardia—Sinus rhythm, rate greater than 100/min.

3. Sinus arrhythmia—Sinus rhythm with cyclic variations in rate usually related to respiration; the rate increases with inspiration and slows with expiration (see Chapter 10).

B. Atrioventricular (AV) Block (see Chapter 11):

1. First-degree—Sinus rhythm, PR interval greater than 0.21 s.

2. Second-degree—At regular or irregular intervals, a P wave is not followed by a QRS complex. The PP interval is constant.

a. Type 1 (Wenckebach)—In a cyclical manner, there is progressive lengthening of the PR interval until a P wave is not followed by a QRS complex.

b. Type II—In a regular sequence (eg, 2:1, 3:1) or in an irregular sequence (eg, 3:2, 4:3), a P wave is not followed by a QRS complex. The PR interval for the conducted P waves is constant.

3. Third-degree—Complete dissociation between atrial and ventricular rhythms. The atrial rhythm may be normal sinus or any atrial arrhythmia. Ventricular depolarization (the QRS complex) is initiated by a subsidiary pacemaker located in the AV junction, resulting in a regular QRS rhythm having a rate of 50–60/min with normal-appearing QRS complexes, or in Purkinje-ventricular tissue, resulting in a regular QRS rhythm having a rate 30–40/min with broad, slurred, or notched QRS complexes.

C. Atrial Arrhythmias (See Chapter 10):

1. Pauses in sinus rate.

a. Sinoatrial (SA) block—Episodes of bradycardia during which P waves are not present. The reappearance of the sinus P wave will occur at a multiple (eg, $2\times$, $3\times$) of the basic sinus rate.

b. SA arrest—Episodes of bradycardia during which P waves are not present. If sinus rhythm resumes, it does so at a PP interval which is not a multiple of the basic sinus rate. If sinus rhythm does not resume, the ventricles will be depolarized from a subsidiary pacemaker in the AV junction (normal-appearing junctional escape complexes) or Purkinje-ventricular tissue (broad ventricular escape complexes).

c. SA Wenckebach—In a cyclical manner, there is progressive shortening of the PP interval until a P wave fails to appear. The PR interval is constant.

2. Atrial premature (ectopic) complexes—A P wave occurs prematurely relative to the basic PP interval. It may be followed by a normal-appearing or aberrant QRS–T complex, or it may fail to be conducted ("blocked" APC), and will not be followed by a QRS complex. The PR interval of the premature P wave may be the same as, longer than, or shorter than the PR interval of the sinus-conducted complexes.

a. High atrial focus of origin—The axis of the P wave is normal (upright in leads I and aVF).

b. Low atrial focus of origin—The P wave is inverted in leads II, III, and aVF. The PR interval is usually shorter than that of the sinus P–QRST complexes. These complexes may be indistinguishable from AV junctional complexes with retrograde conduction to the atria.

   c. Wandering atrial pacemaker—The P waves have varying morphology and the PP and PR intervals vary. The rate is less than 110/min.

3. Atrial tachycardia.

   a. Automatic (ectopic) atrial tachycardia—The PP interval is constant and the atrial rate is 160–220/min. The P wave axis is usually normal. The AV conduction ratio can be 1:1 or higher. The usual AV rates in atrial tachycardia with block is 2:1.

   b. Multifocal atrial tachycardia—The P waves vary in morphology and axis. The PP and PR intervals vary; thus, the ventricular rate varies. The atrial rate exceeds 110/min. P waves may be blocked and thus not followed by QRS complexes. The QRS complexes may be aberrant.

4. Atrial flutter—Regular atrial activity at a rate of 260–320 is present. The P waves have a characteristic "sawtooth" appearance in leads II, III, and aVF. AV block is almost always present. The AV ratio is usually fixed (eg, 2:1, 4:1), resulting in a regular ventricular rate, but may vary (eg, 2:1 followed by 3:1 followed by 2:1), resulting in an irregular ventricular rate. Type I (Wenckebach) block

of some flutter impulses can occur, producing a "regularly irregular" ventricular rate. The QRS complexes may be aberrant.

5. Atrial fibrillation—Atrial activity is totally irregular, resulting in an undulation of the baseline of the ECG and no isoelectric interval. The ventricular rhythm is grossly irregular. The QRS complexes may be aberrant if the ventricular rate is rapid. If the ventricular rhythm is regular, complete AV dissociation is present (see Chapter 12). Normal-appearing QRS complexes indicate an AV junctional focus of origin; the rate is usually 50–100/min. Wide, slurred, or notched QRS complexes indicate a Purkinje-ventricular focus of origin; the rate is usually less than 50/min.

D. AV Junctional Rhythms (see Chapter 10):

1. Junctional ectopic complexes—A QRS complex occurs prematurely relative to the basic RR interval. It may be unassociated with a P wave, dissociated from a sinus P wave, or associated with a retrograde P wave which can precede or follow it.

2. Junctional rhythm—A regular QRS rhythm at a rate of 50–100/min. P waves may not be seen. When they are seen, they are inverted in leads II, III, and aVF. The PR (or RP) interval is usually short. The rhythm may represent an escape rhythm (see Chapter 10) or an

---

Table 21-1. Steps in the analysis of an ECG.

1. Identify the atrial rhythm.	
2. What is its rate?	Establishing the atrial and ventricular rates allows the rhythm to be divided into 3 rate categories: bradycardia (rate less than 60/min), normal (rate between 60 and 100/min), and tachycardia (rate exceeding 100/min) (see Chapters 10–13). If the atrial and ventricular rates are different from each other, atrioventricular dissociation is present (see Chapter 12) and their rates must be determined separately.
3. Is it regular or irregular?	Cardiac rhythms are described as being regular or irregular. Irregular rhythms should be further described as totally irregular ("irregularly" irregular) or regular with periods of irregularity ("regularly" irregular).
4. What is the P wave axis? Normal or abnormal?	The duration, morphology, and axis of P waves can help provide information about the focus or origin of atrial rhythm and about whether the atria are being depolarized antegradely or retrogradely.
5. What is the P wave duration? Normal or abnormal?	
6. Describe the P wave morphology	If the atrial rhythm is sinus, the P wave morphology can suggest the presence of atrial enlargement or hypertrophy (see Chapter 6).
7. What is the ventricular rate?	The duration, morphology, and axis of the QRS complexes can help to define the origin of the ventricular rhythm. Rhythms originating above the ventricles usually utilize the normal His-Purkinje system to active ventricular muscle (see Chapter 11); complexes are narrow and normal-appearing. QRS complexes originating from ventricular tissue, on the other hand, will be broad and bizarre.
8. Is it regular or irregular?	
9. Is it associated with the atrial rhythm? Is there 1 P wave for each QRS complex? Do the P waves precede or follow the QRS complexes? What is the PR interval? Is it constant or does it change?	
10. What is the QRS axis? Normal or abnormally superior and rightward?	
11. What is the QRS duration? Normal or abnormal?	
12. Describe the QRS morphology.	

accelerated one (see Chapter 10); escape rhythms are generally slow whereas accelerated rhythms are generally normal or rapid.

3. Junctional tachycardia—Similar to junctional rhythm, but the rate is 120–250/min. The tachycardia may be automatic or reentrant (see Chapter 10).

E. Ventricular Rhythms (see Chapter 13):
1. Ventricular premature (ectopic) complexes—A wide, notched, or slurred QRS complex, not preceded by a premature P wave, occurs prematurely relative to the RR interval.
   a. Uniform complex—All ventricular premature complexes have the same morphology in a given electrocardiographic lead.
   b. Multiform—The ventricular ectopic complexes vary in morphology and axis in a given electrocardiographic lead.
   c. "R-on-T"—A ventricular premature complex which occurs on the peak or downstroke of the preceding T wave.
2. Ventricular tachycardia—A run of 3 or more consecutive ventricular ectopic complexes. The rate is usually 100–200/min and may be slightly irregular. Usually no P waves are seen; but occasionally independently occurring regular P waves can be identified. Fusion QRS complexes can occur which have a configuration intermediate between the ventricular complex and the sinus-generated QRS complex.
3. "Idioventricular" rhythm—A regular or slightly irregular ventricular rhythm at a rate of 30–40/min. The atrial rhythm is dissociated from it.
4. Accelerated ventricular rhythm—A ventricular rhythm whose rate is 60–120/min.
5. Ventricular fibrillation—A very rapid and irregular ventricular rhythm having no distinct morphology on the electrocardiographic recording (VF arrest).
6. Ventricular asystole—Absence of QRS complexes for seconds to minutes (a systolic cardiac arrest).

F. Ventricular Preexcitation (see Chapter 15):
1. Wolff-Parkinson-White (WPW)—The P waves have normal morphology and axis— The PR interval is short. An initial slurring of the upstroke of the R wave (delta wave) or of the downstroke of a Q wave is present, which prolongs the QRS interval. Concomitant ST depression and T wave inversion are often present.
2. Short PR interval syndromes. The P waves are normal, the PR interval is short, and the QRST complexes are normal. The cause of the short PR interval may be an intra–AV nodal bypass tract (see Chapter 15), an anatomically short AV node, or an atrio-His connection which bypasses the AV node.

III. DETERMINE THE P-QRST MORPHOLOGY.
A. Hypertrophy Patterns (see Chapter 7):
1. Left atrial hypertrophy—The P waves are broad and notched in several frontal plane leads and in V_{4-6}. They are diphasic in lead V_1, with a terminal portion that is negative (at least 1 mm) and broad (at least 0.04 s).
2. Right atrial hypertrophy—The P waves are tall (over 2.5 mm) and peaked in leads II, III, and aVF.
3. Left ventricular hypertrophy.
   a. Voltage criteria (valid only over age 35):
      1) RI + SIII greater than 26 mm.
      2) RaVL greater than 11 mm.
      3) RV_5 or RV_6 greater than 26 mm.
      4) SV_1 + RV_5 (or RV_6) greater than 35 mm.
   b. ST depression and T wave inversion is present in those leads with high QRS voltage.
   c. The frontal plane QRS axis is often superior to $-30°$.
   d. Slight to moderate prolongation of the QRS interval (0.10–0.12 s) may be present.
4. Right ventricular hypertrophy.
   a. Right axis deviation is present, with the mean frontal plane QRS axis greater than $+90°$ in adults over 40 years of age.
   b. Prominent anterior forces (RV_1 greater than 5 mm or R:S ratio greater than 1 in lead V_1 (or both). Right ventricular hypertrophy acquired later in life (eg, cor pulmonale in adults over about age 60) may show small or absent r waves in V_{1-3}.
   c. ST depression and inverted T waves in leads V_{1-3}.
   d. The presence of criteria for left or right atrial hypertrophy aids in the electrocardiographic diagnosis of right ventricular hypertrophy.
5. Biventricular hypertrophy—Voltage criteria for left ventricular hypertrophy with ST depression and T wave inversion in leads V_{5-6}, plus a frontal plane QRS axis of $+90°$ or greater.

B. Intraventricular Conduction Delays (see Chapter 8).
1. Bundle branch block patterns.
   a. Right bundle branch block pattern.
      (1) The QRS interval is 0.12 s or greater.
      (2) Wide, slurred S waves are present in leads I and V_{5-6}.
      (3) Wide, slurred rR′ waves are seen in leads V_{1-2} (V_3).
   b. Left bundle branch block pattern.
      (1) The QRS interval is 0.12 s or greater.
      (2) No q wave is seen in leads I and V_{5-6}.
      (3) The QRS complexes are wide, notched, or slurred.
      (4) The QRS complexes are upright in leads I and V_{5-6}.
      (5) ST depression and T wave inversion are present in leads I and V_{5-6}.
2. Fascicular conduction delays.
   a. Left anterior fascicular block.
      (1) The frontal plane QRS axis is superior to $-30°$.
      (2) There is a dominant R wave in lead I.
      (3) The R:S ratio in lead II is less than 1.
   b. Left posterior fascicular block.

(1) The frontal plane QRS axis is greater than +110°.

(2) A qR pattern is often present in leads II, III, and aVF.

3. Fascicular block patterns.

    a. Right bundle branch block plus left anterior fascicular block: All the criteria for RBBB, plus a frontal plane QRS axis superior to −30°.

    b. Right bundle branch block plus left posterior fascicular block:

        (1) All the criteria given for RBBB, plus a frontal plane QRS axis greater than +110°.

        (2) Absence of clinical evidence of right ventricular hypertrophy or lateral wall infarction.

    c. Right bundle branch block plus first-degree AV block.

    d. Left bundle branch block plus first-degree AV block.

    e. Alternating right and left bundle branch block in single or serial ECGs.

4. Trifascicular block.

    a. RBBB, plus

    b. Left anterior (or posterior) fascicular block.

    c. First-degree AV block.

C. Myocardial Ischemia (see Chapter 9): Myocardial ischemia is recognized by transient, reversible ST segment and T wave abnormalities, which may be nontransmural or transmural. Nontransmural ischemia is characterized by

1. ST segment depression of 1 mm or more in one or more ECG leads.

2. Downsloping, horizontal, or slowly upsloping ST segments. Slowly upsloping ST segments are defined as 2 mm of ST depression 80 msec after the J point.

Transmural myocardial ischemia is characterized by ST segment elevation.

D. Myocardial Infarction (see Chapter 9): The typical sequence of events in acute myocardial infarction is

1. ST segment elevation (minutes to 1–2 weeks).

2. Tall ("giant," "hyperacute"), upright T waves. These are often present in those electrocardiographic leads showing the ST segment elevation, and are usually no longer present at 24 hours.

3. T wave inversion (days to years).

4. Q wave (or QS complex) (hours to years). The pathologic Q wave is

    a. 0.04 or more in duration.

    b. 25% of the R wave height in a given lead (except leads III, aVL, and V_1).

5. The infarct location is established by applying these criteria to specific lead groups:

    a. Anterior infarction: leads V_{2-6}.

    b. Inferior infarction: leads II and aVF.

    c. Lateral infarction: leads I, aVL, and V_6.

    d. Posterior infarction: V_{1-2} (reciprocal ST depression is seen in the anterior precordial leads; an abnormal Q wave is recorded only from the posterior surface of the heart).

E. Mimics of Myocardial Infarction (see Chapter 9): Several technical and clinical conditions can mimic the electrocardiographic patterns of myocardial infarction. They are

1. Technical.

    a. Lead reversal.

    b. Contact of chest leads with electrode paste which has been applied across the chest rather than discretely in the appropriate places.

2. Acquired conditions.

    a. Left ventricular hypertrophy.

    b. Right ventricular hypertrophy.

    c. Left anterior fascicular block.

    d. Pneumothorax.

    e. Cardiomyopathy of any etiology.

    f. Chronic obstructive pulmonary disease.

    g. Acute pulmonary embolism.

    h. Hyperkalemia.

3. Congenital conditions.

    a. Pectus excavatum.

    b. Corrected transposition.

    c. Dextrocardia.

    d. Congenital absence of the left pericardium.

    e. Accessory AV conduction (eg, Wolff-Parkinson-White).

F. Pericarditis:

1. Initially, ST segment elevation is present in all leads except aVR and V_{1-2}. Depression of the PR segment may occur.

2. Electrical alternans, which can involve the P waves, QRS complexes, and T-U waves. Electrical alternans is not a specific finding for pericardial effusion, nor is it a very frequent finding; but, when it occurs, malignant pericardial effusion is usually present. Myocardial disease and acute myocardial ischemia may also produce electrical alternans. Occasionally, a rapid reentrant supraventricular tachycardia may show QRS alternans; this is of no clinical significance.

G. Myocarditis: The wide variety of electrocardiographic abnormalities resulting from myocarditis include

1. Those associated with pericarditis.

2. AV or intraventricular conduction delays.

3. Ventricular (usually left) hypertrophy patterns.

4. Ventricular arrhythmias.

5. Nonspecific ST–T wave changes.

H. Drug Effects:

1. Digitalis (see Chapter 16)–

    a. Effect—The electrocardiographic findings which indicate that the patient is taking digitalis are:

        (1) ST segment depression, often having a "scooped" appearance.

        (2) Slowing of the ventricuar rate in the presence of atrial fibrillation.

        (3) Shortening of QT interval. This effect is usually difficult to measure.

    These features do not correlate with clinical efficacy of the drug.

    b. Toxicity—The electrocardiographic findings which suggest digitalis toxicity are:

(1) Market sinus bradycardia (rate less than 50/min).

(2) First-degree AV block.

(3) Second-degree AV block.

(4) Third-degree AV block.

(5) Ectopic atrial tachycardia, commonly with 2:1 AV conduction.

(6) AV junctional rhythms with or without AV dissociation.

(7) Ventricular ectopic complexes, bigeminy, and trigeminy.

(8) Ventricular tachycardia.

2. Type IA antiarrhythmic agents (eg, quinidine, procainamide) (see Chapter 16).

a. Effect—The following effects on the ECG may or may not represent drug toxicity; clinical evaluation is necessary. There is poor correlation of these effects with plasma drug levels.

(1) ST depression.

(2) T wave flattening.

(3) Prolongation of ventricular repolarization with prominent U waves.

(4) "Giant" U waves (U wave amplitude exceeds T wave amplitude in a given lead).

b. Toxicity—The following are electrocardiographic signs of drug toxicity; there is some correlation with high plasma drug levels.

(1) Prolongation of QRS interval by 50% over the pretreatment interval.

(2) AV block.

(3) AV dissociation.

(4) Ventricular ectopic complexes.

(5) Ventricular tachycardia, often polymorphic.

I. Electrolyte Abnormalities:

1. Hyperkalemia (see Chapter 16)—With increasing levels of serum potassium, the following are seen:

a. Narrow based, peaked T waves. The T waves may or may not be tall, and tall amplitude is not a criterion for the diagnosis.

b. AV conduction delays.

c. Low voltage and eventual disappearance of P waves.

d. Widening of QRS interval.

e. Sine-wave QRS–T pattern.

f. Ventricular tachycardia.

g. Ventricular fibrillation.

2. Hypokalemia (see Chapter 16)—With decreasing levels of serum potassium, the following changes are seen:

a. ST depression.

b. Lowering of T wave amplitude.

c. Prolongation of ventricular repolarization with large, upright U waves (best seen in leads V_{2-4}).

d. "Giant" U waves.

3. Hypercalcemia (see Chapter 16)—Marked shortening of QT interval is seen. The ST segment, as a distinct isoelectric period, is eliminated and the T wave begins immediately at the end of the QRS.

4. Hypocalcemia (see Chapter 16)—Prolongation of the QT interval due to lengthening of the ST segment occurs.

Index

Note: Italicized page numbers refer to electrocardiographic tracings, illustrations, or tables.